MW00611624

BARRON'S

THE TRUSTED NAME IN TEST PREP

Family Nurse Practitioner Certification Exam

Premium

ANCC ▪ AANPCB

Angela Caires, DNP, CRNP, and
Yeow Chye Ng, Ph.D, CRNP, AAHIVE, CPC, FAANP

Acknowledgments

The authors would like to thank Richard and Mike for their unwavering support and help. We would also like to thank our students, whose enthusiasm for learning is the impetus for this book.

Published by Kaplan North America, LLC, dba Barron's Educational Series
1515 W. Cypress Creek Road
Fort Lauderdale, FL 33309
www.barronseduc.com

ISBN: 978-1-4380-1156-1

10 9 8 7 6 5 4 3 2 1

Kaplan North America, LLC, dba Barron's Educational Series print books are available at special quantity discounts to use for sales promotions, employee premiums, or educational purposes. For more information or to purchase books, please call the Simon & Schuster special sales department at 866-506-1949.

About the Authors

Angela Caires, DNP, CRNP (Huntsville, Alabama) has been a Family Nurse Practitioner for more than 15 years, and she is also a Clinical Associate Professor at the University of Alabama in Huntsville (where she has taught numerous FNP-related courses). She has been honored with several awards (including the 2015 State Award for NPAA Outstanding Nurse Practitioner), and she has been published in the *Journal of the Association of Nurses in AIDS Care* and the *Journal of Creative Nursing*.

Yeow Chye Ng, Ph.D, CRNP, AAHIVE, CPC, FAANP (Huntsville, Alabama) has been a Family Nurse Practitioner for more than 10 years, and he is also an Associate Professor at the University of Alabama in Huntsville and an Associate Professor at the University of Alabama Capstone College of Nursing. He has given several presentations at renowned nursing conferences (including the Sigma Theta Tau International's 29th, 30th, and 31st International Nursing Research Congress), received several professional accolades (such as the 2019 Fellow in the American Association of Nurse Practitioners), and was published in the *Journal of the Association of Nurses in AIDS Care*, the *International Nursing Review*, and the *Journal of Urgent Care Medicine*.

Table of Contents

PART VII: RESEARCH AND THEORY (FOR ANCC TEST-TAKERS ONLY)

PART VIII: PRACTICE TESTS

How to Use This Book

It is our pleasure to introduce this test preparation guide to future family nurse practitioners. This book provides the quick review and practice you need to succeed on the Family Nurse Practitioner Certification Exam. This guide covers all of the most frequently tested topics on both versions of the FNP exam, as administered by the American Nurses Credentialing Center (ANCC-BC) and the American Academy of Nurse Practitioners Certification Board (AANPCB). All of the tools you'll need to prepare yourself for either version of the exam are provided in the chapters that follow.

Exam Overview

Begin by reading the Overview, which summarizes both versions of the FNP exam and provides critical information about both credentialing boards.

Review and Practice

Next, review Chapters 1 through 17, which cover all of the content areas on both versions of the exam. These chapters are grouped together according to overarching categories (Systems, Reproduction, Mental Health, Pediatrics and Adolescents, Geriatrics, and Professional Issues). Within each of these chapters, you will find a detailed overview of each topic, key tables and figures when necessary, and "Clinical Pearls" to remember on test day. Each chapter concludes with a series of practice questions designed to test whether you've mastered the content covered in that chapter. Attempt every practice question, and then check the detailed answer explanations at the end of the chapter to see what you know and what you need to study further.

Then, if you are preparing for the ANCC version of the FNP exam, read Chapter 18. This chapter focuses on research, theory, and evidence-based practice. It concludes with a series of practice questions that are similar to those on the actual ANCC-style exam. If you are preparing for the AANPCB version, however, you can proceed directly to the practice tests.

Practice Tests

Once you've worked through all of the review chapters, proceed to Part VIII, which contains two full-length practice tests. One practice test is modeled after the style and format of the ANCC version of the exam, while the other practice test is modeled after the style and format of the AANPCB version. Try to complete the test that matches the one you'll be taking under timed conditions: in the time allotted and with no breaks or interruptions. Once you've completed the practice test, see how many questions you answered correctly and review all of the answer explanations for further clarification. For added practice, you may want to take the second test offered—even though the format will differ from the test you will be taking, completing those questions will still allow you to practice answering actual FNP-style questions.

Online Practice

Finally, in addition to all of the content offered within this book, there are two full-length online practice tests. One reflects the ANCC version of the exam, while the other reflects the AANPCB version of the exam. You may take these tests in practice (untimed) mode or in timed mode. As with the tests in the book, be sure to work through each exam carefully and then review all of the answer explanations to see why one choice is the correct answer and why the remaining choices are incorrect. Refer to the card at the beginning of this book, which provides instructions for accessing these online tests.

One Final Note

Now that you know all of the resources this book has to offer, it's time to begin your review. Remember, you've worked very hard to get to this point, and you have all of the tools to succeed. With discipline and preparation, you are well on your way to passing your certification exam. We wish you all the best on your examination and in your career as a family nurse practitioner!

Overview

Family nurse practitioner (FNP) students are required to pass a national certification examination in order to practice as an FNP in most states within the United States. There are two FNP certifying agencies: the American Nurses Credentialing Center (ANCC) and the American Academy of Nurse Practitioners Certification Board (AANPCB). Both credentialing boards offer computer-based testing (CBT). Thus, all candidates preparing for either version of the FNP exam should be proficient in computer-based testing and able to complete the test in a time-sensitive environment. Overall, both credentialing boards evaluate the candidate's ability to manage care for families and individuals, across the human life span, in a primary care setting. The certification questions are designed to test an FNP's knowledge at the entry level of practice. However, the two versions of the exam vary slightly in terms of the topics covered and the format. Another important aspect is that most payers require national certification in order for an FNP to be credentialed through the various organizations in order to receive reimbursement for care provided.

American Nurses Credentialing Center (ANCC)

The ANCC offers certification examinations for several nursing specialty areas, including nurse practitioner tracks. Candidates who successfully pass the ANCC-style family nurse practitioner certification exam should use the proper credential: FNP-BC (Family Nurse Practitioner-Board Certified).

Exam Format

The ANCC-style family nurse practitioner certification exam contains 175 questions. Of those 175 questions, there will be 25 "pilot" questions that will be used for future exam development items and thus will not be scored. The remaining 150 questions will determine your final score. Note that you will *not* be told which questions are the "pilot" questions. Therefore, be sure to answer *all* of the questions to the best of your ability. The total allocated time for the ANCC-style exam is 3.5 hours.

Scoring

The maximum score for the ANCC-style exam is 500. A minimum score of 350 or higher is required to pass the examination. For example, you will need to correctly answer a minimum of 125 questions out of the given 175 questions to receive a passing score.

Note that the ANCC-style exam also includes a "diagnostic feedback" area that provides information for candidates who do not meet the minimum accepted score for certification. Candidates will receive this feedback from the ANCC in the mail. This feedback will assist test-takers in identifying the areas in which they need more study and preparation prior to retaking the exam. There is a 60-day wait time before a candidate can apply for a retest. However, candidates may not test more than three times within a 12-month time period.

Question Types

The ANCC's FNP exam consists of several question types, including:

- Multiple-choice questions (where test-takers select one correct answer among the choices listed)
- Multiple-select questions (where test-takers select one or more correct answers among the choices listed)
- Drag-and-drop questions (where test-takers must drag an answer from one section of the screen to another)
- "Hot spot" questions (where test-takers must move items around the computer screen or click dedicated areas of the screen to indicate a response)

Domains Tested

ANCC questions are divided into four domains:

1. **Assessment (31 questions):** These questions relate to all aspects of patient assessment, including relevant medical history, the chief complaint, and risk assessment and functional assessment through a holistic approach. Items in this domain test your ability to apply evidence-based health promotion and screening for individuals of all ages.
2. **Diagnosis (39 questions):** These questions evaluate your ability to understand the pathogenesis and clinical manifestations of diseases, understand the differences between normal and abnormal physiologic and psychiatric changes in the human body, develop different diagnoses with appropriate diagnostic test selections, and establish a final definitive diagnosis.
3. **Clinical Management (65 questions):** These questions focus on establishing safe, cost-effective, and evidence-based plans of care and anticipatory guidance for individuals with different cultural beliefs and practices and providing patient education and referrals for specialty care, with an emphasis on motivational interviewing and shared decision making.
4. **Professional Role (15 questions):** These questions evaluate whether you understand the foundations of evidence-based clinical guidelines and standards of care; the ethical and legal principles for patients, populations, and systems; and the concepts of patient advocacy, leadership, and interprofessional collaboration practices.

Certification Renewal Requirements

The ANCC's FNP certification is valid for five years. After this time period, the nurse practitioner may renew his or her certification by meeting the renewal requirements or retesting. According to the latest ANCC Candidate Handbook, the ANCC's renewal requirements include completion of the Category 1 requirement plus completion of one or more of the Category 2–8 options, as described below:

- **Category 1:** Applicants must complete a total of 75 continuing education hours (CH), with a minimum of 25 CH of pharmacotherapeutics as a portion of the mandatory 75 CH.
- **Category 2:** Academic Credits—Five semester credits or six quarter credits of academic courses in the FNP certification specialty.
- **Category 3:** Presentations—Candidates may receive recertification credit for presentations given that they relate to the FNP specialty. A maximum of five hours may be counted toward recertification.
- **Category 4:** Publications, Participation in Evidence-Based Practice (EBP) or Quality Improvement (QI) Projects, or Research—The activity must be related to the FNP certification specialty.

- **Category 5:** 120 Preceptor Hours—These hours could involve mentoring an advanced practice registered nurse, a medical student, a physician assistant student, or a pharmacy student affiliated with an academic program related to their certification specialty.
- **Category 6:** Professional Service—This criteria for recertification may be met by serving on the board of a state, national, or international nursing or specialty organization or participating in state or national task force initiatives, editorial boards, or health care committees at the community, state, or national level. Providing care on medical mission trips may also meet this requirement.
- **Category 7:** Practice Hours—This necessitates a minimum of 1,000 practice hours.
- **Category 8:** Assessment—This necessitates retaking the FNP certification exam.

Be aware that the current ANCC certificate renewal is $275 for ANA members and $375 for nonmembers.

Additional Information

For more information about the ANCC and the ANCC-style FNP exam, visit:

https://www.nursingworld.org/our-certifications/family-nurse-practitioner

American Academy of Nurse Practitioners Certification Board (AANPCB)

The American Academy of Nurse Practitioners Certification Board is another FNP certifying agency. This nonprofit organization operates under the oversight of an elected commission, which provides guidance and input into the certification program design. Following successful completion of the certification examination, nurse practitioners may use the credential NP-C, which signifies Nurse Practitioner-Certified.

Exam Format

The AANPCB-style family nurse practitioner certification exam contains 150 questions. Of those 150 questions, there will be 15 "pilot" questions that will be used for future exams and will not be scored. The remaining 135 questions will determine your final score. Note that you will *not* be told which questions are the "pilot" questions. Therefore, be sure to answer *all* of the questions to the best of your ability. The total allocated time for the AANPCB-style exam is three hours.

Scoring

The scaled score reported on the AANPCB-style exam ranges from 200 to 800. You will need a minimum score of 500 or higher to pass the exam. For example, you will need to correctly answer a minimum of 110 questions out of the given 150 questions.

Candidates who pass the AANPCB-style certification examination will receive an official score letter with their final exam score and their relative performance from strongest to weakest in the testing domains. Candidates who fail the examination will be required to complete a minimum of 15 continuing education (CE) hours before applying for a retest. However, candidates may not test more than two times in a calendar year (January 1st to December 31st).

Question Type

The AANPCB's FNP exam consists of one question type:

- Multiple-choice questions (where test-takers select one correct answer among the choices listed)

Domains Tested

AANPCB questions focus on clinical knowledge areas, including health promotion, growth and development, physical examinations, and assessments, as well as evidence-based practice guidelines and ethical issues related to care. These areas evaluate the test-taker's ability to safely and efficiently manage all aspects of providing comprehensive care to individuals of all ages. The content areas are divided into four basic task areas:

1. **Assessment (48 questions):** These questions relate to all aspects of patient assessment, including relevant medical history, the chief complaint, and a review of systems. Items in this task area test your ability to evaluate health care needs for individuals of all ages.
2. **Diagnosis (33 questions):** These questions evaluate your ability to develop differential diagnoses based on relevant data and establish a final definitive diagnosis.
3. **Plan (31 questions):** These questions focus on establishing safe, effective, evidence-based plans of care for individuals with different diagnoses, providing education and/or counseling to patients, and making referrals for specialty care.
4. **Evaluation (23 questions):** These questions evaluate whether you can determine if a plan of care is working and/or if modifications or adjustments to the plan are needed.

Certification Renewal Requirements

AANPCB certifications are valid for five years. Following the initial certification period, the nurse practitioner may renew his or her certification by completing and submitting all certification agency requirements for recertification. According to the latest AANPCB Candidate Handbook, the AANPCB's renewal requirements include Option 1 or Option 2, as outlined below:

Option 1

1. Complete a total of 100 continuing education (CE) hours, with a minimum of 25 CEs of pharmacotherapeutics as a portion of the mandatory 100 CEs. Note that precepting (mentoring FNP students) is an optional criterion that can be used to replace up to 25 non-pharmacology CE credits.
2. Complete a minimum of 1,000 practice hours.

   (Note that currently AANPCB certificate renewal by CEs and practice hours is $120 for AANP members and $365 for nonmembers.)

Option 2

1. Recertify by retaking the AANPCB-style FNP examination.

   (Note that AANPCB recertification by examination is currently $240 for AANP members and $315 for nonmembers.)

Additional Information

For more information about the AANPCB and the AANPCB-style FNP exam, visit:

https://www.aanpcert.org/certs/fnp

Comparison of the American Nurses Credentialing Center (ANCC) vs. the American Academy of Nurse Practitioners Certification Board (AANPCB)

Table 1. Comparison of the American Nurses Credentialing Center vs. the American Academy of Nurse Practitioners Certification Board

	ANCC	AANPCB
Number of Questions	**175** questions (including 150 questions that are scored and 25 "pilot" questions that are not scored)	**150** questions (including 135 questions that are scored and 15 "pilot" questions that are not scored)
Time Limit	3.5 hours	3 hours
Scoring	■ Total raw scores are converted to a scaled score ranging from 0 to 500 points. ■ Candidates must obtain a score of **350** or higher to pass the exam (350 out of 500 = 70%).	○ Total raw scores are converted to a scaled score ranging from 200 to 800 points. ○ Candidates must obtain a score of **500** or higher to pass (500 out of 800 = 62.5%).
Question Types	■ Multiple-choice ■ Multiple-select ■ Drag-and-drop ■ "Hot spot"	■ Multiple-choice
Knowledge Domains Tested	■ Assessment (21%) ■ Diagnosis (26%) ■ Clinical Management (43%) ■ Professional Role (10%) Population focused: Infant, preschool, school-age, adolescent, adult, young-old, middle-old, and oldest-old	○ Assessment (36%) ○ Diagnosis (24%) ○ Plan (23%) ○ Evaluation (17%) Population focused: Prenatal (3%), pediatric (including newborns and infants) (14%), adolescents (18%), adults (37%), geriatrics (21%), and frail elderly (7%)
Certification Fee	$290–$395*	$240–$365**
Retesting Fee	$270*	$240–$365**
Renewal Fee	$275–$375* (every 5 years)	$120–$365** (every 5 years)

*According to: *https://www.nursingworld.org/our-certifications/family-nurse-practitioner* (as of the date of this publication)

**According to: *https://www.aanpcert.org/resource/documents/2014%20Cert%20Recert%20Flyer%2003%2027%20 2014.pdf* (as of the date of this publication)

Test-Taking Advice

In the Weeks Prior to the Exam

Since there is a lot to review for this exam, it may be best to map out how you want to divide up your test preparation time based on how much time you have before test day. The following study plans assume that you have six weeks left before the exam, but you may want to spread out some of the review if you have more time or work through this schedule a bit faster if the exam date is quickly approaching. One study plan is written specifically for those test-takers who are taking the ANCC version of the exam, while the other is devoted to those test-takers who are taking the AANPCB version of the exam. Keep in mind that these study plans were written with the expectation that the test-taker has already completed his or her graduate coursework and has already met the coursework requirements.

Table 2. ANCC Study Plan

Weeks Left Before the Exam	Goal
5–6 weeks	Review all of Part I (Chapters 1–10)
4 weeks	Review all of Parts II, III, and IV (Chapters 11–14)
3 weeks	Review all of Parts V and VI (Chapters 15–17)
2 weeks	Review all of Part VII (Chapter 18) Complete Practice Test 1 (ANCC-style), and be sure to review all of the answer explanations, especially for any questions that you answered incorrectly
1 week	Complete the online practice test (ANCC-style), and be sure to review all of the answer explanations, especially for any questions that you answered incorrectly

Table 3. AANPCB Study Plan

Weeks Left Before the Exam	Goal
5–6 weeks	Review all of Part I (Chapters 1–10)
4 weeks	Review all of Parts II, III, and IV (Chapters 11–14)
3 weeks	Review all of Parts V and VI (Chapters 15–17)
2 weeks	Complete Practice Test 2 (AANPCB-style), and be sure to review all of the answer explanations, especially for any questions that you answered incorrectly
1 week	Complete the online practice test (AANPCB-style), and be sure to review all of the answer explanations, especially for any questions that you answered incorrectly

When reviewing each section of the book, be sure to take your own notes, which will help you remember key ideas and concepts. If there is a topic that is especially difficult for you to understand or if you feel it would help to learn more about that topic, consult your course textbook in addition to reviewing the content covered in this book. Always attempt all of the practice questions provided at the end of each chapter to see what you know and what you need to study further. Carefully read through all of the answer explanations to see the rationale for why one choice is right and why the remaining choices can be discredited. For any questions that you did not answer correctly, revisit those topics in the chapter once more to make sure that you fully grasp that concept before moving on to the next chapter.

During the Exam

When taking the exam, employ the following strategies:

- Use the provided earplugs. The test center will be quiet, but you will not have control over any external noises (i.e., stroking of the keyboards, clicking sounds from the mouse, noise from the other candidates taking the exam, etc.). Using the earplugs will reduce any minor distractions and keep you focused on reading each question carefully.

- Remind yourself that, since this is an FNP certification, all correct answers should fall within your scope of FNP practice in a primary care setting, not in a specialty setting. For example, if a question asks you to order a diagnostic test, you should only order tests that have a follow-up action plan for the result in a primary care setting.

- Answer ALL of the questions. Do NOT skip any questions or leave any questions unanswered. There is no penalty for guessing on either version of the FNP exam if you are unsure; however, only questions that were answered correctly will be counted toward your final exam score.

- Use the process of elimination if you need to guess at an answer.

- Watch out for opposite answer choices (i.e., *hypo* versus *hyper*, *increase* versus *decrease*, etc.).

- Relax, regroup, and take deep breathing breaks every 25–30 questions. Stretch your arms and legs, and make a note of the time remaining. This technique will allow you to focus your thoughts and concentrate on the remaining questions.

- Treat each individual question as a *single clinical encounter* unless otherwise stated. Do not waste your time thinking about the scenario presented in the previous question. Stay focused on each individual question.

- Remind yourself that this certification only evaluates "minimum" competency and knowledge.

PART I
Systems

1

Disorders of the Eyes, Ears, Nose, and Throat

Disorders of the eyes, ears, nose, and throat (EENT) are common problems in family practice. Expertise in the diagnosis, management, and follow-up of these problems is an essential skill required of the family nurse practitioner (FNP). While being able to diagnose and effectively manage common conditions is important, it is critical that the FNP is able to recognize serious, potentially life-threatening conditions as well. This chapter will review the most common EENT disorders seen in the family practice setting.

Blepharitis

Blepharitis is a chronic, bilateral, inflammatory condition that affects the eyelid margins. Causes include chemical irritants, allergies, chronic dry eye, bacteria such as staphylococcus aureus, and viral inflammation of the eye area. It may be anterior, involving the lids and lashes, or posterior, secondary to obstruction of the Meibomian gland. Blepharitis is a common cause of recurrent conjunctivitis.

Symptoms

Patients with blepharitis present with bilateral tearing, burning, itching, and irritation of the eyes. An examination may reveal dryness and flaking around the eyelids. The patient's vision is not affected, and systemic symptoms are not present.

Management

Management of blepharitis includes improved hygiene of the lid margins, lashes, eyebrows, and scalp. Administering an ophthalmic topical antibiotic may be indicated based on the patient's presentation. For infants, who often present with Meibomian gland obstruction, regular expression of the Meibomian glands by gentle massage twice a day promotes resolution. Chronic blepharitis may require long-term topical antibiotics to control symptoms.

Hordeolum and Chalazion

Hordeolum and chalazion are two separate conditions that affect the eyelids and the lid margins. Although these conditions are separate, they often occur together.

Hordeolum

A **hordeolum**, also known as a "stye," is a pustule that forms along the border of the eyelid. Organisms that may be involved in the development of a hordeolum include *Staphylococcus aureus* (90–95% of cases) and *Staphylococcus epidermidis* (5–10% of cases).

Symptoms

Patients with a hordeolum present with a small pustule at the lid margin with localized inflammation of the eyelashes. Other symptoms include foreign body sensation and localized tenderness.

Management

Management of a hordeolum includes instructing the patient how to perform lid hygiene twice a day. A solution of 1:1 water and baby shampoo works well and does not cause irritation to the eyes. Management also includes the application of warm compresses and antibiotic ointment, if the lesion does not spontaneously resolve with the above measures.

Chalazion

A **chalazion** is a granulomatous inflammation of the Meibomian gland near the eye that may occur after or along with an internal hordeolum.

Symptoms

This condition presents as a painless, hard nodule within the eyelid with possible inflammation of the surrounding tissue.

Management

Management of a chalazion includes the use of warm compresses and lid hygiene, as indicated for the management of a hordeolum.

Conjunctivitis

Conjunctivitis is the inflammation of the mucous membrane that covers the eye (conjunctivae). Conjunctivitis may be acute or chronic. Its etiologies include viral, bacterial, and allergic causes, as outlined in Table 1.1.

Table 1.1. Etiologies, Symptoms, and Management of Different Forms of Conjunctivitis

Etiology	Symptoms	Management
Viral causes: Viral adenovirus Coxsackie virus Herpes simplex virus Enteric cytopathic human orphan (ECHO) viruses	▪ Bilateral, copious, watery discharge ▪ Marked foreign body sensation ▪ Vesicular lesions near, surrounding, or involving the eye (see the Clinical Pearl on HSV that follows)	▪ Apply cool compresses to relieve itching ▪ Avoid touching the eyes

Continued

Table 1.1. Etiologies, Symptoms, and Management of Different Forms of Conjunctivitis (Continued)

Etiology	Symptoms	Management
Bacterial causes: *Staphylococcus* *Streptococcus* *Haemophilus sp.* *Pseudomonas* *Moraxella cat.* *Gonococcus*	▪ Mild discomfort with copious purulent discharge but without blurring of vision ▪ Eyes "stuck together" upon awakening ▪ Severe symptoms suggest gonococcal etiology	▪ Warm compresses with gentle cleansing of the lids ▪ Topical antibiotics or oral antibiotics ▪ Gonococcal etiology may require hospitalization for IV antibiotics or IM ceftriaxone with topical bacitracin ▪ Neonatal gonococcal conjunctivitis necessitates the use of topical bacitracin with oral erythromycin for 14 days
Seasonal or perennial allergies	▪ Bilateral symptoms of itching, increased tearing, and edema of the eyelid ▪ Bilateral hyperemia with no changes in vision	▪ Topical antihistamines ▪ Mast cell stabilizers ▪ Artificial tears, if indicated ▪ Oral 2nd generation antihistamines may alleviate symptoms

Viral conjunctivitis symptoms often accompany a viral upper respiratory infection, and eye symptoms may persist for two weeks. Bacterial conjunctivitis is usually a mild, self-limiting condition in healthy individuals, and symptoms often resolve within one week with lid hygiene alone. Gonococcal conjunctivitis presents with more marked symptoms and requires close follow-up attention.

Cataracts

A cataract is an opacity of the crystalline lens of the eye that causes a progressive, painless loss of vision. It may be unilateral or bilateral. The underlying pathophysiology is age-related changes of the eye that result in thickened, fibrous lenses and decreased vision. Most individuals over the age of 60 have some degree of opacity, and this condition is a leading cause of blindness worldwide. Cataract formation may also be congenital, traumatic, or secondary to chronic disease. Excessive lifetime exposure to UVB sunlight may also lead to cataracts. As cataracts develop, they produce a temporary improvement in near vision, making reading less difficult.

Symptoms

Patients with cataracts usually report a progressive loss of vision, usually in one eye. Individuals with cataracts have difficulty driving at night and report blurry, foggy vision, photophobia, and altered color perception.

Management

The management of cataracts includes increased environmental illumination, a change in prescription lenses as needed, and a referral for surgical cataract removal as the patient's vision worsens.

CLINICAL PEARL

Herpes simplex conjunctivitis (HSV) presents as vesicular lesions near, around, or on the eye and requires an immediate referral to an ophthalmologist to prevent blindness.

Glaucoma

Glaucoma refers to a group of eye disorders that are most commonly associated with increased intraocular pressure (IOP). This increased pressure leads to progressive or acute vision loss, based on the pathophysiology. It may be a primary (chronic) open-angle or acute angle-closure disease, as described in Table 1.2.

Table 1.2. Pathophysiology, Symptoms, and Management of Different Types of Glaucoma

Type of Glaucoma	Pathophysiology	Symptoms	Management
Primary (chronic) open-angle	■ Reduction in the outflow of aqueous humor from the eye ■ IOP is normal or increased	■ Insidious onset of gradual loss of peripheral vision ■ Bilateral involvement of both eyes ■ Central vision is affected in the late stage of this disease	■ Assess the patient's visual acuity at each visit ■ Refer the patient to an ophthalmologist for an evaluation and ongoing management ■ Medical management may include carbonic anhydrase inhibitors, beta blockers, or alpha 2 agonists ■ Monitor the patient's medications for drug interactions
Acute angle-closure	■ An elevated IOP with decreased vascular perfusion of the optic nerve and resultant ischemia, leading to blindness	■ Sudden onset of unilateral ocular pain, blurred vision, and "halos" around lights ■ Headaches, nausea, and vomiting are often present ■ Pupils may be dilated and unresponsive to light ■ The IOP is usually greater than 20 mm Hg ■ Retinal "cupping" as noted upon an exam	■ Oral mannitol or glycerin to rapidly decrease the IOP and preserve vision ■ Ongoing management as per an ophthalmologist

CLINICAL PEARL

Acute angle-closure glaucoma is an ophthalmologic emergency. Immediate referral to an ophthalmologist is required. A delay in treatment may lead to permanent vision loss.

Amblyopia

Amblyopia is a reduction in visual acuity that results from abnormal visual pathway development. Misalignment of the visual axes causes one eye to turn inward or outward. Amblyopia often occurs early in life when the brain detects unequal images. As a result, the brain suppresses one image, enabling the patient to see. Suppression of an image can only occur while there is critical plasticity of neuro-adaptive responses, usually within the first few years of life.

Symptoms

The child often squints one eye in bright light, rubs his or her eyes, and sits close to the television or computer screen. During an exam, one eye turns outward or inward ("wandering" eye). An abnormal corneal light reflex is noted upon examination.

Management

Management for amblyopia includes referring the patient to a pediatric ophthalmologist for further treatment, which may include patching of the stronger eye.

Strabismus

Strabismus is an ocular misalignment due to a problem with the muscular coordination of the eyes. It is commonly identified in childhood, and it may affect the patient's depth perception. The pathophysiology of strabismus may be paralytic or nonparalytic in nature. Paralytic strabismus is caused by paralysis or weakness of specific extraocular muscles. Nonparalytic strabismus is a product of a congenital imbalance of extraocular muscle tone, causing difficulty focusing and unilateral refractive errors or anatomical variance in the eyes.

Symptoms

Patients present with crossed or "turned in" eyes, usually with photophobia and double vision.

Management

Patients with strabismus require a referral to an ophthalmologist for an evaluation. When treating strabismus, some key medical terminology to be familiar with are **esotropia** (inward deviation of the affected eye), **exotropia** (outward deviation of the affected eye), and **pseudo strabismus** (strabismus appears to be present because of a flat, broad nasal bridge, prominent epicanthal folds, or narrow interpupillary space).

Dacryocystitis

Dacrocystitis is an inflammation or infection of the lacrimal sac of the eye due to undeveloped lacrimal glands (present in neonates). This condition may be acute or chronic. Acute dacryocystitis is commonly seen in newborns because the lacrimal gland is immature and unable to clear bacteria from the eye surface effectively. Causative organisms include the *Staphylococcus aureus* and *Streptococcus* species.

Symptoms

Older children will present with unilateral eye pain, redness, and swelling of the lacrimal area. Increased tearing and a fever may be present. Newborns will present with mucus collection at the corner of the eye.

Management

Management techniques include the use of warm, moist compresses four times daily and discarding old makeup. For newborns specifically, management includes gentle massaging of the lacrimal sac four times daily. Management for all patients with dacryocystitis may also include erythromycin or dicloxacillin ophthalmic ointment.

CLINICAL PEARL

Treatment for amblyopia must be initiated early (before the patient is between four and six years old) or else the condition may not be correctable. The treatment may need to be repeated because the condition frequently recurs.

CLINICAL PEARL

Persistent ocular deviation is an abnormal finding at any age. A patient with this finding should be referred to an ophthalmologist for an evaluation immediately.

Age-Related Macular Degeneration (ARMD)

Age-related macular degeneration is the leading cause of irreversible loss of vision in individuals who are 65 years old or older. This disease causes pigmentary changes of the macula that lead to a progressive loss of vision. This condition is not caused by cataracts or other eye diseases and occurs in two forms, dry and wet, as outlined in Table 1.3. Note that dry ARMD often progresses to the wet, proliferative form.

Table 1.3. Pathophysiology, Symptoms, and Management of Different Types of ARMD

Type of ARMD	Pathophysiology	Symptoms	Management
	▪ Atrophic changes of the retina ▪ Degeneration of the outer retina and the retinal pigment epithelium	Sequential, progressive loss of central vision occurring over a period of a few years	Refer the patient to an ophthalmologist for an evaluation
Wet ARMD (exudative, neovascular)	▪ Growth of new choroidal vessels, leading to an accumulation of exudative fluid, hemorrhages, and fibrosis of the retina	▪ Fairly rapid and severe loss of central vision ▪ Patient complains of distorted central vision ▪ Patient may report that straight lines (such as a telephone pole) appear to be crooked ▪ Evidence of Drusen bodies, new vessel growth, and/or exudates during a retinal exam	Refer the patient to an ophthalmologist for growth-inhibiting therapy

Diabetic Retinopathy

Diabetic retinopathy is a condition that produces a progressive loss of vision. This condition is present in around 35% of patients who are diagnosed with diabetes mellitus. This disease affects about four million people and is the leading cause of blindness among individuals between the ages of 20 and 65 years old. The development of diabetic retinopathy is related to how long the patient has had diabetes and is directly related to the level of diabetic control. Screening for development of retinopathy should be included in every comprehensive diabetic examination. It is recommended that all patients with diabetes undergo retinopathy screening every one to two years. Diabetic retinopathy is often divided into three stages: nonproliferative, preproliferative, and proliferative, as outlined in Table 1.4.

Table 1.4. Stages of Diabetic Retinopathy and Their Symptoms and Management

Diabetic Retinopathy Stage	Symptoms	Management
Nonproliferative	<ul><li>Microaneurysms</li><li>Retinal hemorrhages</li><li>Venous beading</li><li>Retinal edema on a fundoscopic exam</li><li>Patient reports decreased vision, needing frequent lens changes for glasses</li></ul>	<ul><li>Strict blood pressure and blood glucose control</li><li>Avoiding smoking</li><li>Close follow-up with an ophthalmologist</li></ul>
Preproliferative	Focal or diffuse macular edema	Follow the same basic management techniques as used for the nonproliferative stage, but management at this stage necessitates tighter control of blood pressure and serum glucose levels
Proliferative	<ul><li>Neovascularization of the optic disk or of the major blood vessels of the retina</li><li>Vitreous hemorrhage</li><li>Retinal detachment</li></ul>	Laser photocoagulation to slow the progression of the disease

Corneal Abrasion

A corneal abrasion is a superficial loss of epithelial tissue from the cornea. Corneal abrasion occurs most often as a result of trauma or foreign body injury to the eye. Airbag deployment during motor vehicle accidents and contact lens use are other common causative factors. Corneal surface foreign bodies are common in individuals who work in dusty environments or around small airborne particles. Assessing a corneal abrasion includes checking visual acuity and blue-light visualization of the cornea with fluorescein dye.

Symptoms

Symptoms include the sudden onset of severe unilateral eye pain, blurred vision, redness, light sensitivity, tearing, eyelid edema, and blepharospasm.

Management

Mild corneal abrasions may be managed with topical antibiotic ointment or oral analgesics. Healing may occur anywhere within a few hours to a few days, at which point the cornea is considered healthy. The patient should follow up with an ophthalmologist if symptoms do not improve rapidly.

CLINICAL PEARL

A corneal injury with an irregular iris and a shallow anterior chamber observed upon examination indicates a full-thickness injury. This type of injury requires an emergency referral to an ophthalmologist.

Acute Otitis Media (AOM)

Acute otitis media is an inflammation or infection of the middle ear structures. It is seen more often during infancy and early childhood, but it may occur at any age. Risk factors include eustachian tube dysfunction, secondhand smoke exposure, chronic mucosal edema, and congestion. Common causative organisms include *Streptococcus pneumoniae*, *Haemophilus influenzae*, *Moraxella catarrhalis*, and viruses.

Symptoms

Patients will present with acute onset otalgia, decreased hearing, and a possible fever. Infants and young children are often seen tugging on their ears. AOM may accompany an upper respiratory infection. Infants may present with poor feeding, irritability, drooling, and a fever. An otoscopic examination will demonstrate erythema and decreased tympanic membrane mobility. Fluid and exudates may be seen behind the tympanic membrane.

Management

CLINICAL PEARL

A tympanic membrane rupture, which is associated with AOM, may provide a relief of pressure and acute pain.

Management of AOM includes amoxicillin as a first-line therapy with erythromycin for a penicillin allergy. Referral to an otolaryngologist is indicated for patients with recurrent infections and/or poor response to treatment. In some instances, the patient may require tympanostomy tube placement.

Hearing Loss

Hearing loss represents the loss of auditory ability. It may be mild, moderate, severe, or profound. Two types of hearing loss (conductive and sensorineural) exist. To assess hearing loss, the provider must administer the Weber and Rinne tests to determine the etiology of the hearing loss. Table 1.5 discusses these two types of hearing losses, the results of the Weber and Rinne tests for each type, and the pathophysiology, symptoms, and management for each type.

Table 1.5. Types of Hearing Loss, the Weber and Rinne Test Results, and the Pathophysiology, Symptoms, and Management for Each Type

Hearing Loss	Results of the Weber Test	Results of the Rinne Test	Pathophysiology	Symptoms	Management
Conductive	Sound is greater in the affected ear	Air conduction equals bone conduction (which indicates conductive hearing loss)	■ External or middle ear dysfunction ■ Cerumen impaction ■ Persistent conductive hearing loss may result from chronic infections, trauma, and/or otosclerosis	■ Gradual, often progressive loss of hearing ■ High-frequency sounds are often lost first	■ Eliminate the cause, if possible ■ Resolve the underlying problem

Continued

Table 1.5. Types of Hearing Loss, the Weber and Rinne Test Results, and the Pathophysiology, Symptoms, and Management for Each Type *(Continued)*

Hearing Loss	Results of the Weber Test	Results of the Rinne Test	Pathophysiology	Symptoms	Management
Sensorineural	Sound is greater in the unaffected ear	Air conduction is greater than bone conduction (which indicates sensorineural hearing loss)	Deterioration of the cochlea (often due to a loss of hair cells from the Organ of Corti), which is usually irreversible	Patient may present with an acute loss of hearing in one or both ears	Evaluation and treatment should be managed by an audiologist

CLINICAL PEARL

Most causes of conductive hearing loss are reversible while many causes of sensorineural hearing loss are irreversible.

Otitis Externa (OE)

Otitis externa is an inflammation and infection of the external auditory canal, including the pinna and auricle. It may be acute or chronic. A small scratch or abrasion in the membranous lining of the ear canal allows bacteria to invade, producing inflammation and edema of the canal. Common causative organisms include *Pseudomonas*, *Proteus*, and *Aspergillus*. This usually benign but extremely painful condition is often associated with repeated water exposure ("swimmer's ear"). This condition is seen most often during summer months. Risk factors for this condition include diabetes mellitus and immunodeficiency. Patients with a chronic disease or immune suppression may develop a malignant, invasive disease, which may be fatal. Those most at risk for an invasive OE include individuals who have a weakened immune response and adults over the age of 65.

Symptoms

A patient with OE presents with erythema and edema of the ear canal (usually unilateral) and purulent, malodorous exudate. There is pain with manipulation of the pinna or tragus, and the tympanic membrane is often erythematous. A fever is often present.

Management

Management of OE includes administering an optic antibiotic solution (usually fluoroquinolone) or suspension, often with a corticosteroid. The medication may be administered to the affected ear canal via a wick if the edema of the canal is severe. If cellulitis of the preauricular tissue is present, administer an oral fluoroquinolone for one week. This condition may evolve into osteomyelitis of the floor of the ear and/or mastoid process if left untreated. To avoid reinfection, protect the ear from additional moisture and promote acidification with a drying agent following water exposure.

Otitis Media with Effusion (OME)

Otitis media with effusion, also called serous otitis media, results from persistent blockage of the Eustachian tube, leading to transudation of fluid into the middle ear space. Eustachian tube dysfunction is often associated with a viral upper respiratory infection and/or allergies.

Symptoms

Exam findings include a retracted tympanic membrane with decreased mobility on pneumatic otoscopy and fluid/air bubbles behind the tympanic membrane. The patient may report muffled hearing, or the patient may be asymptomatic.

CLINICAL PEARL

Be sure to recognize the signs and symptoms (fever, excruciating ear pain, and granulation tissue formation) of "malignant external otitis," which requires an emergency referral to a specialist (otolaryngologist or the emergency department) and may be *fatal*.

Management

Systemic and intranasal decongestants are used to manage OME. The patient should be instructed to "auto-inflate" the Eustachian tube by forced exhalation against closed nostrils. Note that this is contraindicated for patients with an active infection. If symptoms persist for longer than three months, the FNP should recommend a referral to an otolaryngologist.

Tinnitus

Tinnitus is the sensation of sound in the absence of any exogenous source of sound or the perception of abnormal ear or head noises. Persistent tinnitus often indicates sensory hearing loss. Brief episodes of tinnitus are common in adults with normal hearing and are benign.

Symptoms

A patient may report "hearing" his or her own heartbeat. High-pitched sounds are usually associated with sensorineural hearing loss. Low-pitched sounds are associated with idiopathic tinnitus or Meniere's disease.

Management

Persistent tinnitus requires a referral to an audiologist for a complete audiological examination.

Cholesteatoma

Cholesteatoma is an abnormal accumulation or overgrowth of squamous epithelial cells that are usually found within the middle ear. This condition may be congenital or acquired, and it may become secondarily infected by the *Pseudomonas aeruginosa*, *Proteus* species, *Enterobacter*, *Staphylococcus*, or *Streptococcus*. Cholesteatoma may progress and spread into the intratemporal structures, causing hearing loss and facial nerve palsy.

Symptoms

A patient with cholesteatoma may report otorrhea or hearing loss; persistent, purulent ear infections with tinnitus; and/or impaired hearing with vertigo or dizziness from erosion of the labyrinth. Patients may also be asymptomatic, in which case the presence of cholesteatoma may be discovered during an ear examination for another condition, such as acute otitis media. During an otoscopic examination, cholesteatoma appears as a retraction pocket or a marginal tympanic membrane perforation with the presence of granulation tissue.

Management

The management of cholesteatoma includes removing debris from the ear canal, preventing water from entering the ear canal, and/or antibiotics as indicated for an infection. Definitive management of this condition is a referral to an otolaryngologist for surgery.

Vestibular Neuritis (Acute Peripheral Labyrinthitis)

Vestibular neuritis is an acute, unilateral dysfunction of the labyrinth of the ear. This condition may be triggered by a viral inflammation of the vestibular nerve, otitis media, or latent herpes simplex infection of the vestibular ganglia.

Symptoms

Patients with vestibular neuritis usually report episodes of severe acute vertigo, nausea, vomiting, and tinnitus, which is aggravated by head movement. Spontaneous nystagmus may also be present. Severe symptoms often subside within 48–72 hours; however, they may persist for four or five days. About 50% of patients experience dizziness and disequilibrium for months.

Management

The goal of managing vestibular neuritis is to alleviate vertigo, nausea, and vomiting and to improve ventral compensation through vestibular exercises. Symptomatic relief can be achieved with the use of anticholinergics and antihistamines. Administer antiemetics as needed but discontinue these meds after three days since longer use may delay vestibular recovery. Short-term corticosteroid therapy may improve symptoms. Refer the patient to an otolaryngologist for severe infections, signs of meningitis, or severe dehydration.

Allergic Rhinitis

Allergic rhinitis is a disorder that is characterized by sneezing, rhinorrhea, and nasal and pharyngeal itching related to exposure to an allergen. This condition is often seen in the presence of other atopic disorders. When the nasal mucosa is exposed to allergens, an IgE response causes mast cells to release histamine and leukotrienes. These substances are responsible for the mucosal edema and nasal drainage seen with allergic rhinitis.

Symptoms

Patients with allergic rhinitis report seasonal or year-round episodes of sneezing, nasal congestion, disturbances of taste or smell, dry mouth, and postnasal drainage. Other symptoms include fatigue, puffy or watery eyes, and itching. Upon examination, the FNP may notice that the nasal mucosa appears pale with swollen turbinates. The FNP may also observe enlarged nostrils, a postnasal drip, and conjunctival irritation.

Management

Management of allergic rhinitis includes environmental control through the identification and elimination of allergens, pharmacologic therapy with intranasal glucocorticoids, oral antihistamines, intranasal anticholinergics, and/or nasal saline irrigations. If the patient exhibits severe symptoms, he or she may need a referral to an allergist for allergy testing and immunotherapy.

Epistaxis

Epistaxis is bleeding from the nose that involves either the anterior or posterior nasal mucosa. Nosebleeds are common with the highest incidences in individuals younger than 10 years old and those between 70 and 79 years old. Predisposing factors include anticoagulant therapy, nasal trauma, rhinitis, dry mucous membranes, alcohol use, septal deviation, and chemical irritants (such as cocaine). Note that epistaxis is a symptom of another abnormality, not a disease itself.

Symptoms

Symptoms of epistaxis include a sudden or slow onset of bleeding from one or both nostrils. The bleeding is usually painless and may vary from scant amounts to a more severe loss of blood. Patients with epistaxis will usually request medical attention when home measures to stop the nosebleeds are ineffective.

Management

Acute management of epistaxis requires the application of direct pressure over the bleeding site for 15–20 minutes. This is best accomplished by pinching the nose closed, without releasing it, for at least 15–20 minutes. Most nosebleeds respond to this treatment alone. Applying an ice pack over the dorsum of the nose may promote hemostasis. Clinical management of epistaxis (in the event that the patient does not respond to the previously described management measures) includes the application of a topical vasoconstrictor (such as oxymetazoline) and/or cautery of the bleeding site with silver nitrate for approximately 10 seconds. For posterior bleeds (or if you cannot see the source of the bleeding), refer the patient to the emergency department for tamponade with a balloon device and/or posterior packing.

Acute Bacterial Rhinosinusitis (ABRS)

Acute bacterial rhinosinusitis is a bacterial infection that affects the nose and the sinuses. It is a symptomatic inflammation of the paranasal sinuses that lasts less than 4 weeks. The condition is considered subacute when symptoms are present from 4 to 12 weeks, and it is considered chronic if symptoms last longer than 12 weeks. In the pediatric population, most sinuses are not fully developed. Complete development of sinuses does not occur until around the age of 20. Maxillary and ethmoid sinuses present at birth are prone to infection because of their small size. Symptoms are often more subtle in pediatric patients. Typical pathogens for this condition include *Streptococcus pneumoniae*, *Haemophilus influenzae*, *Staphylococcus aureus*, and *Moraxella catarrhalis*.

Symptoms

Patients with ABRS usually report an upper respiratory infection with worsening symptoms after initial improvement, headaches, nasal congestion, otalgia, retro-orbital pain, fever, erythema, edema of the nasal mucosa, and purulent discharge. Upon examination, the FNP may find sinus tenderness to palpation, and transillumination of the sinuses may reveal fluid collection within the sinuses.

Management

Management techniques for ABRS include the use of non-steroidal anti-inflammatory drugs (NSAIDs) for pain relief as indicated with oral and/or nasal decongestants to relieve nasal congestion. Intranasal corticosteroids (such as high-dose mometasone fumarate for 21 days) will assist in reducing facial pain and pressure. Amoxicillin or amoxicillin/clavulanate are first-line antibiotics and may be recommended for 7–10 days. Doxycycline or clindamycin may be recommended for patients with a penicillin allergy. The FNP should monitor the patient for complications such as orbital cellulitis, intracranial extension, or sinus thrombosis, which require immediate hospitalization and referral to the emergency department for urgent care.

Pharyngitis and Tonsillitis

Pharyngitis and tonsillitis represent an inflammation of the pharynx and the tonsils due to an infection or irritation. These disorders may be infectious or noninfectious. The goal of managing these disorders is to identify the presence of a group A beta-hemolytic streptococcal (GABHS) infection in order to prevent complications as well as to avoid an unnecessary use of antibiotics.

Infectious Pharyngitis and Tonsillitis

A viral etiology for infectious pharyngitis and tonsillitis is most common in adults, whereas a bacterial etiology is most common in children and adolescents. The most common bacterial pathogens for infectious pharyngitis and tonsillitis include *Streptococcus pyogenes* (including GABHS), *Mycoplasma pneumoniae*, *Chlamydia trachomatis*, *Neisseria gonorrhoeae*, *Corynebacterium* species, and *anaerobic bacteria*.

Symptoms

Patients with infectious pharyngitis and tonsillitis report the presence of and/or a history of fever with a severe sore throat and hoarseness. Upon examination, the FNP will note tonsillar exudate along with a tender cervical adenopathy, which is seen most often in patients who are younger than 15 years old.

Management

Supportive care for infectious pharyngitis and tonsillitis includes voice rest, humidification, warm saline gargles, and NSAID therapy for pain. Pharmacological management includes the use of penicillin, amoxicillin, amoxicillin-clavulanate, cefuroxime, or cefpodoxime, as well as acetaminophen or ibuprofen for a fever and pain. Children and adolescents with positive GABHS require early treatment with high-dose penicillin to prevent rheumatic fever. The FNP should administer cephalosporin to the patient if he or she has an allergy to penicillin. The patient should be instructed to follow up with the FNP if improvement does not begin within 48 hours or if symptoms worsen.

Noninfectious Pharyngitis and Tonsillitis

Noninfectious pharyngitis and tonsillitis are caused by allergies, trauma, cancer, burns, chemotherapy, irradiation, dust, smoke, dryness, or toxins.

Symptoms

Patients with noninfectious pharyngitis and tonsillitis may experience a sore throat, dryness, a postnasal drip, or rhinorrhea.

Management

The best course of action for managing noninfectious pharyngitis and tonsillitis is the remediation or elimination of all environmental symptom triggers, such as pets, dust, or smoke.

Epiglottitis

Epiglottitis is an acute inflammation of the supraglottic area of the oropharynx. It is a **life-threatening condition** that has not been seen as often in the United States since the advent of the Hib vaccine for children. However, there has been a steady increase in the incidence of epiglottitis in adults in recent years. This illness occurs more often in patients with diabetes mellitus or immunodeficiency. For children under the age of five, *Haemophilus influenzae* type B (Hib) continues to be an important cause of this illness. In addition to this bacterial pathogen, which is most common in children, other common bacterial pathogens include *Streptococcus* groups A, B, and C, *Streptococcus pneumoniae*, *Klebsiella pneumoniae*, *Staphylococcus aureus*, and *Candida albicans*.

Symptoms

Adults with epiglottitis typically present with a severe sore throat, anterior neck tenderness, fever, anxiety, pallor, cyanosis, and/or mental status changes. Children with epiglottitis typically present with respiratory distress, upright posturing with the "sniff" or "tripod" position, a refusal to swallow, and/or drooling.

Management

CLINICAL PEARL

When epiglottitis is suspected, avoid a direct inspection of the oropharyngeal cavity because laryngospasm and obstruction may occur.

The FNP should allow a patient with epiglottitis to sit upright in a quiet environment with humidified oxygen. The FNP should not attempt to visualize the pharynx as this may precipitate airway closure. A lateral neck radiograph may demonstrate the "thumb sign," which is indicative of partial airway obstruction. If epiglottitis is suspected, the FNP should **immediately refer the patient to the emergency department** for further management, which will include airway protection, antibiotics if indicated, and corticosteroids.

Peritonsillar Abscess (PTA)

A peritonsillar abscess is an accumulation of infectious exudate (abscess) within the peritonsillar tissues between the pharyngeal muscle and the tonsil. It is usually unilateral. This condition is a deep infection that is often a complication of acute tonsillitis. A common causative pathogen is group A beta-hemolytic streptococcus (GABHS).

Symptoms

Patients with a peritonsillar abscess will present with a fever, sore throat, dysphagia, trismus, pooling of saliva, and muffled "hot potato" voice. Upon examination, the FNP may see a medial deviation of the uvula and soft palate.

Management

For a more severe occurrence, or if the airway may be compromised, refer the patient to the emergency department immediately, where treatment, may include hospitalization, incision and drainage, aspiration, or a tonsillectomy. For a less severe illness, with no risk of airway compromise, the patient should be given oral antibiotics for 7–10 days.

Practice Questions

1. An 88-year-old female presents with complaints of hearing loss. Upon examination, the FNP notes impacted cerumen in both external ear canals. Based on this physical exam, the FNP should document that the patient is experiencing which type of hearing loss?

   (A) presbycusis
   (B) cholesteatoma
   (C) conductive
   (D) sensorineural

2. A middle-aged female presents with a complaint of sudden vision loss in her right eye. Upon examination, the FNP finds a fixed pupil with a red eye. During a funduscopic examination, there is cupping of the retina. This presentation is most consistent with:

   (A) an acute cerebrovascular accident (CVA).
   (B) a cataract formation.
   (C) acute angle-closure glaucoma.
   (D) primary open-angle glaucoma.

3. A young adult female presents with a chief complaint of "allergies." She reports that her constant rhinitis is bothering her at work and at home. Other than an itchy, runny nose, she reports that she feels well. She has been taking 10 mg of loratadine by mouth daily; however, she is still symptomatic. Which of the following classes of medications has proven to be a more effective maintenance medication for the treatment of allergic rhinitis?

   (A) antihistamines
   (B) leukotriene inhibitors
   (C) intranasal corticosteroids
   (D) oral decongestants

4. A 3-year-old female is brought into the clinic by her mother, who reports that the child had a recent "cold" that resolved itself about a week ago. The mother is concerned because her daughter is still experiencing a lot of drainage from her right nostril only. Based on this patient's age, which of the following is a likely cause of this symptom?

   (A) an unresolved upper respiratory infection
   (B) dental caries
   (C) allergic rhinitis
   (D) a foreign body in the right nostril

5. A 10-month-old infant with a diagnosis of acute otitis media will likely demonstrate all of the following signs and symptoms, EXCEPT:

   (A) nausea, vomiting, and possibly diarrhea.
   (B) persistent crying and irritability.
   (C) increased mobility of the tympanic membrane.
   (D) pulling and tugging at his ears.

6. A 30-year-old male has a chief complaint of "tiredness and headaches." He tells the FNP that he had a "head cold" a couple of weeks ago. He began feeling better, but started feeling worse about two days ago. He reports a low-grade fever, headaches, poor appetite, and malaise. Based on this history, the FNP suspects that the patient has acute bacterial rhinosinusitis (ABRS). Which of the following findings supports a bacterial etiology rather than a viral etiology?

   (A) nasal congestion and rhinorrhea
   (B) worsening of symptoms after initial improvement
   (C) headaches
   (D) yellow nasal drainage

7. When examining the tympanic membrane with an otoscope, the FNP attempts to identify visual landmarks within the ear. Which of the following landmarks is NOT assessed using an otoscope?

   (A) tympanic membrane structure
   (B) cone of light
   (C) ossicles
   (D) Eustachian tube

8. When testing the vision of a three-year-old, the best tool to use is the:

   (A) Ishihara test.
   (B) cover-uncover test.
   (C) Snellen chart.
   (D) E chart.

9. The patient is an infant with a red, slightly edematous, tender area in the medial corner of her left eye. This presentation is most consistent with:

   (A) conjunctivitis.
   (B) dacryocystitis.
   (C) pinguecula.
   (D) an obstructed nasolacrimal duct.

10. A 75-year-old male reports a "problem" with his eyes that he started noticing a few years ago, but it is getting worse. Based on his age, you suspect cataract formation. Which of the following is a common complaint of a patient with cataracts?

   (A) drainage from both eyes
   (B) sensitivity to sunlight
   (C) increased episodes of falling
   (D) unilateral eye pain

11. A 4-year-old boy is brought to the clinic by his father. The father tells the FNP that his son suddenly started complaining of right ear pain. The boy cries when he moves his head and tells the FNP that it makes the pain worse. His temperature is 102°F. During a physical exam, the FNP notes marked tenderness with edema and cellulitis behind the right ear. These findings are suggestive of:

   (A) otitis externa.
   (B) otitis media.
   (C) mastoiditis.
   (D) otosclerosis.

12. A patient with a ruptured tympanic membrane would most likely exhibit which of the following findings during a physical exam?

   (A) bright red blood in the external canal
   (B) purulent, foul-smelling fluid in the external canal
   (C) increased pain in the affected ear
   (D) total loss of hearing in the affected ear

13. Transillumination of the maxillary sinuses can aid in the diagnosis of rhinosinusitis. A reddish glow seen on the hard palate with transillumination is suggestive of:

   (A) an anatomical absence of the maxillary sinuses.
   (B) clear maxillary sinuses.
   (C) thickened mucosa of the sinuses.
   (D) fluid or exudate within the sinuses.

14. Finding a cloudy cornea during a physical exam is characteristic of which of the following diagnoses?

   (A) a corneal abrasion with primary open-angle glaucoma
   (B) macular degeneration with a corneal ulcer
   (C) cataracts and acute angle-closure glaucoma
   (D) conjunctivitis and the presence of a foreign body

15. The cover-uncover and Hirschberg tests are used to detect the presence of:

   (A) amblyopia.
   (B) conjunctivitis.
   (C) refractive error.
   (D) strabismus.

Answer Explanations

1. **(C)** Conductive hearing loss results from dysfunction in the external or middle ear. Mechanisms that impair the transmission of sound waves to the inner ear include obstruction (cerumen impaction), fluid (otitis media with effusion), discontinuity (ossicular damage or disruption), and stiffness of the middle ear structures (otosclerosis). Cerumen impaction is the most common of these mechanisms for the development of conductive hearing loss. Presbycusis (choice (A)) is an age-related sensorineural hearing loss that is bilateral. Cholesteatoma (choice (B)) is a type of chronic otitis media, and the most common cause of cholesteatoma is prolonged dysfunction of the Eustachian tube. This dysfunction creates an epithelium-lined sac within the middle ear. This sac may become obstructed, which can lead to a chronic infection that may eventually cause bone erosion and destruction of the ossicular chain. Sensorineural hearing loss (choice (D)) occurs as a result of a lesion in the organ of Corti or in the central nerve pathways, including the eight cranial nerves (CN VIII). This type of hearing loss is usually irreversible.

2. **(C)** Acute angle-closure glaucoma occurs as a result of a narrow anterior chamber in the eye with increased intraocular pressure (> 25 mm Hg) as a result. Several factors cause individuals to have a narrow (or shallow) anterior chamber, including farsightedness, short stature, family history, ethnicity (Asian and Inuit), and aging. This disorder presents with an acute onset of severe pain in the eye along with profound visual loss. Patients often report seeing "halos" around lights. The eye is red with a cloudy cornea and a fixed pupil. The eye feels firm to palpation. An acute cerebrovascular accident (stroke) (choice (A)) presents with the sudden onset of neurological deficits in the presence of comorbid hypertension, diabetes mellitus, atherosclerosis, atrial fibrillation, and/or smoking. These neurological deficits manifest in the area affected by cerebral ischemia. Cataract formation (choice (B)) presents with a gradual progression of blurred vision due to opacity of the crystalline lens of the eye. This disorder may develop unilaterally, bilaterally, or sequentially. Lens opacities may be grossly visible. Patients report difficulty driving at night and the development of nearsightedness. Patients also often develop double vision. Primary open-angle glaucoma (choice (D)) is sometimes referred to as chronic glaucoma and is asymptomatic in the early stages of the disease. With progression, patients experience an insidious, progressive loss of peripheral vision, resulting in tunnel vision in later stages. Pathologic cupping of the optic disc is seen, and intraocular pressure is usually (though not always) elevated.

3. **(C)** Allergic rhinitis (AR) is also called "hay fever" and is very common in the United States. Symptoms include clear rhinorrhea, tearing, eye irritation, sneezing, and pruritus in the setting of an allergen exposure. The mainstay of treatment is intranasal corticosteroid sprays. Research has demonstrated that these agents are more effective, and are often less expensive, than non-sedating antihistamines. However, patients should be reminded that there is often a delay in improvement of symptoms for two or more weeks. These sprays shrink hypertrophic nasal mucosa and decrease nasal congestion. Second-generation antihistamines (choice (A)) are classified as "non-sedating," although many of these agents have a mild sedating effect. These medications work well for the treatment of allergic rhinitis symptoms because they work quickly (usually within 1.5 to 2 hours), but the antihistamine effect of non-sedating antihistamines is *less* effective than intranasal corticosteroid sprays in relieving nasal congestion. Leukotriene inhibitors (choice (B)) are frequently used for long-term management of atopic disorders, such as asthma. These agents work by decreasing inflammation. Oral decongestants (choice (D)) have several side effects, including nervousness, dizziness, and

headaches. This class of medications has not demonstrated clear efficacy in the treatment of allergic rhinitis and would not be recommended in this situation.

4. **(D)** Young children are prone to inserting foreign objects into body orifices, such as the nose and ear. A nasal foreign body may be discovered right away by the parent, or it may remain hidden until symptoms appear. Often, a persistent or recurrent, unilateral purulent drainage is noted in the presence of a foreign body. The nasal discharge is often foul-smelling. Children will often deny putting something in their nose; however, this symptom should raise suspicion of the presence of a foreign body. Nasal drainage associated with an unresolved upper respiratory infection (choice (A)) is usually bilateral and may persist after other symptoms have resolved, especially in young children. Dental caries (choice (B)) is the most common chronic disease in children. Tooth decay is a bacterial disease that may result in permanent damage and loss of teeth. Lactobacilli are often present, adhering to active cavities, and these organisms may be transmitted from person to person when saliva is shared. Allergic rhinitis (choice (C)) represents a type I IgE-mediated response to allergen exposure. This clinical diagnosis is based on the presence of bilateral rhinorrhea, nasal pruritus, congestion, and sneezing.

5. **(C)** Acute otitis media (AOM) is an infection of the middle ear that usually presents with an abrupt onset of ear pain, irritability, fever, and otorrhea. Infants may have mild nausea, vomiting, and diarrhea, so choice (A) is true. They may also be irritable or cry persistently, making choice (B) true. Infants will also often pull or tug at the affected ear, making choice (D) true as well. However, upon an otoscopic examination, the tympanic membrane will demonstrate *hypo*mobility, not *hyper*mobility, making choice (C) false and thus the right answer.

6. **(B)** Acute sinusitis is a symptomatic inflammation of the paranasal sinuses for less than four weeks. Since rhinitis and sinusitis occur together, *rhinosinusitis* is the preferred term. Nasal congestion and rhinorrhea (choice (A)), headaches (choice (C)), and yellow nasal drainage (choice (D)) may be seen in rhinosinusitis caused by *either* viral or bacterial pathogens. Worsening of symptoms after initial improvement, however, suggests a bacterial infection of the sinuses following an initial viral illness. The most common bacterial pathogens associated with acute bacterial rhinosinusitis include *Streptococcus pneumoniae*, *Haemophilus influenzae*, and *Moraxella catarrhalis*. A fungal infection of the sinuses may occur in individuals who are immunocompromised or as a nosocomial illness.

7. **(D)** When visualizing the internal ear structures using an otoscope, identifying landmarks is helpful in terms of differentiating normal findings from abnormal findings. The Eustachian tube connects the middle ear with the oral cavity. This tube is normally flat and closed but opens briefly with swallowing or yawning and helps to equalize pressure in the middle ear with atmospheric changes. This structure is not visible with an otoscope. The tympanic membrane (choice (A)) separates the external and middle ear and should be seen as a pearly gray membrane with a prominent cone of light (choice (B)) seen on the anteroinferior quadrant. The drum is an oval area that is pulled in at the center by the middle ear ossicles (choice (C)), known as the malleus. Parts of the malleus that may be visualized through the tympanic membrane are the umbo and the manubrium. The small, slack upper portion of the tympanic membrane is called the pars flaccida. The annulus is the outer rim of the drum.

8. **(D)** Use of the E chart with young children facilitates vision screening because children can point to or indicate the direction the letter is pointing. This tool does not require the child to read letters. The Ishihara test (choice (A)) is used to screen for color vision deficiencies. The cover-uncover test (choice (B)) is used to detect ocular misalignment. The Snellen chart (choice (C)) is used for older children and adults.

9. **(B)** Dacrocystitis is an inflammatory condition that affects the lacrimal sac, which is the area between the lower eyelid and the nose. Dacrocystitis presents as a painful, red, and tender area around the eye, especially near the nose and lower eyelid. Conjunctivitis (choice (A)) is an inflammatory or infectious condition that affects the conjunctivae. Findings for conjunctivitis may include tearing, burning, and discharge from the affected eye(s). Pinguecula (choice (C)) is a benign, yellow, triangular-shaped nodule on the bulbar conjunctiva, sometimes extending to the iris. This is a common finding in elderly individuals. An obstructed nasolacrimal duct (choice (D)) results in mucopurulent drainage from the puncta of the eye.

10. **(B)** A cataract is an opacity of the crystalline lens of the eye. This condition is extremely common, affecting most individuals to some degree as they age. Cataracts present with a slow, insidious loss of vision related to hardening and clouding of the lens. Opacity may be partial or total. Patients typically report an increased sensitivity to sunlight as the disease progresses. Cataracts are painless and affect central vision more so than peripheral vision. Drainage from both eyes (choice (A)) is consistent with a diagnosis of conjunctivitis. The discharge from conjunctivitis may be clear and watery or yellow and purulent, depending on the pathophysiology. Increased episodes of falling (choice (C)) are not usually associated with cataract formation unless other conditions that cause the individual to fall are present. Unilateral eye pain (choice (D)) is a symptom of uveitis (inflammation of the uvea) or acute angle-closure glaucoma. Cataract development is not associated with eye pain.

11. **(C)** Mastoiditis is an acute suppurative (pus-forming) condition that usually develops after several weeks of untreated or inadequately treated otitis media. Its symptoms include post-auricular pain and erythema behind the ear along with a high fever. Otitis externa (choice (A)) is an inflammation of the external auditory canal and often the auricle as well. Patients with acute otitis externa complain of severe pain with manipulation of the auricle or tragus of the ear. There is marked edema and purulent discharge from the canal. Otitis media (choice (B)) involves an infection within the middle ear. External symptoms and pain with head movement are not associated with uncomplicated acute otitis media. Otosclerosis (choice (D)) is associated with presbycusis, an age-related hearing loss seen in elderly individuals. Hearing loss with this condition is associated with a hardening or stiffness of the middle ear structures.

12. **(A)** A ruptured tympanic membrane may occur due to an infection, trauma, or excessive pressure when blowing one's nose. A common finding is a small amount of bright red blood in the ear canal. Active bleeding should not be present. Purulent, foul-smelling fluid (choice (B)) should also not be present. Pain may be present in the affected ear only, but it should only be experienced briefly, not increasingly (choice (C)). Hearing may be slightly diminished, but a total loss of hearing (choice (D)) would be due to some other cause. Patients will often report that sounds are "muffled" when the tympanic membrane is ruptured. The membrane usually heals without complication in one to two weeks.

13. **(B)** Transillumination of the sinuses will produce a reddish glow seen on the hard palate when the sinuses are clear and no infection is present. An anatomical absence of maxillary sinuses (choice (A)) would be difficult to demonstrate with transillumination. Thickened mucosa of the sinuses (choice (C)) as well as the presence of fluid or exudate within the sinuses (choice (D)) may be identified by a lack of sinus illumination on an X-ray.

14. **(C)** A cloudy cornea is sometimes described as a "steamy" cornea. This finding is seen in the presence of cataracts and acute angle-closure glaucoma. These conditions obscure normal light reflexes and diminish visual acuity. The diagnoses described in choices (A), (B), and (D) would not produce a cloudy cornea. A corneal abrasion may be identified using fluorescein dye and visualization with a black light. Primary, open-angle glaucoma cannot be identified through a physical assessment of the cornea. Macular degeneration causes changes in the macula of the eye and is associated with progressive vision loss. A corneal ulcer is an extended form of a corneal abrasion in which the total thickness of the cornea is affected. This may be identified via fluorescein dye staining. A patient with this condition should be referred to an ophthalmologist for management. Conjunctivitis often produces redness around the eye, including the conjunctiva. The conjunctiva is the mucus membrane that lines the inside of the eyelids and covers the front of the eye. The cornea is unaffected. A foreign body on the cornea may cause a laceration or an ulceration to occur on the cornea; however, the cornea (the transparent layer covering the eye) would be red and appear inflamed, but it should not be cloudy in appearance.

15. **(D)** Strabismus is a defect in ocular alignment. It may be manifested in children as a phoria or a tropia. A phoria indicates intermittent deviation in ocular alignment, whereas a tropia refers to a constant or intermittent deviation. During the cover-uncover test and the alternating cover test, the examiner rapidly covers and uncovers the eyes while looking for orbital movement that indicates misalignment. The Hirschberg test is also called the "corneal light reflex test." This test evaluates extraocular muscle function and assesses for ocular misalignment. Amblyopia (choice (A)) usually presents as a unilateral defect in the development of the visual pathway. The affected eye is unable to attain central vision. This leads to a refractive error, which may be identified during an optometric exam. Conjunctivitis (choice (B)) is an inflammation or infection of the conjunctival membrane covering the eye. Refractive errors (choice (C)) are alterations in the refractive power of the eye, leading to decreased visual acuity, which may be corrected with prescription lenses. The cover-uncover and Hirschberg tests will only assist in the identification of strabismus.

2

Disorders of the Respiratory System

Respiratory disorders are extremely common and have diverse causes; however, they frequently share pathologic and clinical features. Abnormalities of the respiratory system often manifest as a cough, dyspnea, shortness of breath, and airflow limitations. Illnesses that affect the respiratory system are often described as disorders that affect the upper airway (above the glottis) or lower airway (below the glottis). The location of the abnormality or dysfunction is important in the diagnosis and management of these conditions, which may be life-threatening. This chapter provides an overview of respiratory disorders that are commonly seen in primary care.

Asthma

Asthma is a chronic inflammatory disorder that affects the airways. Components of this disorder include bronchial hyper-responsiveness and airflow obstruction that is associated with an immunohistologic pathology. Strong identifiable risk factors for the development of asthma include atopy and obesity. This condition is considered to be partially reversible. Exacerbations are often triggered by pets, dust mites, indoor molds, cockroaches, cigarette smoke, and exercise. Asthma can be classified as intermittent (mild and lasting less than two days per week) or persistent (mild to severe and lasting more than two days per week). Refer to Table 2.1 for a more in-depth classification of asthma severity. Airway obstruction is at least partially reversible, whereas persistent inflammation may lead to airway remodeling, which is irreversible.

Symptoms

Patients with asthma experience episodes of coughing, wheezing, dyspnea, respiratory distress, bronchospasm, and chest tightness. These symptoms are often worse at night.

Management

Managing asthma includes patient and family education regarding how to manage exacerbations. Medications include inhaled relievers (such as albuterol and oral corticosteroids) and controllers (such as inhaled corticosteroids (ICS), leukotriene modifiers, and a combination of inhaled corticosteroids with a long-acting beta-2 agonist (ICS/LABA)).

Table 2.1. Classification of Asthma Severity

Components of SEVERITY		Age (Years)	Classification of Asthma SEVERITY (Intermittent vs. Persistent)			
			Intermittent	Persistent		
				Mild	Moderate	Severe
Impairment	Symptoms	All	≤ 2 days/week	> 2 days/week but not daily	Daily	Throughout the day
	Nighttime awakenings	0–4	0	1–2x/month	3–4x/month	> 1x/week
		≥ 5	≤ 2x/month	3–4x/month	> 1x/week but not nightly	Often 7x/week
	SABA use for symptom control	All	≤ 2 days/week	> 2 days/week but not daily	Daily	Several times a day
	Interference with normal activity	All	None	Minor limitation	Some limitation	Extremely limited
	Lung function: FEV$_1$ (predicted) or PEF (personal best)	≥ 5	Normal FEV$_1$ between exacerbations > 80%	> 80%	60–80%	< 60%
	FEV$_1$/FVC	5–11	> 85%	> 80%	75–80%	< 60%
		≥ 12	Normal	Normal	Reduced 5%	Reduced > 5%
Risk	Exacerbations requiring oral corticosteroids	0–4	≥ 2x in 6 months or ≥ 4 wheezing episodes/year lasting > 1 day AND risk factors for persistent asthma			
		5–11	≤ 1x/year	≥ 2x/year		
		≥ 12		Consider severity and interval since last exacerbation. Frequency and severity may fluctuate over time for patients in any severity category. Relative annual risk of exacerbations may be related to FEV$_1$.		
Recommended step for starting treatment		0–4	Step 1	Step 2	Step 3	Step 3
		5–11	Step 1	Step 2	Step 3	Step 3 or 4
		≥ 12	Step 1	Step 2	Step 3	Step 4 or 5
		All	Consider short course of oral corticosteroids			
		All	In 2–6 weeks, evaluate level of asthma control that is achieve and adjust therapy accordingly. For children 0–4 years old, if no clear benefit is observed in 4–6 weeks, stop treatment and consider alternative diagnosis or adjusting therapy.			

FEV$_1$, forced expiratory volume in 1 second; FVC, forced vital capacity; PEF, peak expiratory flow; SABA, short-action beta$_2$-agonist

Chronic Obstructive Pulmonary Disease (COPD)

Chronic obstructive pulmonary disease is a preventable and irreversible disease state that is characterized by the presence of airflow obstruction due to chronic bronchitis or emphysema. Airflow limitation, caused by the obstructive pathophysiology of the disease, is progressive and may be accompanied by a degree of airway hyper-responsiveness, which may be partially reversible. COPD is usually categorized as either chronic bronchitis or emphysema, and many patients have a combination of both conditions. Chronic bronchitis presents with a daily productive cough with excessive production of bronchial secretions. Emphysema is a disease in which there is an abnormal, permanent enlargement of the lung spaces. These obstructive disorders impair respirations by preventing adequate oxygenation and by not allowing air out of the lungs. Frequent exacerbations are common for those with COPD and are often caused by atypical pathogens, such as *Klebsiella pneumoniae* or *Mycoplasma* species. Risk factors for COPD include advancing age, male gender, and cigarette smoking. The onset of COPD usually presents in the fifth decade of life.

Symptoms

Most patients who are diagnosed with COPD are asymptomatic for 10–20 years before breathing problems prompt them to seek care. Patients with COPD report shortness of breath, a progressive cough, and excessive sputum production with sputum that is often thick and colored (gray, brown, yellow, or green). As the disease advances, patients develop frequent respiratory infections, such as bronchitis, which become chronic. Pulmonary hypertension may develop with chronic hypoxia. These patients are the "blue bloaters" who have progressive edema and cyanosis. The complete blood count may demonstrate polycythemia. Patients whose disease is primarily emphysema are known as "pink puffers." These individuals have severe dyspnea and are usually very thin with a "barrel-shaped chest" as a result of chronic hyperinflation of the lungs. Many patients with emphysema use pursed lip breathing to help get more air out and oxygen in.

Management

The goals of managing COPD are to improve airflow, control coughing and secretions, and prevent infections and further complications. Smoking cessation is critical to slowing the disease progression. Patients should be encouraged to receive the influenza vaccine annually and the pneumococcal vaccine series based on disease severity and risk for complications of COPD. Management is determined based on the severity of the disease and is also often based on pulmonary function studies. Mainstays include oral corticosteroids for exacerbations, inhaled bronchodilators, oxygen therapy, and inhaled corticosteroids. Oxygen has proven to be effective in improving the quality of life for patients with COPD, as long as it is used for at least 15 hours a day. Antibiotics may be prescribed for exacerbations that are associated with a bacterial superinfection. Adequate hydration and controlling comorbid conditions are also important in managing this disease.

Acute Bronchitis

Acute bronchitis is a nonspecific inflammation that involves the bronchi, the bronchioles, and, in children, the trachea. Bronchitis is most often caused by viral pathogens; however, a bacterial superinfection may occur.

CLINICAL PEARL

Smoking cessation is the single most important action that can be taken to slow the progression of COPD. Oxygen use for severe COPD for at least 15 hours per day may increase the patient's life span. Long-acting beta-2 agonists carry a black-box warning for an increased risk of death. They should always be used with an inhaled corticosteroid.

Symptoms

Patients with acute bronchitis experience the acute development of a persistent cough with sputum production and dyspnea. The patient's mucus membranes are often hyperemic and edematous. Systemic symptoms include malaise, fatigue, and anorexia.

Management

The management of acute bronchitis includes supportive care to minimize symptoms and the administration of antibiotics if pertussis or other bacterial pathogens are suspected. Recommendations for first-line treatment include macrolides, doxycycline, and trimethoprim-sulfamethoxazole.

Community-Acquired Pneumonia (CAP)

Community-acquired pneumonia is an acute infection of the lungs that is frequently associated with symptoms of an active infection in an individual who has not been in a hospital or a resident of a long-term care facility within the past 14 days. This disorder is often classified as typical or atypical based on the causative pathogen. Examples of typical pathogens include *Streptococcus pneumoniae, Haemophilus influenzae,* and *Moraxella catarrhalis.* Examples of atypical pathogens are *Mycoplasma pneumoniae, Legionella pneumophila,* and *Chlamydia pneumoniae.* Vaccines are available to prevent or lessen the severity of several types of pneumonia. The PCV13 protects against 13 types of bacteria that cause pneumonia. This vaccine is recommended for infants, young children, and adults over the age of 65. A newer vaccine, the PPSV23, protects against 23 types of pneumonia-causing bacteria. This vaccine is recommended for adults over the age of 65 and children over the age of 2 who are at an increased risk for this disease.

Symptoms

Patients with pneumonia present with chills, a fever, malaise, and chest discomfort. Infants and young children may present with a cough, the use of accessory muscles for breathing, and hypoxia. Viral pneumonia often presents more insidiously than a bacterial illness.

Management

The management of pneumonia is based on its etiology. Viral pneumonia is managed with supportive care and rest. Bacterial pneumonia is treated with antibiotics such as azithromycin, clarithromycin, or doxycycline for typical pathogens. Patients who have chronic, comorbid conditions and illnesses caused by atypical pathogens often require treatment with respiratory fluoroquinolones, such as levofloxacin, gemifloxacin, or moxifloxacin, or a macrolide plus a beta-lactam agent. The **CURB**-65 criteria is a tool that is used to help the clinician determine the severity of the illness. This objective tool is easy to remember and is a quick method that can be used to assess patients to determine if they can be treated on an outpatient basis or whether they may need hospitalization. The **C** stands for confusion (new onset disorientation). The **U** refers to an elevated blood urea nitrogen (BUN) level over 19 mg per dL. The **R** refers to the respiratory rate, and individuals with a rate of 30 breaths per minute or more are at a higher risk. The **B** stands for a blood pressure measurement of a systolic less than 90 mm Hg or a diastolic of 60 mm Hg or less. In patients who are 65 and older, each positive finding equals one point. Age is also one point. A score of 0–1 represents a low-risk illness that may be treated on an outpatient basis. A score of 2 indicates the need for short inpatient treatment or closely monitored outpatient treatment. A score of 3 or above represents severe pneumonia that requires inpatient, possibly intensive care unit, management. Blood cultures may be performed to determine the bacterial origin of the illness.

In the United States, there are two types of vaccines that protect against pneumococcal disease. These vaccines continue to undergo development to include more protection against a greater number of pathogens that are responsible for pneumonia. The first type of vaccine is the pneumococcal conjugate vaccine (PCV), which is available as PCV7 (which protects against 7 pneumoniae serotypes) and PCV13 (which protects against 13 pneumoniae serotypes). The PCV13 is the newer of these two vaccines and is recommended for all children under the age of 2 as well as adults who are 65 and older. Some individuals who are not within those two age groups may also be eligible for this vaccine because of chronic medical conditions or because they are immunocompromised. The pneumococcal polysaccharide vaccine 23 (PPSV23) offers protections against 23 pneumoniae serotypes and is recommended for all individuals under the age of 2, those who are 65 and older, and for adults who are smokers and are between the ages of 19 and 64 years old.

Pertussis

Pertussis is a respiratory illness that is caused by a Gram-negative bacillus, *Bordetella pertussis*. This infection is also known as whooping cough because of the characteristic high-pitched stridor associated with the coughing spasms. More serious symptoms of illness are seen in neonates and young infants. Transmission occurs via aerosol droplets or close contact. The virus may live for up to 30 minutes on surfaces. Therefore, transmission often occurs through hand-to-hand contact. Pertussis is present in all age groups; however, most cases are asymptomatic, with the highest mortality seen in infants less than one month old. Adult household members are now seen as a vector for transmission of pertussis to very young infants.

Symptoms

Young infants may present with episodes of apnea, seizures, coughing (without "whoop"), poor feeding, and tachypnea. Older infants, children, and adolescents often present with high-pitched inspiratory sounds associated with coughing ("whooping cough"). Leukocytosis with marked elevation of the lymphocytes is common.

Management

To treat pertussis, use macrolide antibiotics, such as azithromycin, and supportive care, such as antipyretics, humidification, and increased fluids. All household members should receive chemoprophylaxis if an infant in the household has pertussis.

Croup (Laryngotracheitis)

Croup is an acute inflammatory disease that affects the larynx and the trachea. It presents with a brassy cough that is bark-like along with some degree of inspiratory stridor. Respiratory distress is often present. Croup is seen in infants and toddlers between 6 and 36 months; however, recurrent croup may occur up to age six in some children. This viral infection causes an inflammatory response in the laryngeal area, which may extend into the subglottic area. If the illness persists beyond five to seven days, a bacterial superinfection is likely. The pathophysiology of croup involves some degree of laryngeal obstruction. Therefore, airway preservation must be considered.

Symptoms

Patients with croup present with a low-grade fever, a cough that is worse at night, poor feeding, and/or periods of apnea.

CLINICAL PEARL

Pneumonia is a common complication of influenza in elderly individuals due to their decreased immune response to illnesses.

CLINICAL PEARL

Most infants who contract pertussis are infected by adults who have asymptomatic pertussis. New guidelines recommend the TDaP vaccination for adults and others who have close contact with infants.

Management

The management of croup involves humidification, nebulized epinephrine, corticosteroids with bronchodilators, and oxygen, if indicated. Infants and young children with respiratory distress should be hospitalized.

Bronchiolitis

Bronchiolitis is also called asthmatic bronchitis, infectious asthma, and virus-induced asthma. This illness causes inflammation, necrosis, and edema of the epithelial cells that line the small airways, along with copious mucus production. It is characterized by the insidious onset of symptoms and is a communicable disease that is seen in infants up to two-year-olds. Bronchiolitis is the leading cause of hospitalization for babies and is commonly diagnosed when an infant presents with a first episode of wheezing. The virus spreads via respiratory secretions or fomites and can live on surfaces for up to 30 minutes. The most frequent mode of transmission is hand carriage of contaminated secretions. Bronchiolitis is primarily caused by the respiratory syncytial virus (RSV) that occurs in outbreaks during the winter.

Symptoms

Infants often present with apnea as the first symptom. These infants may also have a low-grade fever, poor feeding, raspy respirations with coryza, mild conjunctivitis, and otitis media or pharyngitis. Infants with RSV also demonstrate varying degrees of respiratory distress.

Management

Infants with RSV require hospitalization along with supportive care, such as humidification and nebulizer treatments.

Tuberculosis (TB)

Tuberculosis is a state reportable, systemic disease that is caused by *Mycoplasma tuberculosis*. The most common presentation is pulmonary disease, but the genitourinary system, bones, heart, peritoneum, lymphatics, and meninges may also be involved. Individuals who are at a high risk for contracting tuberculosis include those living in crowded conditions, those who are immuno-compromised, and those with diabetes mellitus, renal insufficiency, or malignancy. With exposure to the *Mycoplasma tuberculosis* organism, granulomas are formed as the body tries to encapsulate the pathogen. For individuals with an intact immune system, these granulomas harden and remain latent. However, patients with a compromised immune system develop an active disease. Testing for TB includes the PPD skin test. With this test, the results are determined by the size of the induration at the testing site. An interpretation of the test results is based on the patient's immune and risk status. Newer serum tests include an interferon-γ release assay and a test that uses a T-cell assay to detect infection.

Symptoms

Most patients, even those with an active disease, are usually asymptomatic until the late stages. When symptoms do occur, they usually include weight loss, a low-grade fever, anorexia, night sweats, and a progressive cough.

Management

Treatment for TB includes a minimum of six months of therapy with isoniazid, rifampin, pyrazinamide, and ethambutol. Individuals with a compromised immune system are treated for a minimum of nine months. Medications are administered in combinations due to the high rate of resistance demonstrated by the *Mycobacterium tuberculosis* bacterium. Patient follow-up and reporting are also important components of management for this condition. Patients who have had tuberculosis will subsequently always have a positive PPD skin test. In these individuals, a chest X-ray is recommended for screening for evidence of TB.

Influenza

Influenza is a highly contagious respiratory illness that occurs annually in epidemic patterns across the globe. The virus responsible for most cases of human influenza is classified as type A, which can affect humans and other mammals, such as horses and pigs. Type B and type C primarily affect humans. Epidemics occur in fall or winter. Pandemics are outbreaks that occur for longer periods of time and over a wide geographic area. They are associated with higher mortality. Viruses that cause influenza are transmitted primarily through respiratory secretions, although fomite transmission is possible. The influenza virus causes necrosis of the respiratory epithelial cells, predisposing tissue to the development of a bacterial infection.

Symptoms

This illness begins with an abrupt onset of fever, chills, myalgias, and malaise. Respiratory symptoms include nasal congestion, sore throat, cough, and hoarseness. Gastrointestinal symptoms, such as nausea, vomiting, and diarrhea, are often seen in young children with the type B virus. Elderly individuals may present with malaise and confusion, usually with no fever or cough. Enlarged cervical lymph nodes and a mildly reddened pharyngeal area may be seen upon examination of the oropharynx.

Management

For the treatment of influenza, supportive therapy is indicated to control a fever, any discomfort, and gastrointestinal symptoms. Antiviral therapy is indicated for those with an acute illness, those with a comorbid chronic disease, or those who are immunocompromised. Antiviral therapy should ideally be started within 48 hours of onset of symptoms. Neuraminidase inhibitors, including zanamivir (inhaled), oseltamivir (oral), or peramivir (IV), may reduce the length and severity of the illness and may thus prevent common complications, such as bacterial pneumonia. Adamantines (amantadine and rimantadine) are not recommended for the management of influenza because of high levels of viral resistance to these agents.

Practice Questions

1. The FNP sees a patient who is a 15-year-old male with a diagnosis of asthma. On a follow-up visit, he reports that he has to use his rescue inhaler almost every day. His mother reports nocturnal coughing episodes that require the use of his inhaler and occur two to three times per night. During a physical examination, the FNP notes bilateral wheezing. Based on this information, the FNP would classify his asthma as:

   (A) intermittent.
   (B) mild persistent.
   (C) moderate persistent.
   (D) severe persistent.

2. The FNP sees a 72-year-old male patient with a diagnosis of chronic obstructive pulmonary disease (COPD). He reports to the clinic with complaints of increased symptoms of shortness of breath. The FNP would like to add an inhaled glucocorticoid to his medication regimen. What is the desired therapeutic action of this agent in the management of COPD?

   (A) mucolytic activity
   (B) improvement of the central respiratory drive
   (C) reduction of airway inflammation
   (D) improvement in cardiac output

3. The FNP is treating a 30-year-old male and who is a recent immigrant from a country where tuberculosis is endemic. The patient produces documentation that shows he received the Bacille Calmette-Guérin (BCG) vaccine as a child. A 10 mm or greater area of induration of the skin, where the purified protein derivative (PPD) is applied, for this patient indicates that:

   (A) the patient might have tuberculosis and should be evaluated appropriately.
   (B) Isoniazid therapy should be administered for six months before any follow-up testing is done.
   (C) the patient does not have an active tuberculosis infection at this time.
   (D) the patient needs a chest X-ray every six months to assess for an active disease.

4. A 68-year-old female arrives at the clinic for an annual wellness examination. The FNP plans to discuss recommended immunizations with her during the visit. Which of the following pneumococcal vaccines offers protection against the greatest number of serotypes?

   (A) pneumococcal 7-valent vaccine
   (B) pneumococcal conjugate vaccine (PCV13)
   (C) pneumococcal polysaccharide vaccine (PPSV23)
   (D) live attenuated influenza vaccine (LAIV)

5. The FNP sees a 79-year-old male whom she has treated before. Today, his chief complaints are a loss of appetite and extreme fatigue. After performing a comprehensive history and physical, and after ordering the appropriate diagnostic studies, the FNP determines that this patient has community-acquired pneumonia (CAP). In the treatment of CAP, the CURB-65 criteria are used to:

   (A) distinguish between a viral etiology and a bacterial etiology.
   (B) provide guidelines for pharmacotherapy.
   (C) determine the severity of the illness.
   (D) determine a local pathogen endemicity.

6. Ipratropium bromide is frequently used in the management of COPD. To which class of medications does this agent belong?

    (A) beta-2 adrenergic agonist
    (B) anticholinergic
    (C) corticosteroid
    (D) phosphodiesterase 4 inhibitor

7. The patient is a 40-year-old male with a new diagnosis of pulmonary tuberculosis (TB). The FNP is seeing him in her office to discuss treatment. When planning his care, the FNP understands that the minimum acceptable duration of treatment for patients with latent TB is:

    (A) 3 months.
    (B) 6 months.
    (C) 9 months.
    (D) 12 months.

8. Which of the following is the most common mode of transmission of a viral upper respiratory infection (URI) in an adult patient?

    (A) hand-to-hand transmission
    (B) air pollution
    (C) sharing toothbrushes
    (D) intimate contact

9. Bronchitis and bronchiolitis are respiratory disorders that are frequently seen in primary care. In which of the following age groups is the rate of occurrence of bronchiolitis the highest?

    (A) infancy to two years old
    (B) preschool and school-age children
    (C) adolescents
    (D) adults

10. The management of asthma often involves the use of several pharmacotherapeutic agents in addition to modifying environmental and lifestyle measures to reduce triggers. In patients with persistent asthma, which class of medications is considered the first-line treatment as anti-inflammatory controller therapy?

    (A) short-acting beta-2 agonists (SABA)
    (B) inhaled corticosteroids (ICS)
    (C) leukotriene modifiers
    (D) anticholinergics

11. The patient is a previously healthy two-year-old with a diagnosis of community-acquired pneumonia (CAP). What is most likely the causative pathogen in this patient?

    (A) *Moraxella catarrhalis*
    (B) *Staphylococcus aureus*
    (C) *Mycoplasma pneumoniae*
    (D) a respiratory virus

12. Which of the following antibiotics provides effective treatment against atypical respiratory pathogens?

    (A) amoxicillin
    (B) ceftriaxone
    (C) clarithromycin
    (D) cefadroxil

13. During which age range is a child at the greatest risk of death from pertussis?

    (A) younger than 1 month old
    (B) 2–4 months old
    (C) 6–12 months old
    (D) 12–24 months old

14. Which of the following diagnostic tests is the most helpful in the diagnosis of pertussis?

    (A) chest X-ray
    (B) CT of the chest
    (C) polymerase chain reaction (PCR) testing
    (D) blood culture

15. Presenting symptoms of pneumonia, in all age groups, most often include a cough and which of the following?

    (A) wheezing
    (B) fever
    (C) nausea and vomiting
    (D) upper respiratory symptoms

Answer Explanations

1. **(D)** The patient described in this scenario is having symptoms nightly with two to three episodes each night. Upon auscultation of the chest, the FNP hears wheezing. The patient is using his "rescue inhaler" two or three times a night as well as daily. Based on these findings, the patient could be classified as having severe persistent asthma. This classification requires the following findings: continuous daily symptoms with frequent nighttime symptoms, frequent exacerbations with a limitation of physical activity secondary to asthma, and a forced expiratory volume/1 second (FEV_1) score that is at or less than 60%. Intermittent asthma (choice (A)) presents as intermittent symptoms that occur less than one time per week. A patient with intermittent asthma has brief, short-term exacerbations that do not occur regularly, and the patient is asymptomatic between exacerbations. The patient's FEV1 is greater than 80% of the predicted value. Patients with mild persistent asthma (choice (B)) have symptoms more than twice a week but not every day. Asthma symptoms occur at night more than twice a month, and exacerbations may affect activity and sleep. Moderate persistent asthma (choice (C)) presents as daily symptoms, but those symptoms are not continuous. Symptoms occur at night at least once a week, but not every night. These patients require the use of a daily inhaled short-acting beta-2 agonist to manage symptoms. Remember that patients do not have to have every symptom in each category to qualify for a specific classification.

2. **(C)** When prescribing medication to improve symptoms in a patient with COPD, it is important to follow established guidelines. However, it is equally important to understand the mechanism of action for each agent. Inhaled glucocorticoid agents improve respiratory function by decreasing airway inflammation. These products include budesonide and fluticasone. Dosing should be individualized based on the patient's symptoms, and it is important to make sure the patient is using the inhaler correctly when prescribing an inhaled agent. Patient education and a return demonstration of inhaler use should be addressed at every visit. Many agents, including over-the-counter products such as Robitussin (an expectorant), are usually ineffective in promoting mucus clearance. Hydration and chest physiotherapy are the best ways to promote mucolysis (choice (A)). Inhaled glucocorticoids do not impact the respiratory drive (choice (B)) nor do they impact cardiac output (choice (D)).

3. **(A)** A 10 mm area of induration in a patient, who is a recent immigrant to the United States and has a history of having received the Bacille Calmette-Guérin vaccine, may indicate the presence of active tuberculosis. Therefore, the patient should be evaluated further. The BCG vaccine is given in many countries where there is a high prevalence of tuberculosis. The vaccine is administered to prevent childhood tuberculous meningitis and miliary disease in areas where these diseases occur often. However, the vaccine is not recommended in the United States because of the overall low risk of infection. The BCG vaccine has variable effectiveness in adults and may interfere with TB skin testing, causing false positive results. Further evaluation and/or treatment of an active tuberculosis infection or a latent tuberculosis infection should be considered for individuals with an induration of at least 5 mm who have human immunodeficiency virus (HIV), have had recent exposure to TB, and are immunocompromised. In this situation, the patient is a recent immigrant with a 10 mm area of induration. Further evaluation would include blood testing for tuberculosis with an Interferon-Gamma Release Assay (IGRA). This test can detect latent and active TB. The initial treatment for tuberculosis is a six- or nine-month regimen that includes isoniazid, rifampin, pyrazinamide, and ethambutol. This treatment does not begin until the patient has been positively diagnosed with active TB. Isoniazid is a component that is frequently used with other medications in treating TB. Thus, choice (B)

is incorrect. Due to the 10 mm area of induration of the skin, the patient should be followed up with further evaluation, such as a chest X-ray or a QuantiFERON-TB Gold blood test (gold standard testing for TB). A patient who did not have the presence of TB in the body should not show signs of induration to the test. Thus, choice (C) is incorrect. A chest X-ray can be used to check for the presence of TB and may be used for patients with a history of having received the BCG vaccine. However, the standard of care does not require a chest X-ray to be performed every six months. Thus, choice (D) is also incorrect.

4. **(C)** In the United States, there are two types of vaccines that protect against pneumococcal disease: the pneumococcal conjugate vaccine (PCV) and the pneumococcal polysaccharide vaccine (PPSV). The Centers for Disease Control and Prevention (CDC) recommends the PCV for all children under the age of 2, all adults who are 65 and older, and individuals between the ages of 2 and 64 who have certain medical conditions. The PPSV23 protects against 23 pneumoniae serotypes. The PPSV23 is recommended for adults who are 65 and older, individuals between the ages of 2 and 64, and adults from the ages of 19 to 64 who smoke cigarettes. The PCV7 only protects against seven pneumoniae serotypes (choice (A)). The PCV13 only protects against 13 pneumoniae serotypes (choice (B)). The LAIV does not protect against pneumococcal disease (choice (D)).

5. **(C)** In the treatment of CAP, the CURB-65 criteria are used to help the clinician determine the severity of the illness. To distinguish between a viral etiology and a bacterial etiology (choice (A)), blood cultures may be performed to determine a bacterial origin of an illness. Viral cultures are now available as well. The CURB-65 criteria do not provide pharmacotherapy guidelines (choice (B)) nor do they determine a local pathogen endemicity (choice (D)). Pharmacotherapy decisions will be driven by causative agents. To determine which pathogens are frequently seen in your geographic area, contact your local health department or an infectious disease specialist.

6. **(B)** Ipratropium bromide is used in the management of COPD to increase bronchial ciliary activity, thereby improving airway clearance. This medication is classified as an anticholinergic that also decreases mucus secretions and prevents the release of allergenic mediators from mast cells. Beta-2 adrenergic agonists (choice (A)) relax the airway smooth muscle and cause slight cardiovascular stimulation. The most common short-acting beta-2 agonist is albuterol, which comes in many formulations. These medications work quickly to relieve a bronchospasm and have mild cardiovascular effects, such as tachycardia. Inhaled corticosteroids (choice (C)) work to decrease airway inflammation and are often indicated in the management of COPD. Inhaled steroids are often combined with long-acting beta-2 agonists and work synergistically to reduce the inflammatory response. Examples are formoterol and budesonide, which are used in the long-term management of COPD. Phosphodiesterase 4 (PPD-4) is an enzyme that is commonly found in respiratory inflammatory cells. Phosphodiesterase 4 inhibitors (choice (D)) decrease the inflammatory response in respiratory cells and are used to reduce the risk of exacerbation in patients who are at high risk for serious exacerbations of COPD. An example of a PPD-4 inhibitor is roflumilast, an oral medication that is used once daily. Side effects of this medication include cardiac arrhythmias, weight loss, diarrhea, and anxiety.

7. **(B)** Pharmacotherapy is the basis of treatment for TB. Individuals with an intact immune system may only be required to take medication for six months. However, another treatment regimen that is commonly used is isoniazid, which is used daily for nine months for individuals who have HIV, children who are 2 to 11 years old, and women who are pregnant (choice

(C)). A patient diagnosed with latent TB may be treated with a combination of anti-tubercular drugs for three months (choice (A)). The question is asking for the minimum treatment duration. Thus, 12 months of treatment is not the appropriate (choice (D)).

8. **(A)** URIs are extremely common illnesses that affect all age groups. The common cold is caused by viruses that are transmitted through direct inhalation of airborne droplets and via hand-to-hand transmission after touching contaminated surfaces. Hand-to-hand transmission is the most common mode of spread in adults. Air pollution (choice (B)) can certainly predispose individuals to the development of upper respiratory infections, but it is not directly responsible for the transmission of URIs. While sharing toothbrushes (choice (C)) and intimate contact (choice (D)) with a sick individual are other ways that URIs can be transmitted, the question asked for the *most common mode* of transmission, which is hand-to-hand transmission.

9. **(A)** Bronchiolitis is a respiratory illness that causes inflammation, edema, and necrosis of respiratory epithelial cells. This occurs in the small airways and produces a large amount of mucus. The illness usually develops slowly over two or three days, beginning in the upper airway and progressing to the lower respiratory system. Bronchiolitis may last up to 10 days and is the leading cause for hospitalization of infants. More severe disease is seen in infants, often those between two and three months old. It is at this time that antibodies received from the mother begin to wane, making infants more susceptible to illness. Infants may become severely ill with cyanosis, retractions, air hunger, and other signs of hypoxia. Apnea may occur, requiring mechanical ventilation. Epithelial necrosis is the pathophysiologic event that leads to airway blockage. While the disease may cause illness in other age groups (choices (B), (C), and (D)), it is usually experienced as mild with a rapid resolution of symptoms.

10. **(B)** Inhaled corticosteroids (ICS) are often considered first-line treatment in patients with persistent asthma. They are used to control and reduce inflammation of the airway. All patients with asthma are prescribed a short-acting beta-2 agonist (choice (A)) as rescue therapy for airway restriction and wheezing. These medications work quickly to relieve bronchospasm. Leukotriene modifiers (choice (C)), such as montelukast, work to decrease inflammation and bronchoconstriction. These agents are less effective than inhaled corticosteroids and are used as alternate medications for long-term control of moderate persistent asthma when used with an ICS. Anticholinergics (choice (D)) are not indicated for the treatment of asthma.

11. **(D)** Viral pneumonia is the most common respiratory infection in children under two years old, and it may cause serious illness in infants. Pneumonia is a lower respiratory tract infection that may be caused by several viruses and bacteria. The disease may involve consolidation in the alveolar space (lobar), interstitial patterns of involvement, and atypical areas of consolidation. The most common cause of pneumonia varies by age, but overall viruses are seen most frequently. During the neonatal period, cytomegalovirus (CMV) is the most common pathogen. Pneumonia in infants who are past the neonatal period is usually caused by viruses such as respiratory syncytial virus (RSV), parainfluenza, influenza, and adenoviruses. Preschool and school-age children develop pneumonia most commonly from viruses as well. Bacterial pneumonia may also occur, and it may be a result of an unresolved viral illness. Atypical bacterial pneumonia may be caused by *Chlamydophila pneumoniae* and is called "walking pneumonia." *Moraxella catarrhalis* (choice (A)) and *Staphylococcus aureus* (choice (B)) are frequently seen in the presence of other types of illnesses that affect children, such as acute otitis media and skin infections. *Mycoplasma pneumoniae* (choice (C)) is the most

common cause of pneumonia in individuals from five years old through young adulthood. Another common bacterial cause of pneumonia is *Streptococcus pneumoniae*. It is important to know which organisms occur most frequently based on the patient's age and the location of the infection.

12. **(C)** Clarithromycin is a macrolide antibiotic that is administered orally and is absorbed by the gastrointestinal tract. The spectrum of microbial activity for agents in the macrolide class includes Gram-positive and Gram-negative aerobes as well as atypical organisms, such as *Mycoplasma pneumoniae*, *Chlamydia pneumoniae*, *Legionella*, and spirochete bacteria. Amoxicillin (choice (A)) is in the penicillin class of antibiotics and is effective against *Staphylococcus aureus*, *Streptococcus pneumoniae*, *Enterococcus* species, and some Gram-negative anaerobes. It is not effective against many atypical organisms, such as *Pseudomonas aeruginosa*, *Chlamydia pneumoniae*, and *Legionella*. Ceftriaxone (choice (B)) is a third-generation cephalosporin that is effective against many Gram-positive and Gram-negative organisms. It has weak activity against *Pseudomonas aeruginosa* and no activity against many of the atypical organisms. Cefadroxil (choice (D)) is a first-generation cephalosporin with poor activity against atypical pathogens.

13. **(A)** Pertussis is caused by a Gram-negative bacillus, *Bordetella pertussis*. This illness, also known as "whooping cough," causes a serious respiratory illness in infants under one year old. In older age groups, the illness is less severe and sometimes goes unnoticed. Transmission of this organism occurs by aerosol droplets through coughing or sneezing or by close contact with an infected person. There is an incubation period of 7–10 days, and children are most contagious during the catarrhal stage and within the first two weeks of cough onset. The highest mortality from pertussis occurs in infants younger than one month old. The usual source of infection for infants is an unrecognized infection in a family member with a cough. The pathophysiologic process of pertussis includes the production of thick mucus and necrotic epithelial material, which blocks the airway. There are three stages in this illness: catarrhal, paroxysmal, and convalescence, which can last for months. Macrolide antibiotics are first-line agents in the treatment of pertussis. However, erythromycin has been associated with the development of pyloric stenosis in young infants and is not recommended. The American Academy of Pediatrics (AAP) recommends azithromycin for the treatment of pertussis in young infants, along with supportive care and airway management. Inpatient care is often required for young infants. The age ranges described in choices (B), (C), and (D) are not at as high of a risk of death from pertussis as are children younger than one month old.

14. **(C)** Currently, polymerase chain reaction (PCR) testing is used to diagnose pertussis because of its improved sensitivity (70–99%) and specificity (86–100%). PCR testing is completed by using a nasal swab or nasal wash from the nasopharynx. A chest X-ray (choice (A)) and a CT of the chest (choice (B)) are not recommended for diagnosing pertussis. Both of these tests also involve radiation exposure. Although blood cultures (choice (D)) have been used to diagnose pertussis, there is only a 12–60% sensitivity, leading to missed diagnoses.

15. **(B)** For all age groups, the hallmark signs of pneumonia are a cough and fever. The other signs described in choices (A), (C), and (D) may also be seen but are sometimes absent in the presence of pneumonia.

3

Disorders of the Cardiovascular and Peripheral Vascular Systems

Disorders of the cardiovascular and peripheral vascular systems are some of the most common conditions in the United States and are the leading cause of death for adults. Disorders that affect the cardiovascular system impact every other body system; therefore, their presentation is frequently complex and requires a high index of suspicion for these often lethal disorders. Disorders of the peripheral vascular system occur more frequently in older adults and may be part of the continuum of cardiovascular disease. Disorders of the cardiovascular system and disorders of the peripheral vascular system often occur together, so it is important for family nurse practitioners to be able to quickly evaluate and assess for potentially fatal illnesses in the setting of outpatient care in order to quickly transfer the patient to the emergency department, if need be. Family nurse practitioners will frequently encounter patients who present with various complaints, such as chest pain, dyspnea, and weakness. The list of different diagnoses for these presenting symptoms is extensive and ranges from mild illness to acute coronary syndrome. As a result, familiarity with the most common disorders of these systems is crucial for effectively managing them.

Hypertension

Hypertension (high blood pressure) is one of the most common health problems that family nurse practitioners encounter in primary care, and, along with smoking, it is one of the two leading causes of preventable death. Statistics demonstrate that one in three adults is affected by hypertension. The risk for developing high blood pressure increases with age. In 2017, management guidelines were updated to reflect new evidence regarding hypertension in adults. Hypertension is usually classified as essential (primary) or secondary. The vast majority of individuals with hypertension have essential (or benign) hypertension, which means that a secondary cause (such as another medical condition) cannot be identified. Diagnosing hypertension requires the recording of an elevated blood pressure on two separate occasions. The Eighth Joint National Committee (JNC-8) Guidelines recommend maintaining a blood pressure of less than 140/90 for individuals over age 60 years. New guidelines developed in 2011 define normal blood pressure as less than 120/80. Systolic blood pressure from 120–129 mm Hg, with a diastolic blood pressure less than 80 mm Hg, is now termed "elevated blood pressure" (rather than "prehypertension"). Stage 1 hypertension is defined as an average systolic blood pressure between 130 mm Hg and 139 mm Hg or an average diastolic blood pressure between 80 mm Hg and 89 mm Hg. Stage 2 hypertension is defined as an average systolic blood pressure of at least 140 mm Hg or an average diastolic blood pressure of at least 90 mm Hg. Due to increasing rates of hypertension in children and adolescents, guidelines have been revised for this population. The American Academy of Pediatrics (AAP) updated guidelines on normative blood pressures for children and adolescents based on age, sex, and height (height percentile). Elevated blood pressure is > 90th percentile. Stage 1 hypertension is > 95th percentile, and Stage 2 hypertension is > 95th percentile with +12 mm Hg.

Symptoms

For most individuals, hypertension remains asymptomatic for many years and is discovered incidentally. Patients with markedly elevated blood pressure may report headaches, vision changes, and palpitations. If the hypertension has been present for many years, a physical exam may reveal evidence of target organ damage such as kidney, heart and eyes (retinal changes in the form of edema of the optic disc, "cotton wool spots" on the retina, flame-shaped hemorrhages and arteriovenous nicking).

Management

Depending upon the degree of blood pressure elevation, initial management may include the adoption of a heart-healthy diet, weight loss, and activity changes, or it may include the use of pharmacological agents along with lifestyle changes. Non-pharmacological or lifestyle measures to optimize blood pressure control include recommending patients follow the DASH diet, the Mediterranean diet, and regular aerobic exercise (such as brisk walking for 30 minutes) at least five days per week. Achieving and maintaining a healthy weight is often a challenge for patients but is critical in improving outcomes and preventing cardiovascular events, so this should be emphasized. Recommendations for the initial pharmacological management of hypertension can include the use of angiotensin-converting enzyme (ACE) inhibitors, angiotensin receptor blockers (ARBs), thiazide diuretics, and calcium channel blockers. Beta blockers are not typically considered first-line therapy for essential hypertension, but they may be used if other symptoms (such as tachycardia) are present. While a diagnosis of hypertension requires two separate documented occasions of elevated blood pressure (not measured on the same day), a patient who presents with very high blood pressure for the first time should be started on antihypertensive therapy, with frequent follow-up appointments, until the patient's blood pressure has been restored to a level that is more normal.

Hyperlipidemia

Hyperlipidemia is an elevation of the cholesterol components in the serum and is a significant risk factor for cardiovascular disease. For patients with known heart disease, lowering cholesterol levels decreases the risk for an acute cardiovascular event. For patients without established heart disease, screening and management guidelines have been developed to guide clinicians in practice. Most cases of hyperlipidemia are caused by lifestyle factors, such as poor diet, obesity, and lack of exercise. A diet that is high in fat is the most common cause of elevated cholesterol. Genetics also play a role, since many individuals with a diagnosis of hyperlipidemia have a positive family history for the condition. Secondary hypercholesterolemia may be caused by diabetes, hypothyroidism, nephrotic syndrome, obstructive liver disease, and certain medications such as thiazide diuretics, carbamazepine, and cyclosporine.

Symptoms

Elevated lipids produce no symptoms until an event occurs associated with disruption of lipid plaques within the blood system. This disorder is often discovered through screening programs or incidentally during other laboratory studies. A physical assessment is often normal, but the presence of xanthelasmas (soft, raised, yellow or flesh-colored growths on the eyelids or brow) may indicate elevated cholesterol levels. Occasionally, xanthelasmas occur on the fingers and are suggestive of the familial form of hypercholesterolemia.

Management

Management of this disorder includes weight control, dieting, and exercise as first-line measures. Pharmacotherapy begins with HMG-CoA reductase inhibitors (statins). The American Heart Association's risk calculator can be utilized with the patient to collaboratively discuss overall cardiovascular risk and develop a comprehensive treatment plan.

Atherosclerotic Cardiovascular Disease (ASCVD)

Atherosclerotic cardiovascular disease, also known as ischemic heart disease, is a leading cause of death in the United States. Patient education programs and early recognition of symptoms have decreased the number of deaths from this disorder, but the mortality level remains high. Managing any comorbid, underlying conditions can significantly decrease an individual's risk for developing ASCVD.

Symptoms

Patients with ASCVD are usually asymptomatic for many years, and the presenting symptom may be a catastrophic myocardial infarction or stroke. Symptoms do not usually become apparent until there is at least a 75% occlusion of an artery.

Management

The goals of managing ASCVD are early identification and preventing disease progression and the potentially lethal complications of the disease.

Acute Coronary Syndrome (ACS)

Acute coronary syndrome is an umbrella term that refers to acute conditions that cause myocardial ischemia, including stable angina, unstable angina, variant angina, and myocardial infarctions (MIs). Clinical presentation is variable and may include ECG changes such as ST-segment elevation with a myocardial infarction (STEMI) as well as non-ST segment elevation myocardial infarction (NSTEMI). Stable angina is myocardial ischemia that occurs in a predictable pattern and is often controlled by medication. Unstable angina refers to chest pain that occurs unpredictably and at lower activity levels, sometimes even at rest. Unstable angina is often a precursor to an acute myocardial infarction. Myocardial infarctions are necrosis, or death, of heart tissue as a result of prolonged ischemia. The area of the infarction, the extent of tissue death, and the speed of tissue reperfusion all impact a patient's prognosis. Blockage of the left main cardiac artery produces necrosis and an infarction that affects the entire left side of the heart and is often fatal. Blockage of the right coronary artery affects the right atrium and the inferior wall of the left ventricle. The left circumflex artery provides the blood supply to the lateral and posterior portions of the left ventricle, while the left anterior descending artery supplies blood to the anterior septal wall of the left ventricle.

Symptoms

Patients having an acute MI may present with crushing chest pain or pressure radiating to the jaw, neck, or left arm, along with diaphoresis, nausea, and dizziness. However, approximately 15% of patients have a "silent MI" with no symptoms. Older adults, women, and individuals with diabetes mellitus are more likely to suffer a silent MI or have an atypical presentation. Presenting symptoms in these individuals may include shortness of breath, fatigue, nausea, sweating, but no chest pain. Since these symptoms are atypical, many of these patients delay seeking treatment and thus experience worse outcomes.

CLINICAL PEARL

New cardiovascular guidelines recommend statin therapy for individuals with diabetes mellitus and other risks for cardiovascular disease.

Management

In the outpatient setting, a patient with suspected MI should be stabilized while awaiting EMS transport to the ED. Provide the patient with oxygen, start an IV, and administer an aspirin.

Heart Failure (HF)

Heart failure is any one of a number of conditions in which the heart is unable to effectively pump blood to meet bodily demand for tissue oxygenation. The two main types of heart failure include failure with preserved ejection fraction (HFpEF) and failure with reduced ejection fraction (HFrEF). Ejection fraction (EF) is a measure of cardiac output and reflects the ability of the heart to provide oxygen to body tissues. HF may develop as right ventricular, left ventricular, or biventricular dysfunction, depending on the areas of the heart that are impaired. The most common cause of right-sided heart failure is left-sided failure. HF is most commonly seen in patients over the age of 65 years. Classification of heart failure is accomplished through the use of the American Heart Association (AHA) and the American College of Cardiology (ACC) stages of heart failure guide and the New York Heart Association (NYHA) functional classification system, as seen in Table 3.1.

Table 3.1. New York Heart Association Functional Classification System

Four-Stage Classification System (ACC/AHA)
Stage A: High risk for developing HF, but no structural heart disease
Stage B: Structural damage to the heart, but no symptoms
Stage C: Past or current HF symptoms and evidence of structural heart damage
Stage D: End-stage disease, requiring special interventions
Functional Classification (NYHA)
■ No limitation of physical activity. Ordinary physical activity does not cause undue fatigue, palpitation dyspnea, or angina.
■ Slight limitation of physical activity. Ordinary physical activity results in fatigue, palpitation, dyspnea, or angina.
■ Marked limitation of physical activity. Comfortable at rest, but less than ordinary physical activity results in fatigue, palpitation, dyspnea, or angina.
■ Unable to carry on any physical activity without discomfort. Symptoms are present at rest. With any physical activity, symptoms increase.

These tools are intended to be used together to determine the stage and progression of disease along with functional impact on daily living. Echocardiography, laboratory studies such as basic natriuretic peptide (BNP) levels, and now point-of-care testing with N-terminal proBNP-type natriuretic peptide (NT-proBNP) assist in the diagnosis and monitoring the progression of disease.

Symptoms

Signs and symptoms vary significantly and may occur at any point during the course of disease. For left-sided heart failure, the cause is usually dysfunction of the left ventricle with hypertrophy of the ventricle and symptoms of dyspnea, orthopnea, cough, and rales (crackles). Right-sided heart failure usually results from left-sided HF and demonstrates signs such as jugular venous distention, peripheral edema, hepatomegaly, and splenomegaly.

Management

Management of heart failure includes treating the underlying cause. Pharmacotherapy includes diuretics, beta blockers, and angiotensin-converting enzyme (ACE) inhibitors or angiotensin receptor blockers (ARBs) for patients with HFrEF. Preservation of heart function and management of fluid volume are mainstays of therapy. Automatic internal cardiac defibrillator (AICD) and pacemaker placement are other methods of treatment for patients with severe congestive heart failure (CHF).

Arrhythmias

Cardiac arrhythmias are abnormalities of heart rate and synchronicity. The most commonly encountered arrhythmias in primary care include atrial and ventricular abnormalities. Atrial arrhythmias include atrial fibrillation (AF), premature atrial contractions (PACs), atrial flutter, atrial tachycardia, and supraventricular tachycardia. Atrial fibrillation is a common disorder with incidence increasing with age. Ventricular arrhythmias encountered in primary care include premature ventricular contractions (PVCs) and ventricular tachycardia. First-, second-, and third-degree heart blocks and associated arrhythmias are often seen as well. In primary care, administer the CHADS2 tool to evaluate the patient's risk for stroke.

Symptoms

A patient with a new arrhythmia may be asymptomatic. However, patients often report noticing "palpitations" or may complain of dizziness or weakness. A new arrhythmia may be found incidentally on examination by the provider. Noting when (systolic or diastolic) the murmur occurs and the location (aortic, mitral, etc.) is critical when evaluating a cardiac murmur. Because irregular heartbeats may allow blood to pool in cardiac chambers, there is the possibility of clot development and the potential for an embolus.

Management

Anticoagulant therapy is individually determined based on risk factors. Patients with new arrhythmias should be referred for cardiology evaluation. Management options now include implanted pacemakers and implanted cardioverter defibrillator devices.

Valvular Disorders and Murmurs

Valvular disorders affect the mitral and aortic valves most frequently and may be congenital or acquired. These disorders may be symptomatic or asymptomatic. Heart murmurs are the sounds of turbulent blood moving through the wall of the heart or the great vessels and the valves. Murmurs may be benign or pathologic. Murmurs are often caused by stenosis (reduction in valvular orifice diameter), regurgitation (backup of blood related to incompetent cardiac valve), or prolapse (incomplete closure of a valve during the cardiac cycle).

Symptoms

These disorders may be symptomatic or asymptomatic. Symptoms may include palpitations, light-headedness, shortness of breath, fatigue, or syncope (fainting).

Management

The goal of murmur management is to determine the cause, maintain normal hemodynamic function, and prevent heart failure. Cardiac valvular disease is associated with increased risk for stroke, and management must include comprehensive patient and family education as well as pharmacological and, if indicated, surgical interventions.

Peripheral Vascular Disease (PVD) and Peripheral Artery Disease (PAD)

Peripheral vascular disease affects the vessels of the lower extremity—arteries, veins, or both. Peripheral artery disease is the development of occlusive atherosclerotic lesions in the arteries delivering oxygen to the extremities. PAD is evidence of systemic atherosclerosis. Blockages lead to circulatory problems and impair cellular function. Patients with PAD frequently have other identified cardiovascular disorders, including lipid abnormalities. Recognition and identification of acute occlusion is critical in order to preserve limb function. Chronic PAD is seen more frequently and requires careful management to improve symptoms and quality of life.

Symptoms

Presentation of PAD often includes complaints of leg pain that worsens with activity and improves with rest (intermittent claudication). Patients will often maintain their extremities in a dependent position in order to relieve pain.

CLINICAL PEARL

Six Ps of PAD: Pain, Pulselessness, Paresthesia, Paralysis, Poikilothermia (coolness), and Pallor, which require urgent/ emergent evaluation!

Management

The goal of management for PVD and PAD is to improve blood flow to the extremity, prevent complications, and aggressively manage complications such as leg ulcers. The best management program includes risk factor reduction, optimization of medications, and institution of an exercise regimen. This includes smoking cessation, lipid level control with statin medication, blood pressure control with antihypertensive agents, and weight loss. Focal (or localized) atherosclerotic lesions may be treated with angioplasty and stenting of the affected vessel. Surgical placement of an aortofemoral bypass graft is highly effective as the diseased portion of the vessel is "bypassed," allowing blood to reach needed tissues distal to the occlusion.

Deep Vein Thrombosis (DVT) and Chronic Venous Insufficiency (CVI)

Deep vein thrombosis and chronic venous insufficiency are disorders affecting the venous system, primarily the veins in the lower extremities. A DVT is the presence of a blood clot somewhere within the deep veins of the lower extremities or the pelvis. DVTs are common after surgery, after prolonged immobilization, and in hypercoagulable states, such as pregnancy and malignancy. Chronic venous insufficiency may result from a DVT; however, this disorder usually represents a progressive failure of venous valves, leading to pooling of fluid in the lower extremities. One important condition to screen for when evaluating a patient with a suspected DVT is pulmonary embolism (PE). This life-threatening event occurs when a large clot in a deep vein dislodges from the vessel wall and travels to the lungs, causing an acute event, which may be fatal. Physical assessment alone reveals unreliable accuracy as only 30% of DVTs are identified through physical assessment alone. Diagnostic studies include serum D-dimer (high specificity, poor sensitivity), ultrasound, venous doppler with contrast, and laboratory testing, including complete blood count and clotting studies.

Symptoms

DVTs are usually initially asymptomatic, with slow, progressive development of symptoms, such as edema, warmth, redness, and tenderness of the affected extremity. Upon examination, unilateral edema of extremity with a palpable vein or "cord" over the affected area may be observed. Patients with CVI often report loss of hair on lower extremity, bilateral symptoms, and increasing pain when walking. Dependent edema and rubor are often noted.

Management

Treatment of DVT includes anticoagulant therapy to prevent extension or embolization of the clot. Most patients with DVT may be safely treated in the outpatient setting with administration of warfarin, dabigatran, rivaroxaban, apixaban, or edoxaban. Some agents, such as edoxaban, require 5–10 days of parenteral anticoagulation before starting the patient as an outpatient. Heparin, especially low-molecular-weight heparins (LMWHs), are very effective for the immediate treatment of DVT and are considered first-line management options because of their stable pharmacokinetic properties allowing for once or twice daily dosing via subcutaneous injection. Unlike coumadin, which requires regular blood-level monitoring, these LMWHs do not require this in most patients. Patients with DVT, even if they do not develop PE, require a minimum of three months anticoagulation therapy to decrease the risk for recurrence.

For certain patients with DVT, however, admission for inpatient treatment is appropriate. These patients include those who have substantial risk for development of a PE or who have an increased risk for bleeding if placed on anticoagulant therapy. Other patients who should be admitted for treatment include those with a large iliofemoral DVT, those with poorly controlled pain, those with a high risk for bleeding, or those who are unreliable for follow-up. Patients who have a condition that prohibits administration of anticoagulants may require admission for surgical placement of an IVC filter.

Treatment of chronic venous insufficiency (CVI) includes the use of fitted, graduated, compression stockings (20–30 mm Hg) applied in the morning and worn until bedtime. These stockings, when used regularly, are very effective in preventing disease progression especially when combined with periods of limb elevation during the daytime hours. Severe cases of CVI may require the use of pneumatic compression devices to control swelling and provide for venous return of fluids. Leg ulcers are serious complications of CVI and difficult to treat until peripheral edema is controlled and regular compression of the extremity is instituted.

CLINICAL PEARL

Virchow's triad: venous stasis, vessel injury, and hypercoagulability

If any of these are present, there is increased risk for DVT.

Practice Questions

1. Your patient is a 76-year-old male with a history of an acute myocardial infarction, STEMI, six months ago. He is in the office for a follow-up physical examination. You perform a 12-lead ECG and expect to see which of the following findings, based on this patients' past medical history?

   (A) R-wave larger than 25 mm
   (B) T-wave inversion
   (C) deep Q-wave
   (D) 2 mm ST segment elevation

2. Which of the following factors is the most common cause of heart failure in adults?

   (A) chronic obstructive pulmonary disease
   (B) severe anemia
   (C) high sodium diet
   (D) uncontrolled hypertensive heart disease

3. One significant risk factor for development of DVT is:

   (A) hypertension.
   (B) obesity.
   (C) pelvic surgery.
   (D) heart failure.

4. Several classes of medications are used in the management of heart failure. For a patient in your practice with a diagnosis of heart failure, you would expect their medication regimen would include all of the following classes of drugs, EXCEPT:

   (A) ACE inhibitors.
   (B) beta blockers.
   (C) calcium channel blockers.
   (D) diuretics.

5. The Eighth Joint National Committee (JNC-8) recommendations for blood pressure control in adults aged 60 years or older include which of the following measurements?

   (A) systolic BP < 120/90
   (B) systolic BP < 130/90
   (C) systolic BP < 140/90
   (D) systolic BP < 150/90

6. A physical examination finding that may indicate hyperlipidemia is:

   (A) jaundice.
   (B) xanthelasmas.
   (C) actinic keratoses.
   (D) lipomas.

7. Acute coronary syndrome, or myocardial infarction, causes symptoms and sequelae based on the area of the heart affected by ischemia and infarction. Myocardial infarctions that affect the anterior wall of the heart are usually the result of occlusion of the:

    (A) left main artery.
    (B) right coronary artery.
    (C) left circumflex artery.
    (D) left anterior descending artery.

8. Essential hypertension affects around 95% of individuals with a diagnosis of hypertension. JNC8 initial recommendations for management include lifestyle measures. If blood pressure remains elevated, or is very high on initial presentation, pharmacotherapy should be started. Which of the following classes of medications is NOT indicated for first-line treatment of benign hypertension?

    (A) beta blockers
    (B) calcium channel blockers
    (C) ACE inhibitors
    (D) thiazide diuretics

9. Peripheral vascular disorders may affect arteries, veins, or both. Differentiating the diagnosis is based on a careful patient history and description of symptoms. Which of the following reports is consistent with a diagnosis of peripheral arterial disease (PAD)?

    (A) pain when standing that is not relieved by rest
    (B) redness and edema with pronounced varicose veins
    (C) pain in the calves with walking that subsides with rest
    (D) pain in the legs that is relieved by elevation of the extremities

10. The goal of treatment for hypertension is prevention of target organ (or end organ) damage. Organ systems that may be affected are the vascular, coronary, and renal systems. Retinal changes that may be seen with target organ damage caused by hypertension include:

    (A) deep inner-retinal hemorrhages.
    (B) retinal detachment.
    (C) edema of the optic disc.
    (D) increased cup-to-disc ratio.

11. Heart failure is a complex disorder that often results from a combination of factors. However, uncontrolled hypertension is the leading cause of heart failure. Which of the following conditions is LEAST likely to lead to heart failure?

    (A) aortic stenosis
    (B) ischemic cardiomyopathy
    (C) hypertension
    (D) valvular heart disease (tricuspid and mitral valves)

12. A possible complication of deep vein thrombosis is:

    (A) atrophy of leg muscles.
    (B) paralysis of the affected extremity.
    (C) pulmonary embolism.
    (D) fat embolism.

13. Hyperlipidemia is frequently associated with chronic disorders such as diabetes mellitus and hypertension. Many factors impact lipid production and storage in the body, including genetics and comorbidity disease. The most common factor associated with elevated LDL cholesterol levels is:

    (A) heredity.
    (B) gender.
    (C) cardiovascular disease.
    (D) high-fat diet.

14. Which of the following statements about hypertension is correct?

    (A) Diets high in salt and fats cause hypertension.
    (B) For 95% of individuals diagnosed with hypertension, the cause is unknown.
    (C) Diabetes mellitus is a causative factor for hypertension.
    (D) Obesity is the leading cause of hypertension in adults.

15. Virchow's triad is the name of a characteristic presentation whose presence is used to evaluate the risk for deep vein thrombosis. Components of Virchow's triad include venous stasis, hypercoagulability, and:

    (A) chronic venous insufficiency.
    (B) vessel injury.
    (C) postphlebitic syndrome.
    (D) pulmonary embolism.

Answer Explanations

1. **(C)** You may expect to find deep Q-waves on the ECG following an acute myocardial infarction. These waves represent areas of absence of depolarization in the area of the myocardial infarction. A Q-wave may develop one to three days after the acute event and will persist on the ECG. The R-wave is the first upward deflection after the P-wave and is part of the QRS complex seen on ECG. A prominent R-wave in lead V1 may indicate right ventricular hypertrophy, septal hypertrophy, right bundle branch block, or Wolff-Parkinson-White syndrome. Normally, the R-wave begins small and progressively gets taller throughout the precordial leads (choice (A)). An inverted T-wave noted on an ECG may represent a pulmonary embolism, left bundle branch block, left ventricular hypertrophy, unstable angina, or myocardial ischemia (choice (B)). An ST segment elevation, especially if a new finding, may indicate an acute myocardial infarction (choice (D)).

2. **(D)** The most common cause of heart failure in adults is hypertensive heart disease, particularly poorly controlled hypertension. Over time, high blood pressure causes damage to coronary vessels and valves as well as end organ damage to the kidneys, eyes, and other organ systems. Hypertension is seen in epidemic numbers in adults, and strict control is needed to prevent eventual heart failure in these patients. Chronic obstructive pulmonary disease may be found in patients with cardiovascular disease but affects the pulmonary system and is not a cause of heart failure (choice (A)). Anemia may cause stress on the cardiac system, as the body attempts to compensate for low hemoglobin and hematocrit. Cardiac murmurs and hyperdynamic pulses may be noted, but heart failure is only rarely a cause of heart failure (choice (B)). A high-sodium diet may exacerbate hypertensive heart disease, as well as heart failure but alone cannot directly cause heart failure (choice (C)).

3. **(C)** Deep vein thrombosis may occur as a result of vessel injury, inflammation, or venous stasis. Risk factors include pelvic, hip, and knee surgery and hypercoagulable states such as those that occur during pregnancy and malignancy and stasis of blood for any reason, such as immobility. Inherited coagulation disorders, such as Factor C deficiency and Leiden, also predispose individuals to developing DVT. External causes of DVT include oral contraceptive use, bone fractures, and trauma. Hypertension is associated with intrinsic cardiovascular properties controlling volume and vessel constriction and is not considered to be a potential risk factor for DVT development (choice (A)). Obesity is a risk factor for development of diabetes mellitus, a chronic disease that may predispose individuals to hypercoagulable states, however it is not considered an independent risk factor (choice (B)). While heart failure affects tissue oxygenation and increases the potential for lower extremity edema, it has not been found to be associated with a higher incidence of DVT (choice (D)).

4. **(C)** Calcium channel blockers are generally not recommended in the treatment of heart failure. Exceptions are amlodipine and felodipine, which have specific indications. In addition to supportive measures, individuals with a diagnosis of heart failure will be prescribed several classes of medication that have proven beneficial in the management of this condition. ACE inhibitors are indicated for patients with any degree of left ventricular dysfunction and have demonstrated efficacy in the treatment of heart failure in patients with preserved ejection fraction (choice (A)). Beta blockers (choice (B)) to reduce cardiac workload and diuretics (choice (D)) help the body eliminate excess fluid, both of which are indicated with this diagnosis.

5. **(D)** JNC8 guidelines propose several new guidelines in management of hypertension. For patients younger than 60 years, the goal BP is < 140/90. In adult patients with chronic kidney disease or diabetes mellitus, the goal is also < 140/90. However, in patients aged 60 years and

older, JNC8 recommends treating a goal of a systolic blood pressure equal to 150 and a diastolic of > 90 (choice (D)). Recommendations are to treat until the patient's blood pressure is below these thresholds.

6. **(B)** Xanthelasmas are benign growths that appear as raised, yellowish plaques on the eyelids. These growths are composed of a lipid matrix and are often associated with hyperlipidemia. Jaundice is a yellowish discoloration of the skin, sclera, and mucous membranes. It is caused by elevated levels of bilirubin in the blood and is frequently seen in patients with liver disease or hemolytic conditions (choice (A)). Actinic keratoses are slow-growing lesions that appear as discrete, slightly raised areas on sun-exposed skin. These growths are considered premalignant, and excision is recommended (choice (C)). Lipomas are benign tumors that are made up of fat cells (choice (D)).

7. **(D)** When there is occlusion of the left anterior descending artery, the area of infarction includes the anterior septal wall and the left ventricle. Based on the position of the heart in the chest, the left ventricle is positioned anteriorly. Infarctions in these areas may result in severe dysfunction of the left ventricle and could lead to pulmonary edema. Conduction abnormalities may also be seen with occlusion of this artery and present as a second- or third-degree block. The left main artery supplies blood to the entire left side of the heart, and occlusion here is often fatal (choice (A)). The right coronary artery supplies the inferior wall of the left ventricle as well as the right atrium, SA and AV nodes, and muscles of the mitral valve (choice (B)). The left circumflex artery supplies blood to the lateral and posterior walls of the left ventricle (choice (C)).

8. **(A)** Beta blockers are not considered first-line or monotherapy agents for management of hypertension in adults. Traditional beta blockers, such as atenolol, do not cause vasodilation and are not effective antihypertensive agents. Other beta blockers, such as carvedilol and nebivolol, work by reducing systemic vascular resistance through systemic vasodilation. Much of the controversy surrounding beta blocker use in hypertension relates to findings of suboptimal decrease in stroke risk and a possible increase in diabetes mellitus occurrence. Other drug classes show stronger evidence for decreasing blood pressure with less side effects than beta blockers. Beta blockers may be used as antihypertensive therapy but are not first-line agents. JNC-8 recommendations for initiating therapy for benign (essential) hypertension include thiazide diuretics (choice (D)), ACE inhibitors (choice (C)), and calcium channel blockers (choice (B)).

9. **(C)** Peripheral artery disease is caused by partial occlusion of the veins supplying blood to the extremities. When there is not enough oxygen being delivered to tissues, pain occurs with walking or exercise. This pain report is called intermittent claudication and is pathognomonic for PAD. Pain when standing that is not relieved by rest may be caused by stenosis of the lumbar spine or other neurologic abnormality (choice (A)). Redness and edema with pronounced varicose veins are often seen with chronic venous insufficiency (choice (B)). Pain that is relieved by elevation of the extremities may also be a sign of diminished venous return (choice (D)).

10. **(C)** Evidence of retinal changes produced by uncontrolled hypertension include edema or swelling of the optic disc, the appearance of "cotton wool" spots, flame-shaped hemorrhages, hard yellow exudates, and arteriovenous nicking. Inner-retinal hemorrhages are caused by vessel occlusion often seen in patients with diabetes mellitus (choice (A)). Grayish lesions are sometimes seen on the retina. These are choroidal nevi, which may appear on the retina as grayish-brown pigmented lesions. These lesions should be distinguished from a melanoma, which can appear on the retina and be fatal. Retinal detachment often occurs spontaneously

and is seen most often in individuals who are over 50 years old and in those who are near-sighted (choice (B)). Penetrating trauma or a blunt trauma injury to the eye may also cause retinal detachment. In the event of retinal detachment, the patient may report "a curtain falling over the eye," which occurs acutely. Retinal detachment may be seen on an ophthalmologic exam. An increased cup-to-disc ratio is seen with glaucomatous eye disease (choice (D)).

11. **(D)** Valvular heart disease (tricuspid and mitral valves) is less likely to lead to heart failure than the other conditions listed. Aortic stenosis (choice (A)), ischemic cardiomyopathy (choice (B)), and hypertension (choice (C)) are all considered causative factors in the development of heart failure.

12. **(C)** Pulmonary embolism is a possible complication of deep vein thrombosis. DVT may result in generalized edema of the affected extremity, as well as warmth and tenderness over the affected area. The patient may complain of calf pain that is exacerbated by walking. Postphlebitic syndrome is a serious, chronic sequelae of deep vein thrombosis that results in pain and progressive venous insufficiency in the affected extremity. Leg muscle atrophy (choice (A)), paralysis (choice (B)), and production of fat emboli (choice (D)) are not associated with a diagnosis of deep vein thrombosis.

13. **(D)** Although genetics, environment, weight, and activity levels affect lipid levels, a diet that is high in saturated fats is the most common cause of high LDL cholesterol levels. Gender does not play a significant role in the development of elevated LDL cholesterol (choice (B)). Although hyperlipidemia may be seen in conjunction with cardiovascular disease, it is not *caused by* cardiovascular disease (choice (C)).

14. **(B)** In approximately 95% of individuals with a diagnosis of hypertension, the exact cause is unknown. This form of hypertension is called essential (or benign) hypertension, although the condition is not benign in nature and can lead to serious sequelae. A diet high in sodium and saturated fats may contribute to risk factors for cardiovascular disease and may exacerbate hypertension, but it is not the cause of hypertension (choice (A)). Diabetes mellitus (choice (C)) and obesity (choice (D)) are often comorbid conditions associated with hypertension but are not causative factors.

15. **(B)** Virchow's triad is a risk factor assessment tool used to help clinicians evaluate a patient's risk for DVT. Components of the triad include venous stasis, hypercoagulability, and vessel injury. When two of these three factors are present, the patient is at high risk for DVT, especially if the patient is recovering from surgery. Chronic venous insufficiency (CVI) is a disorder primarily caused by progressive dysfunction of the valves present in veins (choice (A)). These valves normally allow and promote one-way movement of fluids from the extremities back toward the heart. When the valves do not close properly, they allow fluid to pool in the lower extremities, leading to CVI. CVI may also be a complication of DVT, especially with recurrent episodes. Postphlebitic syndrome occurs as a complication of DVT and/or CVI and is demonstrated by irreversible damage to veins leading to chronic pain, edema, and the development of venous ulcers (choice (C)). Pulmonary embolism (PE) develops when a large thrombus in a deep vein breaks away from the vessel wall and travels to the circulation of the lung (choice (D)). A large portion of the lung may become unoxygenated with resultant ventilation/perfusion mismatch and possibly death.

Disorders of the Endocrine System

The endocrine system is integral for all regulatory functions and is made up of glands located throughout the body. These glands include the pituitary, thyroid, adrenals, hypothalamus, pineal, thymus, pancreas, ovaries, and testes. These glands synthesize and secrete hormones that serve a number of functions, including causing a developing fetus to become either male or female, stimulating growth and development throughout infancy and childhood, maintaining a homeostatic internal environment, facilitating reproduction, and initiating corrective adaptations when emergencies occur. The endocrine system works intimately with the nervous system to promote communication and the control of hormones throughout the body.

Diabetes Mellitus (DM)

Diabetes mellitus is a multisystem disorder of carbohydrate, fat, and protein metabolism often associated with lack of or decreased insulin production. Hyperglycemia is the physical outcome of absent or low insulin production. Uncontrolled DM may result in micro- and macro-vascular damage, which may lead to multiple organ failure. Diabetes is divided into two types: type 1 and type 2.

Type 1 diabetes is an autoimmune destruction of insulin-producing cells in the pancreas. The etiology of type 1 diabetes is not completely understood but is believed to be a combination of genetic variants along with environmental triggers. Patients with type 1 diabetes do not produce insulin at all, which can lead to profound hyperglycemia and death, if left untreated. Type 1 diabetes is commonly found in children who may have had a recent viral illness.

Most individuals who have been diagnosed with DM have type 2 diabetes. In fact, incidences of type 2 diabetes are increasing in conjunction with the epidemic of obesity in the United States. With this disease, there is a progressive reduction in the production and secretion of insulin, which can result in hyperglycemia. The etiology of type 2 diabetes consists of a strong genetic component as well as lifestyle factors. Risk factors for type 2 diabetes include obesity, physical inactivity, metabolic syndrome, insulin resistance, family history of the disease, maternal history of diabetes, and gestational diabetes. Unlike type 1 diabetes, the symptoms of type 2 diabetes are often less acute in presentation. Insulin resistance is demonstrated by tissue resistance to the effects of insulin and is often seen with type 2 DM. Diagnosis of diabetes has been revised over the past several years as researchers are increasingly focused on the period just prior to overt symptom development. The hemoglobin A1c is a serum measurement used to evaluate diabetes control. Prediabetes is considered when the A1c is between 5.7% and 6.4%, or FPG between 100 and 125 mg/dL, or the 2-hour oral glucose tolerance test (OGTT) of $\leq$140 mg/dL. An A1c $\geq$ 6.5%, or FPG $\geq$ 126 mg/dL, or 2-hour OGTT of $\geq$ 200 with symptoms is pathognomonic for diabetes. Screening for type 2 DM is recommended once every three years for adults who are asymptomatic and have a BMI of $\geq$ 25 or other risk factors. Screening for asymptomatic children is recommended once every three years when the BMI is greater than the 85th percentile with two or more risk factors.

Symptoms

Children with type 1 diabetes often present with signs and symptoms of the three Ps: polyuria, polydipsia, and polyphagia. Other symptoms include fruity odor to breath, nausea, vomiting, abdominal pain, and sudden weight loss. Often large amounts of ketones are found in the urine upon presentation for medical care.

Patients with type 2 diabetes present with nonspecific symptoms. The individual is usually overweight with hypertension, hypercholesterolemia, and hyperinsulinemia. The classic symptoms of polyuria and polydipsia may or may not be present. Patients will often report fatigue, visual changes, recurrent infections, pruritus, or paresthesia and weakness of extremities. Type 2 diabetes is often diagnosed after target organ damage has occurred, indicating a significant lag time in identifying the disease.

Management

Type 1: Basal insulin; adjustment is needed for snacks, meals, and illness. Insulin type, onset, peak, and duration of action: short-acting (15–30 mins, give within 5–10 mins before meal, or give within 15 mins right after meal, peak at 1–3 hrs, duration of 3–5 hrs), intermediate-acting (1–2 hrs, peak at 6–14 hrs, duration of 16–24 hrs), long-acting (1–2 hrs, peak at 6–8 hrs, duration of > -24 hrs).

Type 2: First-line monotherapy treatment is a biguanide: metformin (Glucophage), followed by dual therapy, triple therapy, or combination injectable therapy as indicated by patient response. Basal and mealtime insulins are often used in early stages of disease to gain control of blood sugar and prevent complications of hyperglycemia. Refer to Figure 4.1 below.

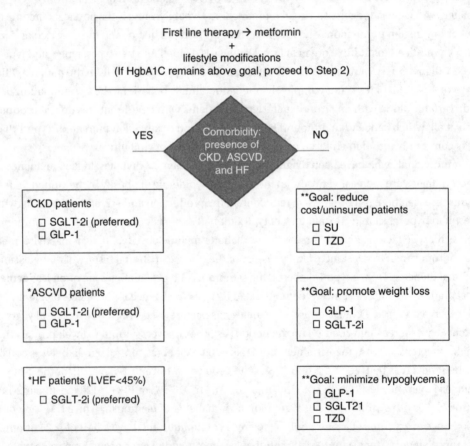

For more options, please refer to the *Pharmacologic Approaches to Glycemic Treatment: Standards of Medical Care in Diabetes—2021*

**If HgbA1C remains above goal, may increase dosage to the recommended dosage by the manufacturer.

After 3 months:
If HgbA1C remains above goal, may initiate triple therapy (addition to suggested drug classes

***Chronic kidney disease (CKD); atherosclerotic cardiovascular disease (ASCVD); Heart failure (HF); left ventricular ejection fraction (LVEF); Glucagon-like peptide (SGLT2i); Dipeptidyl peptidase 4 inhibitors (DPP-4i); Thiazolidinediones (TZD); Sulfonylureas (SU)

Figure 4.1. Metformin Therapy

Guidelines for adult DM care: BP (goal < 140/< 90), annual eye and foot exam, kidney function test, fasting lipids profile, and diet and physical activity (if not contraindicated, minimum of 150 mins per week of moderate physical activity). Routine monitoring is aimed at early identification and management of target organ damage, such as renal impairment and retinopathy. Basic labs should include a comprehensive metabolic panel with careful attention to renal function studies. Diabetic patients who require contrast for imaging studies should be monitored closely for complications. If the patient takes metformin, this medication should be held before testing and labs should be ordered within 48 hours after imaging to assess for signs of renal failure or impairment.

Thyroid Disorders

The thyroid gland is located anteriorly within the neck and is composed of two lobes connected by isthmus at the level of the cricoid cartilage. This gland produces and stores thyroxine (T4), triiodothyronine (T3), and calcitonin, which are necessary for all basic metabolic processes in the body. Normal thyroid lobes (which are butterfly-shaped) should move up and down when swallowing. Observations of nodules, masses, and/or abnormal sizes and shapes of these glands warrant an ultrasound and could potentially be an indication of a thyroid disorder. Disorders of the thyroid gland may occur as a result of disease or dysfunction of the gland; these disorders could also be a secondary result of any alterations of the pituitary gland and the hypothalamic gland. Disorders of the parathyroid glands often accompany thyroid disorders. The parathyroid glands lie behind the thyroid gland and secrete the parathyroid hormone (PTH). This hormone works together with vitamin D to increase serum calcium concentrations and decrease serum phosphate levels. Since calcium is necessary for normal bone growth and development, alterations in the functioning of the parathyroid glands are often manifested in the musculoskeletal system. For a patient with suspected hypoparathyroidism, the FNP should check for a positive Chvostek's sign, which may assist in making the diagnosis.

Hypothyroidism

Hypothyroidism is a common thyroid disorder frequently seen in primary care. Symptoms occur as a result of underfunctioning of the thyroid gland. The disorder may be autoimmune in etiology, such as with Hashimoto's thyroiditis.

Symptoms

Patients with hypothyroidism often present with symptoms of cold intolerance, alopecia, constipation, arthralgia, fatigue, dry skin, goiter, and weight gain. Common lab findings include an elevated TSH, low T4, elevated phosphate level, and decreased serum calcium level.

Management

Management includes levothyroxine 25 to 50 mcg per day, usually for life. The TSH should be rechecked every four to six weeks until the TSH has normalized. Pregnant patients with a diagnosis of hypothyroidism should continue levothyroxine therapy, although most women will need an increase in the dosage, sometimes up to 30% of the original dose.

Hyperthyroidism

Hyperthyroidism results from increased secretion of thyroid hormone. Common causes of primary hyperthyroidism include Graves' disease, a toxic adenoma, toxic multinodular goiter, or carcinoma. Secondary hyperthyroidism is less common but may be caused by a TSH-secreting

CLINICAL PEARL

Per 2021 ADA recommendations, statin therapy should be suggested for patients over 40 years of age with diabetes.

CLINICAL PEARL

Serum TSH level is a good indicator of the function of a thyroid with a normal range 0.404.5 u/mL. T4: normal range is 4.512.0 (↓T4 and ↑TSH confirms hypothyroidism, while ↑T4 and ↓TSH confirms hyperthyroidism).

CLINICAL PEARL

Order TSH-receptor antibodies to confirm Hashimoto's disease.

pituitary adenoma. Hyperthyroidism is also seen post–viral illness and postpartum. An elevated TSH level without thyroid disease produces a subclinical hyperthyroidism and may result from subacute thyroiditis or ingestion of excess thyroid hormone.

Symptoms

Symptoms of hyperthyroidism include heat intolerance (sweating), nervousness, insomnia, amenorrhea, increased bowel movements, and unintentional weight loss. Lab studies will demonstrate a low TSH with an elevated T4.

Management

Management consists of ablation therapy or oral propylthiouracil or methimazole. Ablation is the therapy of choice. Medications shrink thyroid tissue and decrease production of thyroid hormone. The other management alternative is a total or partial thyroidectomy.

Addison's Disease

Addison's disease is a slow progressive disease that commonly occurs in middle-aged adults due to deficiency of adrenal hormones (cortisol and aldosterone).

Primary adrenal insufficiency: malfunction of adrenal gland, autoimmune infections, tuberculosis, or cancer.

Secondary adrenal insufficiency: failure of pituitary gland to regulate ACTH.

Symptoms

Symptoms include hyperpigmentation of the skin (on areas of the body that are not exposed to the sun), fatigue, muscle weakness, hypotension, weight loss, hypoglycemia, salt craving, and nausea/vomiting.

Management

Labs: ACTH stimulation test and antibody testing to assess for autoimmune origin. Referral to an endocrinologist for further evaluation and management.

Cushing's Syndrome and Cushing's Disease

Usually caused by long-term exposure to cortisol steroids (both exogenous/endogenous). For example, frequent long-term steroids taken for managing chronic disease (asthma, rheumatoid arthritis, and systemic lupus) or adrenal adenomas/carcinomas (overproduction of ACTH by the adrenal gland itself). First-line diagnostic testing includes a 24-hour urinary test for free cortisol or dexamethasone suppression test. Second-line testing includes ACTH test, high-dose DST testing, CRH stimulation test, or pituitary CT/MRI.

Symptoms

Patients present with unintentional progressive weight gain, metabolic syndrome, fatigue, muscle weakness, depression, anxiety, hirsutism, and irregular or absence of menstrual cycle for women.

Management

Management begins with identification and amelioration of underlying etiology. Gradual discontinuation of exogenous corticosteroids should be undertaken to avoid triggering an adrenal crisis.

> **CLINICAL PEARL**
>
> Levothyroxine doses > 200 mcg per day are seldom required. Patients given > 200 mcg with no improvement on the lab report may indicate poor compliance, malabsorption, drug interactions, or a combination of these factors.

> **CLINICAL PEARL**
>
> Stressful life events could precipitate Addisonian crisis, which may be life-threatening.

> **CLINICAL PEARL**
>
> Tapering dosage should be initiated for patients who present with Cushing's syndrome and are currently taking long-term corticosteroid therapy.

Practice Questions

1. How frequently should the nurse practitioner implement laboratory testing to screen for prediabetes in an asymptomatic healthy patient?

   (A) at least once every three months
   (B) at least once every six months
   (C) at least once each year
   (D) at least once every three years

2. Which of the following laboratory tests should be used to screen for prediabetes?

   (A) comprehensive metabolic panel
   (B) in-office glucose finger-stick test
   (C) Hgb hemoglobin A1c test, FPG, or two-hour post-75-gram OGTT
   (D) CBC, CMP, or lipid panel

3. Which of the following tests does not require a confirmation testing for a diagnosis of diabetes mellitus?

   (A) A1c of 6.8% and FPG of 130 mg/dL
   (B) FPG of 130 mg/dL and random glucose of 180
   (C) random glucose of 180 and a two-hour post-75-gram OGTT of 200 mg/dL
   (D) two-hour post-75-gram OGTT of 200 mg/dL and an A1c of 6.4%

4. What treatment plan should an FNP employ for a patient with type 2 diabetes who has adhered to dual therapy (metformin and sulfonylurea) for the past year and has an A1c of 12.1%?

   (A) increase metformin to 2 grams per day
   (B) replace metformin and sulfonylurea with thiazolidinedione
   (C) stop the current dual therapy and initiate insulin therapy
   (D) initiate adjunct insulin therapy into current dual therapy regimen

5. Which of the following statements about diabetes is true?

   (A) Patients with diabetes mellitus are at a higher risk for developing cataracts and glaucoma.
   (B) The first-line treatment of choice for a patient with type 2 DM is a thiazolidione medication.
   (C) Insulin therapy should only be initiated in patients with type 1 diabetes.
   (D) With appropriate management and lifestyle changes, a patient with type 2 diabetes will reverse previous target organ damage.

6. An FNP is treating a 38-year-old female with a BMI of 32. Since her diagnosis of type 2 diabetes two months ago, she has been trying to lose weight. When discussing pharmacotherapeutic agents with the patient, the FNP should consider her desire (and need) to lose weight. This impacts potential medication options. Which of the following oral antidiabetic medications causes weight gain?

   (A) bile acid sequestrant (Welchol)
   (B) incretin mimetic (Byetta)
   (C) biguanide (metformin)
   (D) sulfonylurea (glipizide)

7. You suspect a thyroid disorder in your patient who reports weight gain, cold intolerance, and fatigue. You decide to order labs to assist in the diagnosis. Which of the following lab results indicate hypothyroidism?

    (A) low TSH, low T4, elevated phosphate level, and decreased serum calcium level
    (B) low TSH, low T4, low phosphate level, and increased serum calcium level
    (C) elevated TSH, elevated T4, elevated phosphate level, and decreased serum calcium level
    (D) elevated TSH, low T4, elevated phosphate level, and decreased serum calcium level

8. What does the thyroid-stimulating hormone (TSH) test measure?

    (A) serum level of free thyroxine (T4)
    (B) total thyroxine (T4) level
    (C) peripheral level of thyroid hormone produced by the pituitary gland
    (D) serum levels of triiodothyronine (T3) and thyroxine (T4)

9. During a routine annual physical exam on a 17-year-old female, the FNP palpates an irregular 2 cm nodule on the right side of the trachea. Which of the following is an appropriate action to further evaluate the nodule?

    (A) request that the patient return to the clinic for follow-up in one week
    (B) order an ultrasound of the thyroid
    (C) order a computed tomography (CT) scan of the thyroid
    (D) order a kidney, ureter, and bladder (KUB) study

10. How soon should a newly diagnosed patient with hypothyroidism be reevaluated for possible dose adjustment of levothyroxine (Synthroid)?

    (A) reevaluate TSH between six to eight weeks
    (B) reevaluate TSH between four to six weeks
    (C) reevaluate TSH between one to two weeks
    (D) reevaluate TSH between two to four weeks

11. A patient presents with heat intolerance, nervousness, amenorrhea, insomnia, and unintentional weight loss. These symptoms are consistent with:

    (A) hypothyroidism.
    (B) hyperthyroidism.
    (C) Hashimoto's thyroiditis.
    (D) myxedema.

12. While renewing a prescription for a cortisol steroid treatment for an elderly woman with a diagnosis of systemic lupus, the advanced FNP will also consider the patient to be at risk for:

    (A) Cushing's disease.
    (B) hepatic cirrhosis.
    (C) intraperitoneal hemorrhage.
    (D) Graves' disease.

13. Upon diagnostic confirmation by fine needle aspiration, what is the most common treatment for a benign thyroid nodule in a primary care setting?

    (A) radioactive iodine therapy
    (B) surgery
    (C) watchful waiting with an annual evaluation
    (D) levothyroxine therapy

14. A patient, who is pregnant, is currently taking levothyroxine for hypothyroidism. What action should the FNP take when managing her hypothyroidism?

    (A) stop prescribing levothyroxine
    (B) refer the patient to an endocrine specialist
    (C) increase her dosage of levothyroxine
    (D) continue with the current dosage of levothyroxine

15. Which of the following tests can be implemented for a patient with suspected hypoparathyroidism?

    (A) Mini-Cog
    (B) Homan's sign
    (C) Tinel's sign
    (D) Chvostek's sign

Answer Explanations

1. **(D)** Per the ADA guidelines, all patients should be screened for diabetes at three-year intervals beginning at age 45. Other recommendations include testing for patients with a BMI > 25 (including children or adolescents who are overweight/obese) and for those who have two or more of the risk factors for diabetes.

2. **(C)** Prediabetes screening can be done using a hemoglobin A1c test, an FPG test, or a two-hour post-75 gram OGTT test. A comprehensive metabolic panel (CMP) evaluates serum electrolyte levels and assesses renal and liver function (choice (A)). This test would not be helpful in ruling out prediabetes. A glucose finger stick done in the office provides a "snapshot" of the patient's glucose level at that time (choice (B)). This test is helpful in the outpatient setting to determine for follow-up testing, but it is not a reliable method for diagnosing prediabetes. A complete blood count (CBC) test evaluates for anemia and infection, and a lipid panel checks cholesterol levels in the serum (choice (D)). These tests are not useful in diagnosing prediabetes.

3. **(A)** Confirmation testing is not necessary for patients who present with two or more of the following positive test results: an A1c $\geq$ 6.5%, an FPG $\geq$ 126 mg/dL, a two-hour post-75 gram OGTT of $\geq$ 200 mg/dL, or a random glucose of $\geq$ 200 *with* symptoms (the three Ps). A random glucose of 180 is not reliable as an indicator of diabetes (choices (B) and (C)).

4. **(D)** A diabetic patient who failed dual oral therapy and presents with an A1c of 12.1% should have adjunct insulin therapy added to their regimen (triple therapy). The patient is considered a high risk for glucose toxicity. Basal insulin is commonly used in primary care for type 2 DM. Oral medications may be continued along with insulin therapy, if indicated and if there is evidence of its efficacy. Increasing the metformin to 2 grams per day is unlikely to produce any increase in hypoglycemic effects (choice (A)). Metformin works by decreasing liver production of glucose (by enhancing hepatic sensitivity) and increasing the peripheral uptake of glucose by peripheral tissues. Sulfonylurea medications stimulate pancreatic secretion of insulin (choice (B)). Because of this, these medications often cause hypoglycemic episodes. Thiazolidinediones (glitazones) enhance insulin sensitivity in the liver, fat, and muscle tissues of the body. For these medications to be effective, insulin must be present in sufficient quantities (choice (C)). This is not usually the case for patients with long-standing disease. Current ADA recommendations are to initiate adjunct insulin therapy when oral medications are not effectively controlling serum glucose levels.

5. **(A)** Patients with diabetes mellitus are at a higher risk for developing cataracts, glaucoma, diabetic retinopathy, and blindness. Oral antidiabetic drugs are not indicated in the management of type 1 diabetes due to the lack of insulin production (choice (B)). Insulin therapy may cause weight gain (choice (C)). Newly diagnosed type 2 DM patients should try lifestyle changes and diet modification before any oral antidiabetic therapy (choice (D)). First-line pharmacotherapeutic recommendation for management of type 2 diabetes is metformin (a biguanide medication). Target organ damage due to secondary to uncontrolled hyperglycemia is not reversible.

6. **(D)** Sulfonylureas, thiazolidinediones, and insulin cause weight gain. Meglitinides and bile acid sequestrants are weight-neutral (choice (A)). Incretin (choice (B)) mimetics, biguanides (choice (C)), and amylin analogs cause weight *loss*. Providing patient-centered care requires collaboration between the patient and clinician. Carefully listening to the patient and eliciting goals for treatment are important components of care. Since this patient is obese and

wants to lose weight, the clinician should be supportive in this with all aspects of disease management.

7. **(D)** Hypothyroidism includes elevated TSH, low T4, elevated phosphate level, and decreased serum calcium level. If the TSH is low, consider a diagnosis of hyperthyroidism. Thyroid hormone is secreted by the hypothalamus through a closed-system feedback loop. If the thyroid gland is producing too much thyroid hormone, the gland will secrete less thyroid stimulating hormone. Although abnormal calcium and phosphate levels may be present, these are usually a result of parathyroid dysfunction.

8. **(C)** The thyroid-stimulating hormone test measures the peripheral level of thyroid hormone produced by the pituitary gland. A free thyroxine (T4) (choice (A)) test measures only the free T4 in the blood cell, while a total T4 test (choice (B)) measures both kinds of T4 (T4 that is bound to protein and also T4 that is unbound in the blood).

9. **(B)** Thyroid ultrasound should be ordered for evaluation of any abnormality in the size and shape of the gland. Waiting a week and having the patient return for a follow-up exam would not be appropriate management (choice (A)). All thyroid nodules should be evaluated at the time they are discovered. A CT scan of the thyroid may be ordered if other testing demonstrates an abnormality (choice (C)). An MRI would likely be ordered to evaluate nodules as well as a PET scan. Most nodules undergo needle aspiration to determine pathology. A KUB study is used to assess for problems with the renal system and would not be helpful in evaluating a thyroid nodule (choice (D)).

10. **(B)** The standard adjustment period for levothyroxine (Synthroid) is every four to six weeks until the patient is clinically euthyroid and the serum TSH returns to normal. The TSH level should be measured every four to eight weeks after initiating therapy and before each dosage increase. It is important to allow enough time for the serum level steady state to be reached; therefore, testing again in one to two levels would not be helpful.

11. **(B)** Patients with hyperthyroidism experience intolerance to heat, nervousness, amenorrhea, insomnia, and unintentional weight loss. Hypothyroidism presents with hypofunction of the thyroid gland, and all body functions are slowed, including metabolic processes (choice (A)). Symptoms of hypothyroidism include cold intolerance, alopecia, constipation, arthralgia, fatigue, dry skin, goiter, and weight gain. Hashimoto's thyroiditis and myxedema are conditions seen in patients who have hypothyroidism (choice (C)). Myxedema is a cutaneous edema associated with Graves' disease and hypothyroidism (choice (D)). It is caused by deposition of connective tissue and is associated with untreated thyroid disease. Patients present with dry skin, pretibial myxedema, mental deterioration, slowed metabolic rate, and edema of the nose and lips. Myxedema may lead to coma, which can be fatal.

12. **(A)** Cushing's syndrome is usually caused by long-term exposure to cortisol steroids, which this patient is taking. Cushing's syndrome is characterized by unintentional, progressive weight gain, headaches, skin changes, muscle weakness, menstrual irregularities and hirsutism in women. Patients will present with generalized or central obesity. Fat deposition around the face produces the "moon face" characteristic that is seen with this disorder. Atrophy of the epidermis is common, along with fungal infections of the skin and nails. Hypertension is often seen as a result of water retention. Hepatic cirrhosis is the irreversible end stage of chronic liver injury (choice (B)). Morphological and functional changes occur in the organ, leading to progressive dysfunction. Chronic alcohol misuse is commonly associated with hepatic cirrhosis; however, other causes include obstructive biliary disease or acute

liver injury. Intraperitoneal hemorrhage is bleeding into the peritoneal space of the abdomen (choice (C)). Causes include acute injury, ruptured appendix, ruptured aortic aneurysm, among others. It is not associated with long-term corticosteroid use. Graves' disease is a disorder of the thyroid gland caused by autoimmune destruction of thyroid tissue (choice (D)).

13. **(C)** Benign thyroid nodules do not require further management. However, it is important for the patient to have an annual follow-up to evaluate the site for any changes in the size or shape of the nodule. Radioactive iodine therapy is sometimes used as ablation therapy for hyperthyroidism (choice (A)). Patients undergoing ablation will require lifelong exogenous insulin administration. Surgery is not indicated for benign thyroid nodules unless they are growing rapidly or causing discomfort or obstruction of surrounding tissues (choice (B)). Levothyroxine therapy is indicated for management of hypothyroidism (choice (D)).

14. **(C)** Pregnant patients may need an additional 30% increase in levothyroxine dosage. This is only a temporary dosage adjustment. The patient should be able to continue her previous dosage immediately after delivery. Serum TSH level should be checked before increasing any dosage. Levothyroxine is safe to take during pregnancy, and the FNP can manage the dosing adjustment in conjunction with the obstetrician, thus eliminating choices (A), (B), and (D).

15. **(D)** Chvostek's sign is used to assess for hypoparathyroidism. The examiner taps on one side of the face over the cranial nerve, triggering a spasm of the face. Trousseau's sign may be used. Other hypoparathyroidism symptoms include tetany, carpopedal spasms, and tingling of the lips and hands. Laboratory results: low serum calcium level, high serum phosphate level, and reduced urine calcium excretion. Mini-Cog is used for evaluating cognitive impairment (choice (A)). Homan's sign is a test that is used for evaluating possible deep vein thrombosis (choice (B)). Tinel's sign is a test that is used to evaluate for carpal tunnel syndrome (choice (C)).

5

Disorders of the Renal System

The renal system consists of the kidneys, ureters, bladder, and the urethra. The kidneys are located in the retroperitoneal space and are responsible for the regulation of fluids and electrolytes. They also produce approximately 1,500 mL of urine daily. Note that, due to organ displacement caused by the liver, the right kidney is slightly lower than the left kidney. The kidneys also play a role in the production of erythropoietin (red blood cells), hormones (renin, bradykinin, prostaglandin, and calcitriol), and vitamin D_3. Any untreated injury, blockage, or infection of the kidneys may cause multiple organs to fail.

LAB FACTS

Serum Creatinine

(Male 0.7–1.3 mg/dL, Female 0.6–1.1 mg/dL): Serum creatinine is a breakdown product of metabolism of the muscles. It has an inverse relationship with renal function. For example, when creatinine level ↑, renal function is ↓. In general, age, gender, race, medication intake, and body muscle mass will affect serum creatinine concentration.

Serum Creatinine Clearance

This is a more sensitive test than serum creatinine because it estimates the glomerular filtration rate (GFR). The GFR measures the amount of fluids filtered by the glomerulus within a minute. The normal range of the estimated glomerular filtration rate (eGFR) for a healthy adult is approximately 90 mL/min. As renal function declines, the creatinine clearance is also reduced. Therefore, some medication adjustments may be needed based on the patient's GFR. A low GFR or creatinine clearance may suggest possible kidney disease. Patients with a large body mass may benefit from a 24-hour urine collection test for creatinine clearance.

Blood Urea Nitrogen (BUN)

BUN measures the kidney's ability to metabolize protein in the urine (excrete urea). Healthy kidneys should be able to filter urea from the bloodstream. A high BUN level should prompt a follow-up with a GFR evaluation.

Urinalysis

Urine is normally sterile and does not contain blood cells. On a urinalysis report, the presence of some epithelial cells and red blood cells (fewer than five cells) is considered normal. If presence of > 5 RBC, ask the patient for history of recent removal of catheter or last menstrual cycle. Leukocyte esterase detects WBCs via esterase produced by WBC. The presence of WBC may be seen with infections, protein indicates possible chronic kidney disease, and the presence of nitrites could be due to *E. coli* (most common), *Klebsiella*, or *Proteus* infections, as they produce nitrite from nitrate.

Proteinuria

An alternate name for proteinuria is albuminuria. Albumin is a protein found in the blood. Healthy kidneys will filter albumin from the urine. The presence of albumin in the urine may suggest additional testing is needed for an undiagnosed patient. In primary care, the measurement of GFR and albumin could serve as a monitoring tool to determine the progression of chronic kidney disease.

Urinary Tract Infection (UTI)

UTI is defined by the presence of 10,000 or more colony-forming units (CFUs)/mL present in the urine. However, if there is a report of dysuria or other symptoms for UTI, the presence of 100 CFU/mL or more will also confirm the UTI diagnosis. The majority of UTIs are caused by *E. coli* bacteria. Risk factors that could lead to a UTI include poor personal hygiene, immunocompromised health status, diabetes mellitus, a change in body pH (caused by a new body wash, a new bubble bath, participating in outdoor water sports for an extended period of time, etc.), and pregnancy. Note that women are more prone to developing UTIs. UTIs are considered recurrent if the patient has developed three or more UTIs in one year or two or more infections within six months.

Symptoms

Symptoms of a UTI include low-grade fever, dysuria, polyuria or urgency, nocturia, hematuria, lower back pain or suprapubic pain, pelvic discomfort, urinary incontinence, and cloudy and foul-smelling urine. Elderly patients may also present with an altered mental status, and that may be the only sign of a UTI.

Management

Management options for a UTI may include the use of any of the following medications: nitrofurantoin monohydrate/macrocrystals, sulfamethoxazole/trimethoprim (SMX/TMP), or fosfomycin. Beta-lactam antibiotics may be prescribed when other recommended agents cannot be used. The treatment time frame for a UTI is generally a three-day regimen for an uncomplicated UTI and a three-day or longer regimen for a complicated UTI. A UTI in an adult male should prompt a urological evaluation as these illnesses are uncommon in men. Infant males with symptoms indicative of a UTI should be evaluated by a pediatric urologist because the most common cause of a UTI in this age group is an anatomical abnormality.

Asymptomatic Bacteriuria

Asymptomatic bacteriuria may occur in healthy patients, and in general, is seen more often in women. According to the Infectious Disease Society of America (IDSA), diagnosing asymptomatic bacteriuria in men is based on a *single* clean catch voided urine specimen with isolation of a single organism in quantitative counts of $\geq$ 10,000 cfu/mL with the absence of symptoms. Asymptomatic bacteriuria in women is based on *two consecutive* clean catch voided urine specimens with isolation of the same organism in quantitative counts of $\geq$ 10,000 cfu/mL with the absence of symptoms.

Symptoms

Asymptomatic bacteriuria does not generate any symptoms.

Management

Currently, there are no recommendations for the screening and management of asymptomatic bacteriuria among men and women, *except* for pregnant women. Asymptomatic bacteriuria occurs in 5% of pregnant women. If left untreated in a pregnant woman, the bacteria could have a strong propensity to develop into a systemic urinary tract infection, including pyelonephritis, which is a serious illness in this population. Management includes the use of nitrofurantoin, fosfomycin and penicillin (with or without beta-lactamase inhibitors), cephalosporins, and aztreonam. Because trimethoprim-sulfamethoxazole (TMP-SMX) is a folic acid antagonist, this medication should not be used in the first trimester of pregnancy due to the risk to fetal development.

Urinary Bladder Inflammation (Cystitis)

Urinary bladder inflammation is a commonly seen condition in primary care. Bladder inflammation is usually associated with infection of the lower urinary tract and, in fact, may be a component of the illness. Note that UTIs in young children and pregnant women require treatment as these are more likely to progress to pyelonephritis if left untreated.

Symptoms

Symptoms of cystitis are similar to those of a UTI with dysuria, bladder spasms, and lower abdominal discomfort. Patients will also report urinary urgency and frequency.

Management

Management of uncomplicated acute cystitis in women includes nitrofurantoin monohydrate/macrocrystals, sulfamethoxazole/trimethoprim (SMX/TMP), or fosfomycin. Beta-lactam antibiotics may be used when other recommended agents cannot be used. Patients should be instructed to increase water intake, limit intake of colas and caffeine, and complete all antibiotics as ordered.

Acute Pyelonephritis

Acute pyelonephritis is inflammation of the kidney typically due to a bacterial infection. The most common causative organisms are *Escherichia coli*, *Proteus mirabilis*, and *Klebsiella pneumoniae*. Pyelonephritis is a serious illness that can lead to multiple organ failure if untreated.

Symptoms

Patients will present with fever above 100.4°F, costovertebral angle tenderness, a urine analysis with elevated number of leukocytes, hematuria, albuminuria/proteinuria, and white blood cell casts.

Management

The usual treatment for uncomplicated pyelonephritis includes ceftriaxone IM, ciprofloxacin PO, levofloxacin, or sulfamethoxazole/trimethoprim (SMX/TMP). Some patients may require short-term hospitalization for IV antibiotic therapy.

Acute Kidney Injury (AKI)

Acute kidney injury is also known as acute renal failure (ARF). AKI may be diagnosed when one of the following criteria is present:

- The patient's serum creatinine level increases to 26 μmol/L or above within 48 hours of injury or is 1.5-fold or greater than the reference value.
- The patient's urine output is less than 0.5 mL/kg/hr for more than six consecutive hours.

The most common causes of AKI are associated with intrarenal injury as a result of renal hypoperfusion or exposure to nephrotoxic agents or blood components.

Symptoms

Patients with AKI may present with acute onset of fatigue, malaise, nausea, vomiting, pruritus, and altered mental status. Symptoms may vary with each patient. Symptoms are more common due to uremia or other underlying causes.

Management

CLINICAL PEARL

The key to managing AKI is to eliminate the underlying cause.

Patients should be referred to an endocrinologist. In primary care, blood chemistries should be monitored during each follow-up visit (basic metabolic panel, complete blood count). The FNP should assess the patient for signs of fluid overload, elevated blood pressure, jugular vein distention, peripheral edema, shortness of breath, and unintentional weight gain.

Chronic Kidney Disease (CKD)

Chronic kidney disease is characterized by a progressive loss of function of the nephrons that has been present for more than three months. The natural progression of CKD is end-stage renal disease (ESRD). The major underlying causes of ESRD are uncontrolled diabetes mellitus and primary hypertension (as much as 70% of cases). This is followed by glomerulonephritis, cystic disease, and other urological diseases. The peak onset of ESRD is between 65 and 75 years of age. In patients 50 years of age and older, renal artery stenosis and chronic ischemic renovascular disease accounts for up to 20% of CKD cases. Hypertension is present in 85% of patients with CKD. Risk factors for developing CKD include analgesic overuse, cigarette smoking, collagen vascular disease, cirrhosis, AIDS-related nephropathies, and hereditary renal diseases. A comprehensive medication history should be obtained to rule out the presence of nephrotoxic medications that may be contributing to the disease.

Symptoms

Patients may present with uremic frost appearance to the skin, bruising, asterixis, peripheral neuropathy, altered mental status, peripheral edema, ascites, and elevated blood pressure with rapid pulse.

Management

CKD patients should be referred to an endocrinologist for management. General principles of managing CKD in primary care include determination and control of the underlying etiology, monitoring changes in renal function, conservatively treating the physiological effects of CKD, and reinforcing the importance of dietary and nutrition education.

Staging of Chronic Kidney Disease

The Kidney Disease: Improving Global Outcomes (KDIGO) work group recommends that CKD is classified based on cause, GFR category, and albuminuria (CGA) category.

GFR and ACR categories and risk of adverse outcomes			ACR categories (mg/mmol), description and range		
			< 3 Normal to mildly increased	3–30 Moderately increased	> 30 Severely increased
			A1	A2	A3
GFR categories (mL/min/1.73 m²), description and range	≥ 90 Normal and high	G1	No CKD in the absence of markers of kidney damage		
	60–89 Mild reduction related to normal range for a young adult	G2			
	45–59 Mild–moderate reduction	G3a*			
	30–44 Moderate–servere reduction	G3b			
	15–29 Severe reduction	G4			
	< 15 Kidney failure	G5			

Increasing risk →

*Consider using eGFRcystatinC for people with CKD G3aA1 (see recommendations 1.1.14 and 1.1.15)

Abbreviations: ACR, albumin:creatinine ratio; CKD, chronic kidney disease; GFR, glomerular filtration rate

Adapted with permission from Kidney Disease: Improving Global Outcomes (KDIGO) CKD Work Group (2013). KDIGO 2012 clinical practice guideline for the evaluation and management of chronic kidney disease. *Kidney International* (Suppl. 3): 1–150.

Figure 5.1. Classification of Chronic Kidney Disease Using GFR and ACR Categories

CLINICAL PEARL

Anemia is commonly seen in patients with chronic renal failure due to a reduction of erythropoietin production by the kidney.

Nephrolithiasis

Nephrolithiasis is the formation of kidney stones. Alternate terms for nephrolithiasis include *kidney stones, renal stones,* and *renal lithiasis*. There are different types of stones and causes:

Table 5.1. Types of Stones and Their Etiologies

Type of Stone	Etiology
Calcium oxalate stones	High levels of urine calcium and oxalate excretion
Calcium phosphate stones	High levels of urine calcium and alkaline urine
Oxalate stones	Occurs naturally in some fruits, vegetables, nuts, and chocolates
Uric acid stones	Urine is persistently acidic
Struvite stones	Kidney infection
Cystine stones	Genetic disorder

Risk factors that contribute to nephrolithiasis include male sex, a family history of kidney stones, obesity, and health conditions such as hypercalciuria, cystic kidney disease, renal tubular acidosis, gout, and hyperparathyroidism.

Symptoms

Symptoms include costovertebral angle tenderness, a sudden onset of fever up to 103°F, shaking, chills, nausea, vomiting, and unilateral flank or localized back pain over the affected kidney. Imaging with X-rays or CT scan can assist in determining the location of the stones.

Management

Management includes analgesics that may be prescribed to alleviate the pain. Small stones are usually passed uneventfully with urine. An alpha blocker may be prescribed to relax the muscle to facilitate the passing of the stone(s). Proper hydration with 2–3 liters of fluids per day is recommended. For patients with larger stones, a referral is required for other management options, including shock wave lithotripsy, ureteroscopy, or insertion of a nephrostomy tube to drain urine and stone fragments. Patients will require a referral for the management of complicated stone disease.

Wilms Tumor

Wilms tumor (also known as nephroblastoma) is the most common childhood cancer in children between the ages of three and eight. About 9 of 10 of all kidney-related cancers in children are diagnosed as Wilms tumors. It usually presents unilaterally in one kidney with significant increase in size (larger than the kidney) before diagnosis. Risk factors include missing iris of the eye (aniridia) at birth and enlargement of one side of the body (hemihypertrophy). Wilms tumor is also more common among siblings and twins. A clinical assessment of the patient may yield a firm, non-tender mass in the upper quadrant of the abdomen.

Symptoms

Abdominal pain could indicate the rapid growth of the tumor, which increases the pressure on the abdominal wall. The rapid growth of the tumor may result in constipation, vomiting, abdominal distress, anorexia, dyspnea, and weight loss.

Management

Initially, abdominal ultrasound, chest X-ray, and CT scan may be ordered to identify areas of involvement. Urine will be positive for blood, but with no increase in vanillylmandelic acid and homovanillic acid levels as occurs with neuroblastoma. A complete blood count, liver function test, renal function test, serum electrolytes, and uric acid may be ordered for baseline measurement. The FNP should also refer the patient to an oncologist.

Practice Questions

1. The most common cause of sepsis in a wheelchair bound patient is:

   (A) Decubitus ulcers
   (B) kidney stones.
   (C) folliculitis.
   (D) urinary tract infection.

2. Which of the following drugs has an analgesic effect and may be used to treat dysuria?

   (A) hyoscyamine (Levsin)
   (B) oxybutynin (Ditropan)
   (C) metronidazole (Flagyl)
   (D) phenazopyridine (Pyridium)

3. Which of the following would be an appropriate plan for a 40-year-old, healthy male patient who presents with persistent proteinuria during two previous office visits?

   (A) order an abdominal CT scan
   (B) provide the patient with two specimen cups, and have the patient collect one urine specimen on first arising in the morning, and then another sample two hours later
   (C) order an abdominal X-ray
   (D) initiate a fasting blood glucose test

4. Sally presents with her six-year-old son with concerns of occasional enuresis. The patient is shy, and his vitals are within normal range. A focused exam is unremarkable. What should the FNP do next?

   (A) Provide parental education about growth & development.
   (B) send the patient's urine for culture
   (C) report the parent for possible child abuse
   (D) order a comprehensive metabolic panel (CMP)

5. Most kidney stones are composed of which of the following substances?

   (A) calcium
   (B) sodium
   (C) magnesium
   (D) iron

6. Which of the following medications is the first choice of treatment to relieve pain caused by kidney stones in a pregnant woman, who is also complaining of nausea and vomiting?

   (A) NSAIDs
   (B) acetaminophen
   (C) oxycodone
   (D) hydrocodone

7. Which of the following is the most common causative organism of urinary tract infections?

   (A) *Klebsiella pneumoniae*
   (B) *Escherichia coli*
   (C) *Staphylococcus saprophyticus*
   (D) *Proteus mirabilis*

8. A 26-year-old male recently diagnosed with a kidney stone presents to the clinic with a complaint of dysuria. The family nurse practitioner should consider all of the following, EXCEPT:

   (A) prescribing an analgesic.
   (B) prescribing a diuretic.
   (C) prescribing an alpha blocker.
   (D) increasing fluids to 2–3 liters per day.

9. A 49-year-old woman, who has type 2 diabetes, is concerned about her kidneys. She has a history of four urinary tract infections within the past nine months. She denies any discharges, dysuria, or polyuria. Which of the following actions is the best initial course of management to follow?

   (A) recheck her urine and order a urine culture and sensitivity test
   (B) order an intravenous pyelogram (IVP)
   (C) refer the patient to a urologist.
   (D) evaluate the patient for a possible kidney infection

10. All of the following are differential diagnoses associated with microscopic hematuria, EXCEPT:

    (A) kidney stones.
    (B) bladder cancer.
    (C) acute pyelonephritis.
    (D) renal stenosis.

11. All of the following statements about Wilms tumor are true, EXCEPT:

    (A) The most frequent clinical sign is a palpable abdominal mass.
    (B) It usually presents in children between the ages of three and eight years old.
    (C) Microscopic or gross hematuria is sometimes present.
    (D) The most frequent clinical sign is changes in vision acuity.

12. A six-year-old patient presents with a chief complaint of nocturia for the past week. His vital signs are stable, and a physical assessment indicates no costovertebral angle tenderness. An in-house urinalysis is negative for blood and nitrites, but is positive for leukocytes, ketones, and protein. Which of the following is the best test to order next?

    (A) a urine culture and sensitivity
    (B) a 24-hour urine test for protein and creatinine clearance
    (C) a 24-hour urine test for microalbumin
    (D) an intravenous pyelogram (IVP)

13. A 45-year-old truck driver presents with a one-week history of fever and lower back pain. He denies any urine frequency, dysuria, nausea, or vomiting. A focused assessment reveals costovertebral angle tenderness. An in-house urinalysis demonstrates 2+ large leukocytes, hematuria, albuminuria/proteinuria, and WBC casts. What is the most likely diagnosis?

    (A) acute urinary tract infection
    (B) acute orchitis
    (C) acute pyelonephritis
    (D) acute epididymitis

14. All of the following are correct regarding physiological changes in the elderly, EXCEPT:

    (A) an increase in the fat-to-lean body ratio.
    (B) a decrease in the liver's ability to metabolize drugs.
    (C) an increase in renal function.
    (D) presbycusis.

15. An elderly man with a history of rheumatoid arthritis reports to the FNP that his arthritis is getting worse. He had been taking ibuprofen TID as directed on the label for the past eight years. Which of the following organ systems has the highest risk of damage from chronic non-steroidal anti-inflammatory drug (NSAID) use?

    (A) gastrointestinal system
    (B) cardiovascular system
    (C) neurological system
    (D) musculoskeletal system

Answer Explanations

1. **(D)** Urinary tract infections are the most common cause of sepsis in individuals who are wheelchair confined or otherwise immobile. Decubitus ulcers (choice A) are common complications of immobility and may lead to sepsis, however UTIs are the most common etiology in this population. or kidney stones (choice (B)) may precipitate a UTI, but they are not as common as UTIs. Folliculitis could be due to secondary infection from uncontrolled diabetes, poor personal hygiene, superficial skin injury, or shaving (choice (C)). Folliculitis rarely causes sepsis.

2. **(D)** Phenazopyridine (Pyridium) has an analgesic effect and is commonly used as an adjunct therapy along with antibiotics in the treatment of urinary tract infections. An FNP should advise patients that phenazopyridine changes the urine color to orange. Hyoscyamine (choice (A)) and oxybutynin (choice (B)) are anticholinergics used for overactive bladder. Metronidazole is an antibiotic and an antiprotozoal medication (choice (C)). It is used either alone or with other antibiotics to treat pelvic inflammatory disease, endocarditis, and bacterial vaginosis.

3. **(B)** Postural proteinuria should be ruled out before ordering an extensive workup. Urine is collected first thing in the morning and another specimen after two hours. If the first specimen does not show any protein, and the second specimen shows + protein, then postural proteinuria is confirmed. Postural proteinuria does not increase the risk factors for other renal diseases, and the prognosis is excellent. Choices (A), (C), and (D) are not appropriate plans.

4. **(A)** Providing education about growth and development to concerned parents is an important component of primary care. Concerns about voiding disturbances are very common in this setting. Most children with voiding disturbances do not have anatomical or neurological disease. Assessment and vital signs are within normal limits. There is no justification for sending urine for culture (choice (B)). Maturational delay could be a probable cause associated with delay in increase in bladder size that occurs as children grow and develop. Most children can be monitored along with parental involvement, such as restricting fluids prior to bedtime and initiating bladder voiding training with voiding schedules. There is nothing stated in the question that would warrant a report of possible child abuse on the part of the mother (choice (C)). There is also nothing stated in the question that would justify the need for a CMP (choice (D)).

5. **(A)** Calcium oxalate stones are the most common type of kidney stone. Sodium (choice (B)), magnesium (choice (C)), and iron (choice (D)) do not form kidney stones.

6. **(B)** Acetaminophen is a non-opioid analgesic that is effective in relieving mild to moderate pain, and it also can be used during pregnancy. However, it has no peripheral anti-inflammatory effects. NSAIDs are not recommended for pregnant patients nor for managing kidney stone pain since they are associated with side effects, such as renal impairment, acute renal failure, and gastritis in patients who use these medications for pain and inflammation relief (choice (A)). Codeine (oxycodone (choice (C)) and hydrocodone (choice (D)) are not appropriate choices for a pregnant patient. Also, codeine will exacerbate nausea and vomiting symptoms.

7. **(B)** Although UTIs are caused by enteric Gram-negative rods from the *Enterobacteriaceae* group, including *E. coli* and *P. mirabilis* (choice (D)), a five-year research study revealed that *Escherichia coli* accounts for more than 90% of uropathogens. All of the *Klebsiella* species are less commonly seen in the presence of UTIs (choice (A)). *Staphylococcus saprophyticus* is a Gram-positive organism (choice (C)).

8. **(B)** Diuretics can increase the risk for renal stones, so they would not be recommended for this patient. Prescribing an analgesic (choice (A)), prescribing an alpha blocker (choice (C)), and recommending that the patient increase fluid consumption to 2–3 liters per day (choice (D)) are all appropriate choices to promote the passing of stones.

9. **(A)** Check urine and order a urine test for culture and sensitivity. A patient, such as the one described, with a history of UTIs requires frequent evaluation, especially if there is a history of other chronic medical conditions, such as diabetes or hypertension. The definition of UTI is the presence of 100,000 organisms per mL of urine in symptomatic patients or greater than 100 organisms per mL of urine with pyuria (more than 7 WBCs/mL) in asymptomatic patients. Choices (B), (C), and (D) would not be the first line to consider.

10. **(D)** Renal stenosis is a narrowing of the renal artery resulting in the depletion of blood flow to the kidney. This could cause renovascular hypertension (a secondary type of high blood pressure). However, it does not cause the presence of blood in the urine. Evidence of microscopic hematuria can be seen with kidney stones (choice (A)), bladder cancer (choice (B)), and acute pyelonephritis (choice (C)).

11. **(D)** Wilms tumor (also known as nephroblastoma) is a congenital tumor of the kidney; it does not affect the eyes. *Neuroblastoma* is related to vision loss. Once a diagnosis is confirmed, the abdomen should NOT be palpated to prevent the spread of the tumor cells (choice (A)). Microscopic or gross hematuria (choice (C)) may be present, and Wilms tumor commonly presents in children between ages three and eight (choice (B)).

12. **(A)** A urine culture and sensitivity (C&S) is the best evaluation for diagnosing a urinary tract infection. Unless there are other comorbidities or symptoms, an order for a 24-hour urine test for protein and creatinine clearance (choice (B)) or intravenous pyelogram (IVP) (choice (D)) is not warranted. Microalbumin is albumin that is excreted in the urine and is a sensitive marker of nephropathy. A 24-hour urine test for microalbumin is used to screen for early renal disease in diabetic patients (choice (C)).

13. **(C)** Acute pyelonephritis is usually associated with fever above 100.4°F, costovertebral angle tenderness, urine analysis of large leukocytes, hematuria, albuminuria/proteinuria, and WBC casts. A UTI usually does not provoke costovertebral angle tenderness and is less common in men (choice (A)). Acute orchitis symptoms include testicular pain and edema and are usually associated with the mumps, but it does not present with urine frequency and dysuria (choice (B)). Acute epididymitis usually presents with complaints of pain in the scrotum area (choice (D)). It is accompanied by urine frequency and dysuria. The scrotum may be edematous and tender to touch. Pain may be relieved with scrotal support briefs.

14. **(C)** There are many physiological changes that occur in the elderly population. For example: there is an increase in body fat (choice (A)), a loss in detecting high-pitch frequency sound (choice (D)), a decrease in basal metabolic rate, a decrease in absorption rate (choice (B), and a *decrease* in renal perfusion (choice (C)).

15. **(A)** NSAIDs have been known to cause adverse effects of the gastrointestinal systems. NSAIDs cause GI irritation and ulceration. This class of medication also causes different forms of acute kidney injury. For example: hemodynamically mediated acute kidney injury and acute interstitial nephritis, which is often accompanied by nephrotic syndrome. Choices (B), (C), and (D) are organ systems that are not associated with complications of chronic NSAID use.

6

Disorders of the Gastrointestinal System

The gastrointestinal (GI) system includes the mouth, esophagus, stomach, and intestines, as well as accessory organs of the liver, gallbladder, and exocrine pancreas. These structures and organs enable the body to ingest, break down, and metabolize food for energy and body processes. GI complaints are common in primary care and may be challenging to diagnose.

A common complaint in primary care is abdominal pain. Obtaining the appropriate patient history and developing an understanding of the anatomy of the body is the key to conducting an accurate physical examination and initiating appropriate diagnostic tests and management measures.

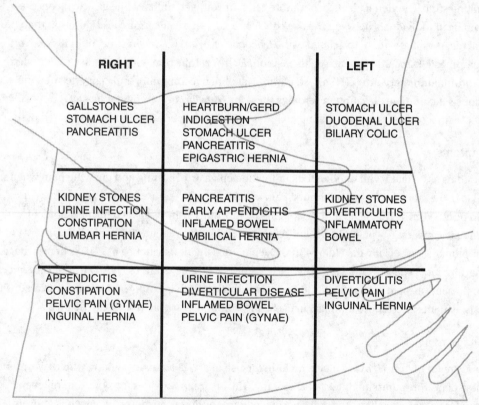

RIGHT

LEFT

GALLSTONES
STOMACH ULCER
PANCREATITIS

HEARTBURN/GERD
INDIGESTION
STOMACH ULCER
PANCREATITIS
EPIGASTRIC HERNIA

STOMACH ULCER
DUODENAL ULCER
BILIARY COLIC

KIDNEY STONES
URINE INFECTION
CONSTIPATION
LUMBAR HERNIA

PANCREATITIS
EARLY APPENDICITIS
INFLAMED BOWEL
UMBILICAL HERNIA

KIDNEY STONES
DIVERTICULITIS
INFLAMMATORY
BOWEL

APPENDICITIS
CONSTIPATION
PELVIC PAIN (GYNAE)
INGUINAL HERNIA

URINE INFECTION
DIVERTICULAR DISEASE
INFLAMED BOWEL
PELVIC PAIN (GYNAE)

DIVERTICULITIS
PELVIC PAIN
INGUINAL HERNIA

Figure 6.1. Know Your Abdominal Pain

Gastroesophageal Reflux Disease (GERD)

GERD is a commonly encountered condition in primary care. GERD is an esophageal inflammatory condition that develops when gastric acid and pepsin reflux from the stomach into the esophagus. Individuals with GERD often have a lower transient resting tone of the lower esophageal sphincter (LES), which allows reflux to occur. Risk factors for developing GERD include certain medications that may lower LES resting tone (such as anticholinergics, nitrates, nicotine, and calcium channel blockers), obesity, and hiatal hernia. Symptoms of GERD may also trigger chronic cough and asthma. Chronic GERD could result in Barrett's esophagus (Barrett's epithelium, a metaplastic change in epithelial lining) through the erosion of the squamous epithelium of the stomach. The gold standard testing for GERD is esophageal motility study.

CLINICAL PEARL

Barrett's esophagus (Barrett's epithelium) may be diagnosed with an upper endoscopy biopsy.

Symptoms

Symptoms include burning in the mid-sternum area after large meals or during sleep, sour odor to breath, chronic sore throat, and chronic nighttime cough.

Management

Management includes a histamine (H2) blocker (such as ranitidine or famotidine) and a two-month course of proton-pump inhibitor (PPI) therapy. This course of treatment will often provide relief of symptoms and promote the healing of the esophageal lining. Follow-up is important, as patients who have not responded adequately to treatment should be referred to gastroenterology for further evaluation.

Peptic Ulcer Disease (PUD)

Peptic ulcers are erosions that develop in the protective lining of the gastric mucosa within areas that are exposed to acidic peptic secretions, such as the esophagus, stomach, duodenum, and small intestine. Duodenal ulcers occur more often in younger adults, while gastric ulcers predominate in individuals between the ages of 55 and 65. Gastric ulcers are less common than duodenal ulcers and are often associated with *Helicobacter pylori* (*H. pylori*) infection. Risk factors for developing PUD include genetic predisposition, *H. pylori* infection, long-term use of non-steroidal anti-inflammatory drugs (NSAIDs), chronic alcohol consumption, and cigarette smoking. Lab diagnosis includes an elevation in serology titers for *H. pylori* immunoglobulin (IgG) or positive urea breath test. Gold standard testing includes upper endoscopy and biopsy of affected tissue.

Symptoms

Symptoms associated with duodenal ulcer include epigastric burning and gnawing pain when no food is in the stomach for several hours. Pain often begins 30 minutes to two hours after eating, often occurs during the night, and disappears by morning. Pain is relieved by ingestion of food or antacids, creating a "pain-food-relief" cycle. Occasionally, patients with duodenal ulcers are asymptomatic, especially the elderly. In these patients, the first evidence of PUD is hemorrhage or perforation, especially if the patient has a history of anticoagulant or NSAID use. Gastric ulcer pain presents as pain in the epigastric area when the stomach is empty and is not associated with meals. Patients also report anorexia, nausea, and vomiting associated with gastric ulcers.

Management

Management of non-*H. pylori* ulcers include the use of an H2 antagonist along with a two-month course of proton-pump inhibitor (PPI) therapy. This regimen provides for symptom relief and allows for mucosal healing. Another pharmacological option is misoprostol, which is appropriate for short-term treatment of uncomplicated PUD. This agent decreases gastric acid production and facilitates mucosal healing. Management of confirmed *H. pylori* ulcers consists of quadruple therapy with bismuth subsalicylate, metronidazole, tetracycline, and a PPI. Some patients benefit from triple therapy, which includes clarithromycin, amoxicillin, and a PPI. Both regimens extend medication therapy for eight weeks to allow for healing.

Acute Pancreatitis

Acute pancreatitis is an acute, inflammatory process that affects the pancreas. It can sometimes be a mild disorder that resolves spontaneously. However, around 20% of patients with acute pancreatitis develop a severe illness requiring hospitalization. Pancreatitis often occurs secondary to an obstruction in the pancreatic system, causing the activation and release of enzymes (including trypsin, lipase, and elastase). An enzyme release causes the autodigestion of cells and tissue within the pancreas, provoking an inflammatory response. Risk factors for developing acute pancreatitis include obstructive biliary tract disease, alcoholism, peptic ulcers, abdominal trauma, elevated lipid levels, genetic factors, thiazide diuretic use, and hyperlipidemia. Laboratory evaluation should include serum amylase and lipase, which have a high sensitivity and specificity for pancreatitis. Other labs may include CBC, CMP, C-reactive protein, blood urea nitrogen, and procalcitonin level. Imaging should include ultrasound, CT scan, and MRI. The American College of Gastroenterology Guidelines state that two of the following criteria should be present for a diagnosis of acute pancreatitis:

1. A characteristic presentation of abdominal pain
2. Elevation of three times higher than normal serum amylase or lipase level
3. Confirmation of acute pancreatitis by abdominal imaging

Symptoms

The cardinal symptom of acute pancreatitis is epigastric or mid-abdominal pain, which is often severe and may be refractory to narcotic analgesics. Fever, nausea and vomiting, bowel hypermotility, and abdominal distension also point to a diagnosis of acute pancreatitis. A positive Cullen's sign, which is noted as an area of bluish discoloration in the umbilical area, is also commonly seen with acute pancreatitis.

Management

There are no specific clinical guidelines for the management of pancreatitis; however, the goal is to halt the inflammation and autodigestion processes and to prevent systemic complications. Management often includes hemodynamic monitoring, IV fluids, and narcotic agents for pain relief.

Acute Cholecystitis

Acute cholecystitis is an inflammation of the gallbladder that is usually caused by a stone (or stones) lodged in the cystic duct. Risk factors include overweight/obesity, high consumption of fatty foods, and pregnancy. The use of ultrasound (diagnostic test of choice) and MRI may demonstrate nonspecific morphological changes to the gallbladder; however, both tests have a substantial margin of error. A hepatoiminodiacetic acid (HIDA) scan is a more sensitive and specific test in identifying cystic duct obstruction. Serum alkaline phosphatase and bilirubin levels may be elevated, but this is a nonspecific finding. Leukocytosis, elevated alanine aminotransferase (ALT) levels, elevated aspartate aminotransferase (AST) levels, and elevated gamma-glutamyl transferase (GGT) levels point to a possible diagnosis of acute cholecystitis. The challenge of diagnosis is to differentiate acute cholecystitis from other disorders presenting similarly.

Symptoms

Symptoms include right upper quadrant abdominal pain with possible radiation to the right shoulder. Pain is often triggered by ingestion of a high-fat meal. Patients may experience vomiting and fever. A positive Murphy's sign (inspiratory arrest with deep palpation of RUQ) is suggestive of acute cholecystitis.

CLINICAL PEARL

For patients with acute pancreatitis, pain relief is managed by administration of meperidine hydrochloride (Demerol) instead of morphine. Morphine may cause spasm of the sphincter of Oddi, thereby exacerbating symptoms.

CLINICAL PEARL

Acute pancreatitis should not be managed in an outpatient, primary care setting. Refer the patient to the ED for evaluation.

Management

Management includes pain control, fluid and electrolyte replacement, and fasting. Antibiotic therapy is often initiated to manage bacterial infection of the gallbladder. Cholecystectomy is indicated for persistent or recurrent symptoms or for complications, such as peritonitis, which is secondary to gallbladder rupture.

Acute Appendicitis

Appendicitis is an inflammation of the vermiform appendix and is often triggered by an obstruction or infection. Acute appendicitis is most commonly seen in individuals between the ages of 10 and 30 years. Evaluation for acute appendicitis includes a physical examination, where positive rebound tenderness is predictive, but not specific, and there is a positive psoas sign. A CT is the diagnostic test of choice; however, an initial evaluation may include an ultrasound for a pediatric patient to prevent exposure to radiation. Laboratory findings consistent with acute appendicitis include total white blood cell count with a differential demonstrating a "left shift," which is a term indicating the presence of a bacterial infection. The presence of *bands* in the differential indicates severe infection and requires immediate emergency department referral.

Symptoms

Early symptoms of acute appendicitis include abdominal pain around the umbilicus. Symptoms are often vague and colicky in nature. Later, the pain moves to the right lower quadrant, with pronounced tenderness of the area and a steady ache that is made worse by walking or coughing. Patients will often experience anorexia, nausea and vomiting, obstipation (a sense of constipation), and low-grade fever. Upon examination, there is often localized rigidity or tenderness at McBurney's point.

Management

Management includes urgent surgical removal of the appendix.

Viral Hepatitis

There are multiple types of viral hepatitis; however, three types (hepatitis A, hepatitis B, and hepatitis C) are commonly seen in primary care. All viral hepatitis illnesses have extremely variable presentation, ranging from asymptomatic infection with no jaundice to rapidly fulminating disease with death occurring within a few days. Serum antibody levels are used to determine the presence of active or resolved hepatitis.

Hepatitis A

Hepatitis A is a self-limiting inflammation of the liver. It is transmitted via the fecal-oral route and is facilitated by crowded conditions and poor sanitation. Since the hepatitis A vaccine (HAV) was introduced in the United States in 1995, incidence has declined dramatically. Currently, the primary risk factor for developing hepatitis A is international travel. Common outbreaks also occur occasionally as a result of exposure to contaminated water or food, including inadequately cooked shellfish.

Symptoms

Individuals with hepatitis A often report a prodromal period of anorexia, malaise, nausea, vomiting, and an aversion to smoking. White count may be mildly elevated, and the patient may report fever and right upper quadrant abdominal pain. Jaundice may be present.

Management

The clinical symptoms of hepatitis A usually resolve themselves over two to three weeks without any intervention. Bed rest is recommended for patients with more severe symptoms. A full clinical recovery usually occurs within three months.

Hepatitis B

Acute hepatitis B is caused by a DNA double-stranded virus known as the hepatitis B virus (HBV). HBV is transmitted through exposure to blood or body fluids, including saliva, vaginal secretions, and semen. It may also be transmitted vertically from mother to fetus. Universal vaccination programs began in 1992, and incidences of hepatitis B have decreased among individuals who are 18 years old or younger. HBV is seen more often in intravenous drug users, those who engage in sexual activity with a person who has hepatitis B, and men who have sex with other men. Other groups at risk include health care workers, dentists, lab personnel, and blood banks. Incarceration is a significant risk factor. Hepatitis B may be acute or chronic, with chronic disease associated with the development of cirrhosis, liver cancer, or liver failure. The appearance of hepatitis B surface antigen (HBsAg) is the first evidence of hepatic infection and is seen before biochemical evidence of disease is present. Specific antibodies to HBsAg (anti-HBs) can be detected in most patients after clearance of HBsAG and following vaccination.

Table 6.1. Serological Test Findings for Hepatitis B

HBsAg	Anti-HBs	HBeAg	Anti-HBe	Anti-HBc	Interpretation
(+)	(−)	(+)	(−)	(IgM)	Confirms a diagnosis of acute hepatitis B
(−)	(−)	(+) or (−)	(−)	(IgM)	Acute hepatitis B*
(−)	(+)	(−)	(+) or (−)	(IgG)	Body developed immunity or recovery from hepatitis B infection
(−)	(+)	(−)	(−)	(IgG)	Body developed immunity via vaccination
(+)	(−)	(+)	(−)	(IgG)	Chronic hepatitis B infection with high viral replication (high risk for transmission)
(−)	(−)	(−)	(+)	(IgG)	Chronic hepatitis B infection with low viral replication activity (low risk for transmission)

*Additional tests (such as an AST test and an ALT test) are required to confirm this diagnosis.

Symptoms

Just like individuals who have hepatitis A, patients who have hepatitis B will often experience a prodromal period of anorexia, malaise, nausea, vomiting, and an aversion to smoking. A fever may be present and the liver may be enlarged.

CLINICAL PEARL

- HBsAg of the hepatitis B surface antigen; detection of a positive HBsAg on a serologic test confirms a diagnosis of acute hepatitis B
- Anti-HBs = an antibody to the hepatitis B surface antigen
- HBeAg = an antigen of the hepatitis B virus that is sometimes present in the blood during an acute infection
- Anti-HBe = an antibody to the e antigen of the hepatitis B virus; someone that has been exposed/ recovered/ initiated hepatitis B vaccination
- Anti-HBc = antibody to the hepatitis B core antigen; the presence of anti-HBc in a sample of serum provides information of infection (past or present) with hepatitis B virus. For example, IgM = acute cases, IgG = recovery stage, or chronic stage

Management

Immunization is available with three doses, given at zero, one, and six months. The ENGERIX-B vaccine and the RECOMBIVAX HB vaccine are included as part of the recommended immunization schedule for all ages. The first dose is now usually given at birth. Management is supportive care with hospitalization for individuals who are severely ill.

Hepatitis C

Hepatitis C is caused by a single-stranded RNA virus. Transmission is via needle sharing associated with injection drug use, organ transplants before 1992, and a history of frequent blood transfusion prior to 1987. Risk factors include injection drug use, body piercing, tattoos, hemodialysis, immune deficiency, having multiple sexual partners, and anal intercourse. The disease often coexists with HIV infection. Of the aforementioned types of viral hepatitis, hepatitis C is the type most likely to become chronic and lead to cirrhosis.

Symptoms

Clinical illness is usually mild and may be asymptomatic. Variable aminotransferase elevations are associated with a high rate ($> 80\%$) of chronic infection.

Management

Management options include alpha-interferon injection, ribavirin, simeprevir, sofosbuvir, and a combination pill (Harvoni) containing sofosbuvir with ledipasvir. Recent studies have demonstrated limited, but significant, success in curing HCV with newer combination medications.

Acute Diverticulitis

Acute diverticulitis is inflammation of the colonic diverticulum and is seen most often in individuals aged 50 years and older. The disease ranges from mild to severe and is related to the level of inflammatory involvement within the colon and surrounding tissues. Patients with acute symptoms are managed empirically with imaging performed after resolution of infection.

Symptoms

Symptoms include left lower quadrant abdominal pain, nausea and vomiting, anorexia, fever, and diarrhea. Left lower abdominal tenderness and a palpable mass may be found on exam. A positive Rovsing's sign (RLQ pain triggered by deep palpation of LLQ), along with rebound tenderness and rigid abdomen, may signal more severe illness. If diverticulitis is suspected, a CT of the abdomen and pelvis should be ordered to rule out abscess development or intestinal perforation, both of which require emergency evaluation.

Management

Management begins conservatively for mild cases with a clear liquid diet, hydration, and, often, broad-spectrum oral antibiotics, such as amoxicillin and clavulanate potassium or metronidazole.

Irritable Bowel Syndrome (IBS)

IBS is a chronic functional gastrointestinal disorder that is characterized by alterations in bowel patterns and is often accompanied by abdominal pain. Approximately 12% of the population in the United States has IBS, and women are affected three times as often as men. Diagnosis of

---

CLINICAL PEARL

Individuals who have been successfully treated for hepatitis C will continue to demonstrate a positive serum-HCV. If there are concerns about relapse, hepatitis C RNA PCR (polymerase chain reaction) quantitative testing should be done.

CLINICAL PEARL

Endoscopic evaluation of the colon or barium enema should not be ordered during acute diverticulitis illness. Insufflation of air at this time could exacerbate and cause perforation of diverticula with resultant peritonitis.

IBS is based on characteristic symptom clusters without evidence of structural or biochemical abnormalities and is a subjective one after ruling out other possible etiologies. Rome III criteria are used in the diagnosis of IBS: At least three days/month over the previous three months associated with two or more of the following symptoms: abdominal discomfort relieved by defecation, change in stool frequency, or a change in stool form or appearance.

Symptoms

Symptoms usually begin during the late teen or early adult years. Individuals with IBS commonly report tenderness in the left lower quadrant of the abdomen. During exacerbation, an alteration in bowel pattern is seen that is uncharacteristic for that patient. This may be more frequent bowel movements or constipation. Often, relief of pain is obtained after defecation.

Management

When treating a patient with IBS, the FNP may recommend that the patient increase his or her daily fiber intake, avoid gas-producing foods, take an over-the-counter fiber supplement (such as psyllium), and/or take short-term antispasmodic agents (such as dicyclomine or hyoscyamine).

Colorectal Cancer (CRC)

Colorectal cancer is now the second leading cause of cancer-related deaths in the United States and the fourth most common cancer diagnosis in adults. Risk factors include lifestyle factors, such as smoking, inactivity, excess body weight, high alcohol consumption, red meat consumption, and processed meat ingestion along with low consumption of dietary fiber, calcium, fruits, and vegetables. Other risk factors include family history of one of several hereditary CRC conditions, including inflammatory bowel disease or adenomatous polyposis or a personal history of inflammatory bowel disease. Health promotion recommendations to prevent colon cancer include eating low-fat meals, reducing red meat consumption, increasing calcium intake, and taking low-dose aspirin daily. Colorectal screening has increased over the past three decades with a corresponding decrease in mortality for CRC in adults who have been screened. However, there has been a noted increase in incidences of this disease in individuals who are younger than 50 years of age. These findings led to new CRC screening recommendations by the American Cancer Society (2018). Current recommendation is that adults 45 years of age or older, who have an average risk of cancer, should undergo regular screening with a high-sensitivity stool-based test or visual examination. All positive non-colonoscopic test results should be followed up with colonoscopy in a timely manner. Strong evidence remains for colonoscopy screening every 10 years for adults who are 50 years old or older and are at average risk. However, screening intervals heavily depend upon the patient's prior screening results, and thus may be needed earlier and more often. Once the patient has reached 75 years old, screening recommendations add the caveat of at least a 10-year predicted life span. Such screenings are not recommended for individuals who are over the age of 85.

Symptoms

CRC is often asymptomatic until late stages, at which point the individual may report blood in the stool, constipation, a change in stool shape, and pressure within the rectal area.

Management

Management in primary care requires timely referral to oncology for evaluation. Visit the CDC website for the complete CRC guidelines.

Practice Questions

1. A positive Cullen's sign is most commonly associated with which of the following conditions?

    (A) acute appendicitis
    (B) gastroesophageal reflux disease
    (C) peptic ulcer disease
    (D) acute pancreatitis

2. Which of the following lab results may help confirm a diagnosis of appendicitis in patients with an atypical presentation?

    (A) total WBCs, 5,000/mm^3; neutrophils, 30%; lymphocytes, 40%; bands 2%
    (B) total WBCs, 17,000/mm^3; neutrophils, 75%; lymphocytes, 20%; bands 9%
    (C) total WBCs, 12,000/mm^3; neutrophils, 50%; lymphocytes, 45%; bands 3%
    (D) total WBCs, 18,000/mm^3; neutrophils, 55%; lymphocytes, 30%; bands 4%

3. Which of the following is NOT a risk factor for acute pancreatitis?

    (A) hypertriglyceridemia
    (B) hypothyroidism
    (C) thiazide diuretic use
    (D) smoking

4. A 56-year-old Caucasian woman presents with a BMI of 35 and complaints of intermittent right upper quadrant abdominal pain over the past few weeks that is precipitated by eating fried foods and popcorn. Upon examination, her heart and lungs are within normal range, bowel sounds are present in all quadrants, and no costovertebral angle tenderness is noted. During abdominal palpation, the patient states that she feels sharp pain during inspiration on the right upper quadrant. Which of the following diagnoses best fits these findings?

    (A) acute gastroenteritis
    (B) acute diverticulitis
    (C) acute cholecystitis
    (D) acute appendicitis

5. Which of the following lab orders will support the diagnosis of acute pancreatitis with a high level of sensitivity and specificity?

    (A) serum lipase and amylase
    (B) alanine aminotransferase (ALT) and aspartate aminotransferase (AST)
    (C) basic metabolic panel
    (D) serum uric acid measurement

6. A 10-year-old male athlete presents to the clinic. He is crying and presents with abdominal pain and guarding at McBurney's point. He tells you that the symptoms began while he was running track at school. During his second lap, he felt a sharp, stabbing pain in his stomach and had to discontinue his activity. What is your diagnosis?

    (A) acute appendicitis
    (B) acute cholecystitis
    (C) acute gastroenteritis
    (D) acute diverticulitis

7. A 64-year-old woman presents with left lower quadrant abdominal pain and fever for the past
    four days. She is pleasant and alert, has no recent history of injury, and denies any nausea,
    vomiting, or diarrhea. Her vitals are as follows: temperature of 100.5°F, BP of 130/80, pulse
    of 90 BPM, and respirations of 16 BPM. A focused assessment reveals that bowel sounds
    are present in all quadrants, her abdomen is soft, she has tenderness in the left lower
    quadrant, and her Rovsing's sign is negative. Which of the following diagnoses will support
    the findings?

    (A) gastroesophageal reflux disease (GERD)
    (B) celiac disease
    (C) pancreatitis
    (D) diverticulitis

8. Which of the following represents an appropriate treatment plan for a mild case of acute
    diverticulitis?

    (A) The FNP should refer the patient to a gastroenterologist for an endoscopic evaluation as
         soon as possible.
    (B) Use conservative management techniques, such as recommending that the patient go
         on a clear liquid diet and increase hydration and take antibiotics for as long as his symp-
         toms last.
    (C) The patient needs to be admitted to the hospital for IV antibiotics.
    (D) The patient should be referred to the emergency department as soon as possible.

9. Risk factors for developing colon cancer include:

    (A) family history of adenomatous polyposis.
    (B) a sibling who has had colorectal cancer.
    (C) a personal history of inflammatory bowel disease.
    (D) all of the above.

10. All of the following options are modifiable lifestyle measures that may relieve symptoms of
    GERD, EXCEPT:

    (A) eliminating caffeine intake.
    (B) family history of GERD.
    (C) eliminating alcohol intake.
    (D) eating small, frequent meals instead of three big meals.

11. A 60-year-old man presents with complaints of GERD. He informs the FNP that he was previ-
    ously prescribed a one-month supply of lansoprazole (Prevacid) from another facility with-
    out any relief. The patient is pleasant and alert. His vitals are normal. His current medications
    include amlodipine, metformin, rosuvastatin, and baby aspirin. Based on this information,
    which of the following medications could be exacerbating his symptoms of GERD?

    (A) amlodipine
    (B) metformin
    (C) rosuvastatin
    (D) baby aspirin

12. The gold standard test that is used to evaluate for peptic ulcer disease is:

   (A) a urea breath test.
   (B) a CT scan of the abdomen.
   (C) an upper endoscopy and biopsy of affected tissue.
   (D) all of the above.

13. Which of the following medications is indicated for the initial treatment of an uncomplicated case of *H. pylori*-negative peptic ulcer disease in a 45-year-old patient who recently recovered from pneumonia?

   (A) cetirizine (Zyrtec)
   (B) misoprostol (Cytotec)
   (C) ranitidine (Zantac)
   (D) Pepto-Bismol tablets

14. A 24-year-old woman presents with recurrent abdominal cramping associated with loose stools that occurs four to five days per month for the past four months. During the flare-up, bathroom frequency increases to five to six times per day. The patient denies fever, has no nausea or vomiting, and has not recently traveled or camped outdoors. Based on this presentation, which of the following conditions does this patient most likely have?

   (A) giardiasis
   (B) irritable bowel syndrome (IBS)
   (C) diverticulitis
   (D) ulcerative colitis

15. A 27-year-old female presents to the clinic with concerns about a possible reinfection with hepatitis C because of recent needle-sharing practices. According to the medical records, she had successfully completed a treatment for hepatitis C in the past year. Based on this information, what is the appropriate next step to further evaluate this patient?

   (A) Order a hepatitis C RNA PCR (polymerase chain reaction) quantitative test and an HIV-1/HIV-2 antibody immunoassay.
   (B) Order a comprehensive STD panel and an HIV-1/HIV-2 antibody immunoassay.
   (C) Order an anti-HCV test and an HIV-1/HIV-2 antibody immunoassay.
   (D) Only order an HIV-1/HIV-2 antibody immunoassay since the patient is now immune to the hepatitis C virus.

Answer Explanations

1. **(D)** Cullen's sign appears in the umbilical area of the abdomen. It usually looks like a patch of ecchymosis (yellowish-green bruising). Cullen's sign is commonly seen with acute pancreatitis. However, other differential diagnoses should be considered, such as severe hemorrhage, duodenal ulcer rupture, blunt abdominal trauma, and ruptured ectopic pregnancy. Choices (A), (B), and (C) are not linked to a positive Cullen's sign.

2. **(B)** A white blood cell (WBC) with a differential will provide better data to support a diagnosis of acute appendicitis. During an episode of acute appendicitis, elevation of leucocytes, neutrophilia, and bands will be observed. Research shows that 80–85% of adults with appendicitis have a WBC count greater than 10,500 cells/μL. Approximately 80% of patients will also have neutrophilia greater than 75%. Less than 4% of patients with appendicitis have a WBC count less than 10,500 cells/μL and neutrophils less than 75%. The presence of bands indicates severe infection, and this finding would require that the patient be immediately referred to the emergency department. Since appendicitis is also an inflammatory disease, a C-reactive protein (CRP) test is another exam that can be used to determine the presence of inflammation, which would support the diagnosis.

3. **(B)** Risk factors for developing pancreatitis include gallstones, alcohol use, elevated triglycerides (choice (A)), thiazide diuretic use (choice (C)), smoking (choice (D)), and drug-induced acute pancreatitis (antibiotics, immunosuppressive agents, blood pressure medications, aminosalicylates, diuretics, corticosteroids, estrogen, diabetes medications, valproate, general anesthetics, and antidepressants).

4. **(C)** Acute cholecystitis is suggested with a finding of a positive Murphy's sign (which is inspiratory arrest during deep palpation of the right upper quadrant of the abdomen). Physical assessment findings associated with gastroenteritis may include mild, generalized tenderness to hyperactive bowel sounds (choice (A)). Examination findings that are consistent with acute diverticulitis include left lower quadrant abdominal pain along with a palpable mass (choice (B)). A patient with acute appendicitis presents with periumbilical pain that moves to the right lower quadrant of the abdomen (choice (D)). Rebound tenderness and guarding are also often noted during a physical exam.

5. **(A)** Patients with acute pancreatitis often have elevated serum lipase and amylase levels. Alanine aminotransferase (ALT) enzymes are most concentrated in the liver. The liver will release the enzyme into the bloodstream when there is damage. Therefore, an ALT test is a more specific indicator that is used to determine the well-being of a patient's liver. Aspartate aminotransferase (AST) enzymes are normally found in a variety of tissues, including the liver, heart, muscles, kidneys, and brain. They are released into the serum when any one of these tissues is damaged. Thus, it is not a specific indicator that can be used to determine the well-being of a patient's liver (choice (B)). A basic metabolic panel evaluates the status of the kidneys, level of blood glucose, and also serum electrolyte levels (choice (C)). A serum uric acid measurement (also known as a uric acid blood test) determines how much uric acid is present inside the bloodstream (choice (D)). This test is usually ordered to support a diagnosis of gout.

6. **(A)** Physical examination findings consistent with acute appendicitis include tenderness or rigidity over the right rectus muscle (McBurney's point). Other findings include rebound tenderness and guarding. Pain and tenderness associated with cholecystitis occurs in the mid-epigastric or right upper quadrant area of the abdomen (choice (B)). Acute gastroenteri-

tis may be associated with mild, generalized abdominal tenderness (choice (C)). Acute diverticulitis is usually localized to the left lower quadrant of the abdomen (choice (D)).

7. **(D)** Symptoms of diverticulitis include left lower quadrant abdominal pain, nausea and vomiting, anorexia, fever, and diarrhea. Symptoms that are associated with gastroesophageal reflux disease include burning in the mid-sternum area after large meals or during sleep, sour odor to breath, chronic sore throat (that is not associated with postnasal drip, strep culture shows negative), or chronic cough at night (choice (A)). Symptoms of celiac disease include a history of chronic diarrhea and flatulence and multiple nutrient deficiencies due to malabsorption and lactose intolerance (choice (B)). Symptoms of pancreatitis include the acute onset of fever, anorexia, weight loss, nausea, vomiting, followed by abdominal pain that radiates to the epigastric region (choice (C)).

8. **(B)** Mild cases of diverticulitis can be managed in a primary care setting with conservative management techniques. The FNP should recommend that the patient begin a clear liquid diet, stay adequately hydrated, and take antibiotics (such as metronidazole or amoxicillin and clavulanate potassium) for the duration of his illness. Frequent follow-up visits are also needed, and the patient should be instructed to go to the emergency department if symptoms worsen. Choices (A), (C), and (D) are not appropriate treatment plans for a mild case of diverticulitis.

9. **(D)** Risk factors for developing colorectal cancer include a family history (choice (A)) of one of several hereditary CRC conditions (such as adenomatous polyposis or inflammatory bowel disease), having a first-degree family member (sibling, parent, or child) who has had colorectal cancer (choice (B)), and/or a personal history of inflammatory bowel disease (choice (C)).

10. **(B)** A family history of GERD is a non-modifiable risk factor for developing GERD. If the patient decreases her caffeine intake (choice (A)), avoids consuming alcohol (choice (C)), and eats small, frequent meals (rather than three large meals) (choice (D)), she may relieve her symptoms of GERD.

11. **(A)** Amlodipine is a calcium channel blocker (CCB). CCBs prevent calcium from entering cells of blood vessels. This mechanism will relax and widen the blood vessel, which results in lower blood pressure. The lower esophageal sphincter (LES) requires calcium to control the contractility of the muscle. Thus, this medication may trigger the symptoms of GERD. Therefore, calcium channel blockers should be avoided in patients with chronic GERD. Metformin is a biguanide medication used in the management of diabetes mellitus (choice (B)). Common side effects include abdominal discomfort, upset stomach, diarrhea, and anorexia. This medication does not affect the LES tone and will not directly exacerbate the symptoms of GERD. Rosuvastatin is classified as an HMG-CoA reductase inhibitor and is used in the management of hypercholesterolemia (choice (C)). Constipation occurs in less than 10% of individuals who take HMG-CoA reductase inhibitors, like rosuvastatin; however, these medications should have no direct effect on one's symptoms of GERD. Aspirin has been shown to decrease the risk of death or myocardial infarction in patients who are at risk (choice (D)). Side effects of baby aspirin include GI upset and bruising. Although long-term use of baby aspirin could lead to erosions in the lining of the stomach, this medication has not been associated with exacerbations of GERD.

12. **(C)** The gold standard in the diagnosis of peptic ulcer disease includes upper endoscopy and biopsy of affected tissue. A urea breath test is a point-of-care test that checks for the presence of urease activity normally associated with the presence of *H. pylori* bacteria (choice (A)). This test, however, has lower sensitivity and specificity than endoscopy and biopsy. A CT scan of the abdomen would not determine the presence of peptic ulcer disease, as it is best used to look for major structural or bony abnormalities (choice (B)).

13. **(B)** Misoprostol (Cytotec) is an appropriate option for short-term treatment for uncomplicated PUD. Misoprostol will decrease gastric acid production and enhance the mucosal healing on the injured tissues. Misoprostol should not be prescribed to women who are pregnant. Cetirizine (Zantac), which is an antihistamine, is used for the treatment of seasonal allergies (choice (A)). Since it is known to increase the risk of developing pneumonia, it would not be indicated for this patient. Ranitidine (Zantac) is an over-the-counter medication used to prevent and treat symptoms of heartburn associated with acid indigestion and sour stomach (choice (C)). Pepto-Bismol is an active antibiotic against *H. pylori* but requires additional medication (adjunct therapy) (choice (D)).

14. **(B)** Based on this presentation, the most likely diagnosis is irritable bowel syndrome. Giardiasis is one of the most common causes of travelers' diarrhea (choice (A)). Risks for developing giardiasis include drinking contaminated water, fecal-oral contamination, and coming into contact with a childcare center, health care workers, and children. Diverticulitis presents with pain, tenderness, or sensitivity in the left lower side of the abdomen (choice (C)). Ulcerative colitis usually presents with bloody stools that are covered with mucus and pus along with systemic symptoms such as fatigue and low-grade fever (choice (D)).

15. **(A)** Because the patient has a history of hepatitis C (regardless of her current viral status), the lab tests ordered should include hepatitis C RNA PCR (polymerase chain reaction) quantitative test and an HIV-1/HIV-2 antibody immunoassay. Anti-HCV test measures immune response to hepatitis C antibodies and not the virus itself. If there are concerns for relapse, the provider should order hepatitis C RNA PCR quantitative testing. Hepatitis C and HIV can also be transmitted with needle sharing. Current recommendation for HIV testing is the HIV-1/2 antigen/antibody immunoassay. Choices (B), (C), and (D) are not appropriate next steps for evaluation of this patient.

7

Disorders of the Neurologic System

The neurologic system controls and "drives" all functions within the human body and allows the body to interact with and respond to the environment. The neurologic network is composed of complex structures that transmit chemical and electrical messages between the brain and body organs and systems. Disorders and disruptions of the neurologic system have widespread effects throughout the body.

Headaches

Headaches are a common complaint in primary care. Headaches are defined as a pain or ache within the head and may be benign and self-limiting or a symptom of severe neurologic pathology. Headaches are classified into categories based on their pathophysiology: vascular headaches (migraines and cluster headaches), muscular (tension-type) headaches, inflammatory (traction-type) headaches, or a combination of one or more of the first three types.

Vascular Headaches

Vascular headaches, which include migraines and cluster headaches, may occur with or without an aura (a characteristic set of symptoms that occur before the headache begins).

Migraines

Migraine headaches are more common in women and may begin during childhood, usually between the ages of five and eight. Migraine headaches are often hereditary and have also been linked to hormonal shifts related to the menstrual cycle. These headaches are often disabling, leading to missed work and school days. Common triggers of migraine headaches include low estrogen levels, bright lights, strong odors, weather changes, alcohol, caffeine, products containing tyramine, red wine, chocolates, foods containing monosodium glutamate, stress, sleep deprivation, dehydration, and smoking.

Symptoms

A migraine headache usually presents with a progressive or abrupt development of unilateral throbbing pain behind one eye, nausea, vomiting, photophobia, and phonophobia. A migraine with aura may also present with scotomas, halos, changes in vision, and flashes of light.

Management

Management of migraines encompasses lifestyle measures, such as identifying and avoiding triggers and beginning treatment early in the headache cycle. Resting in a darkened room and applying ice or cool compresses to the face and head are often helpful. Pharmacotherapeutic agents include triptans (gold standard) such as sumatriptan, which should not be used within 24 hours of ergot medications such as dihydroergotamine nasal spray. Ergot derivatives are another option for managing migraines. NSAIDs and antiemetics are also used to manage symptoms and may be recommended as first-line depending on patient presentation and severity of headaches. Prophylaxis is recommended for patients who have severe and frequent migraine attacks that jeopardize activities of daily living and is accomplished through the use of beta blockers, anticonvulsants, and antidepressants.

CLINICAL PEARL

Patients over age 50 who present with new onset headache, especially if accompanied by systemic symptoms or neurologic deficits, should be evaluated emergently!

Cluster Headaches

The second type of vascular headache is the cluster headache. These headaches are so named because they tend to occur in clusters lasting several weeks to months. They then disappear for months or years before returning. This type of headache occurs most often in men and is considered to be the most painful type of headache. Onset of cluster headaches is usually between ages 20 and 30 with clusters occurring seasonally with anywhere from 3 to 18 months between episodes. This type of headache pain is caused by hypersensitization of the optic nerve and seems to be triggered by an abnormality in the circadian pacemaker located in the hypothalamus.

Symptoms

This type of headache often presents with the abrupt onset of severe pain located behind one eye (sometimes behind both eyes, and patients may complain of a hot poker sensation). There are ipsilateral autonomic signs such as lacrimation, nasal stuffiness, conjunctival injection, and ptosis.

Management

Management includes oxygen at 7–12 L/min for 10–20 mins and administration of triptans, ergots, or Zomig. Prophylaxis may be managed with verapamil, Depakote, and Topamax.

Muscular (Tension-Type) Headaches

Muscular (tension-type) headaches are the most commonly reported headaches in primary care and are often chronic. This type of headache usually occurs several times during the month and may last for hours or even days. The female to male ratio is 5:4. Symptoms of a muscular headache are believed to result from muscular tension and spasms, usually of the neck and shoulders. Interestingly, these types of headaches are not caused by muscular tension but by hypersensitized neural circuitry within the head and neck.

Symptoms

Patients will report mild to moderate, constant pain that is usually bilateral, pressing, nonpulsatile pain in the head, without nausea or vomiting. Patients may also report a "bandlike" pain around the head. These headaches usually occur several times during the month and may last for hours to days.

Management

Management of this chronic type of headache should be individualized based on presentation and effect of the headache on daily living activities. Goals for managing muscular headaches include identifying and avoiding triggers to decrease occurrence. Analgesics that may be recommended for this condition include aspirin, NSAIDs, and triptans for prophylaxis if needed. Recent studies indicate tricyclic antidepressants are modestly effective in reducing occurrence of this type of headache.

Inflammatory (Traction-Type) Headaches

Inflammatory or traction-type headaches are usually associated with neurologic or cerebrovascular pathology and are seen in patients over the age of 35.

Symptoms

Patients with this type of headache often report an abrupt onset of severe, constant, progressive headache and may describe it as "the worst headache of my life."

Management

This type of headache requires immediate referral for neurologic evaluation.

Polymyalgia Rheumatica Giant Cell Arteritis (Temporal Arteritis)

Polymyalgia rheumatica giant cell arteritis involves the ophthalmic, temporal, and carotid systems. It occurs most commonly in patients who are between 50 and 85 years old. Laboratory tests include erythrocyte sedimentation rate (ESR) test and C-reactive protein (CRP) test. The ESR may be elevated to 100 mm/hr or higher.

Symptoms

Symptoms include acute onset of unilateral headache around the temple region, fever, fatigue, and tongue claudication.

Management

Patients should be referred for a temporal artery biopsy (gold standard) for diagnosis, which is performed by an ophthalmologist. Management includes high-dose steroids 40–60 mg PO daily (first-line treatment). **Untreated giant cell arteritis could result in blindness.** Patients with temporal arteritis should be referred to a specialist's care for management.

> **CLINICAL PEARL**
>
> **Patients with polymyalgia rheumatica (PMR) are associated with a high risk for giant cell arteritis.**

Transient Ischemic Attack (TIA)

A transient ischemic attack is a brief episode of cerebral ischemia that produces a neurological deficit. If it is short-lived, any neurological symptoms usually resolve within one hour. When these neurological symptoms do not improve within four hours, some cell death has occurred. A TIA is often a precursor to a stroke. Risk factors include untreated atrial fibrillation, carotid artery disease, uncontrolled hypertension, combined oral contraceptives, and illicit drug use.

Symptoms

Symptoms include numbness or weakness in upper/lower/all extremities, difficulty speaking, and visual changes. If symptoms persist beyond 24 hours, the diagnosis of stroke should be considered.

Management

If it is suspected that a patient has had a TIA, he or she should immediately be referred to the emergency department for further evaluation and management. Interventions include committing to lifestyle changes (quitting smoking, dieting, and exercising), controlling/managing other chronic vascular diseases, taking a daily aspirin or clopidogrel, and managing underlying conditions, such as uncontrolled hypertension or atrial fibrillation.

Stroke (Cerebrovascular Accident, CVA)

A stroke, or a cerebrovascular accident, is an acute loss of blood supply to part of the brain, resulting in ischemia, infarction, and neurological deficits. Obstruction of blood flow is caused by thrombi, emboli, atherosclerosis, hemorrhage, or vasospasm. Insufficient blood flow to the cerebrum (embolism, thrombosis) causes 80% of acute strokes, and the other 20% are the result of hemorrhagic aneurysms.

Symptoms

The signs and symptoms of a stroke depend upon its severity and the area of the brain affected. For example, a left-hemispheric stroke may affect the patient's ability to swallow, impair memory, and cause paralysis or weakness on the right side of the body.

Management

Patients who have had an embolic stroke may need long-term anticoagulation with warfarin to keep the INR level between 2.0 and 3.0 to decrease the risk of further injury. Patients experiencing a CVA require immediate referral to the ED and will be managed by a neurology specialist.

Bacterial Meningitis

Bacterial meningitis is an acute purulent bacterial infection of the meninges, cerebrospinal fluid (CSF), subarachnoid space, and spinal cord. Common pathogens of bacterial meningitis in adults include *Streptococcus pneumoniae*, *Neisseria meningitidis*, *Staphylococcus* species, and *Haemophilus influenzae* type b. Bacterial meningitis primarily occurs in infants and young children, whose blood-brain barrier is not fully developed. The bacteria that cause this type of meningitis are often colonized within the nasopharynx of the affected individual, causing inflammation. The bacteria are then able to enter the bloodstream through compromised mucosa. From the bloodstream, the bacteria enter the CSF through the choroid plexuses in the ventricles as well as through leaky or injured portions of the blood-brain barrier. Lab tests that can be used to diagnose bacterial meningitis include a lumbar puncture (CSF cloudy, high numbers of WBCs), Gram staining, culture and sensitivity testing, and a CBC. Vaccines that are used to prevent bacterial meningitis include the pneumococcal conjugate vaccine (PCV13), the pneumococcal polysaccharide vaccine (PPSV23), and meningococcal vaccines (MCV4 and MPSV4).

Symptoms

Symptoms of bacterial meningitis include headaches, fever, neck pain and stiffness (nuchal rigidity), photophobia, and rapid changes in the patient's mental status. Lethargy and confusion may also be present, and coma could possibly occur.

Management

Management occurs in a hospital setting with IV antibiotics and supportive care.

Trigeminal Neuralgia

Trigeminal neuralgia is a chronic neurological pain disorder that affects the trigeminal nerve. The disorder is caused by demyelination of axons in the fifth cranial nerve (CN V). Trigeminal neuralgia is seen most often in individuals with hypertension and multiple sclerosis. Severity of symptoms is often disabling to affected individuals and most will do anything possible to avoid triggering an attack. Lab imaging should include an MRI or CT scan to rule out possible tumor or nerve compression.

Symptoms

Common symptoms include excruciating, episodic, burning or shock-like facial pain lasting a few seconds to minutes. Pain may be triggered by chewing, eating foods that are at cold temperatures, and being exposed to cold air.

Management

This disorder is commonly treated with carbamazepine or phenytoin.

Bell's Palsy

Bell's palsy is an acute paralysis of the facial nerve or the seventh cranial nerve (CN VII). The disorder may be triggered by an acute viral infection of the herpes simplex virus, herpes zoster virus, Epstein-Barr virus, cytomegalovirus (CMV), or adenoviruses. Risk factors include a weakened immune system or pathology that causes inflammation or compression of the nerve. Lyme disease is also frequently associated with development of Bell's palsy, so an evaluation should include screening for this condition.

Symptoms

Patients present with an acute onset of partial or total paralysis of one side of the face. Ocular movements are usually normal and facial sensation is intact. Individuals may complain of loss of taste, abnormal sensitivity to sound, and postauricular pain. Loss of the protective blink reflex on the affected side is seen as well and may lead to corneal ulcers if not managed appropriately with patching and the use of moisturizing drops.

Management

Most cases of Bell's palsy resolve themselves spontaneously. Treatment involves the use of corticosteroids and antivirals.

Guillain-Barré Syndrome (GBS)

Guillain-Barré syndrome is a rare immune disorder in which antibodies attack part of the peripheral nervous system. GBS usually occurs a few days after an acute infection (such as a respiratory infection or a gastrointestinal infection). The disorder may be self-limiting over the course of several days, or it may become permanent. The period of greatest weakness is usually around two weeks after symptoms begin.

Symptoms

Symptoms of GBS include symmetrical weakness or tingling sensation first beginning in the lower legs, with progressive spread to the arms and upper body. There have been reports of cases of patients becoming totally paralyzed.

Management

The two main management options for treating GBS are plasmapheresis and high-dose immunoglobulin therapy.

Alzheimer's Disease (AD)

Alzheimer's disease is a permanent, progressive neurodegenerative disorder and is the most common cause of dementia in elderly individuals. Around 50% of patients with AD have a family history of the disorder. Incidence is greatest between ages 65 and 69 years, with an average life span of eight years after diagnosis. Risk factors include aging, smoking, having a family history of AD, and having positive genetic markers for AD. Pathophysiological findings consistently include senile plaques and neurofibrillary tangles within the cerebral cortex, cerebellar cortex, and basal ganglia. The Mini-Mental State Exam (MMSE) is a quick, easy-to-administer screen for cognitive deficits.

Symptoms

Patients usually present with reports of memory problems. Occasionally, the memory problems are noticed by family members before the patient recognizes a deficit. As the disease progresses, patients may begin to have trouble with directions, may get lost while walking or driving, and may demonstrate increasing difficulty with word-finding.

Management

Behavior and cognition declines until most individuals require total care and supervision. These individuals are managed in collaboration with physicians specializing in AD care.

CLINICAL PEARL

If a patient with Bell's palsy presents with impaired eye closure, evidence of corneal abrasion or injury, or abnormal tear duct flow, refer the patient to an ophthalmologist for further evaluation and management.

METHODS OF EVALUATING THE CRANIAL NERVES

When treating disorders of the neurologic system, it is important to have a strong working knowledge of all of the cranial nerves and how they can be tested for optimal functionality. Table 7.1 reviews all of the cranial nerves, how they are tested, and tips for memorizing each type.

Table 7.1. Evaluating Cranial Nerves

Cranial Nerve (CN)	Test of Optimal Functionality	Memorization Tip
CN I—Olfactory	Identify scents	You have **1** nose.
CN II—Optic	Vision screen	You have **2** eyes.
CN III—Oculomotor	Cardinal directions of gaze	You will need **3** muscles to make "funny eyes" (CN III, IV, and VI).
CN IV—Trochlear	Move eyes down and inward	
CN V—Trigeminal	Check for facial sensation and symmetric jaw movement	The shape of your jaw is a "V."
CN VI—Abducens	Move eyes laterally in both directions and check for symmetric eye movement	
CN VII—Facial	Have the patient close his or her eyes, close his or her mouth, and try to frown	The sad face emoji
CN VIII—Acoustic	Check hearing	h**ear**ing, **e**ar, **e** = eight
CN IX—Glossopharyngeal	Check swallow	
CN X—Vagus	Ask the patient to say "ah," and observe if the palate rises equally on both sides	
CN XI—Spinal Accessory	Ask patient to turn head to one side, while pushing the examiner's hand sternocleidomastoid muscle	Both hands attached under the shoulders, representing the **11**, while shrugging the shoulder
CN XII—Hypoglossal	Ask the patient to protrude the tongue and push the tongue against cheek	Eating an ice-cream cone; tongue movement

TESTS OF THE NEUROLOGIC SYSTEM

Various diagnostic tests are used to check for disorders of the neurologic system. Table 7.2 reviews the most commonly used tests for diagnosing these disorders.

Table 7.2. Types of Neurologic Tests

To Check the Patient's	Use This Test/These Tests
Mental status	■ Mini-mental state exam (MMSE) ■ Cranial nerve exam
Cerebellar system	■ Romberg test ■ Tandem gait ■ Rapid alternating movements (diadochokinesis) ■ Heel-to-shin test
Auditory status	■ Rinne test ■ Weber test
Sensory status	■ Vibration sense testing (using a 128-Hz tuning fork) ■ Sharp-dull touch ■ Stereognosis test ■ Graphesthesia test
Motor status	■ Gait ■ Pronator drift test
Reflex status	■ Quadriceps reflex ■ Achilles reflex ■ Plantar reflex (Babinski's sign) Grading reflexes: 0 = no response 1+ = low response 2+ = normal/average response 3+ = brisk, below average response 4+ = sustained clonus
Meningitis status	■ Kernig's sign ■ Brudzinski's sign
Carpal tunnel status	■ Tinel's sign ■ Phalen's sign

Weber versus Rinne Hearing Test

	Weber Test	Rinne Test
Normal	Patient able to perceive tuning fork sound coming from the midline	Air conduction > bone conduction
Possible conduction deafness	Sound perceived coming from the conductive hearing loss ear (affected side)	Bone conduction > air conduction on the affected ear
Possible sensorineural deafness	Sound perceived coming from the normal ear	Air conduction > bone conduction

Practice Questions

1. The Weber and Rinne tests may be used to assess which of the following cranial nerves?

   (A) CN III
   (B) CN V
   (C) CN VIII
   (D) CN X

2. Which of the following cranial nerves is evaluated when an FNP is assessing the strength of a patient's trapezius muscle?

   (A) CN II
   (B) CN III
   (C) CN IX
   (D) CN XI

3. Which of the following is the best initial method for assessing suspected Alzheimer's disease in a 55-year-old patient?

   (A) Mini-Mental State Exam (MMSE)
   (B) computed tomography (CT) scan of the brain
   (C) patient health questionnaire (PHQ 9)
   (D) electroencephalography (EEG)

4. Which of the following tests is conducted to check for balance?

   (A) tandem gait
   (B) rapid alternating movements
   (C) heel-to-shin test
   (D) Romberg test

5. What types of food should a 32-year-old patient newly diagnosed with migraine headaches without aura avoid in order to reduce her risk of headaches?

   (A) foods with aspartame
   (B) foods with magnesium
   (C) foods with complex carbohydrates
   (D) foods with caffeine

6. Which of the following would be an appropriate prophylactic migraine headache treatment for a commercial pilot?

   (A) prochlorperazine
   (B) naproxen sodium
   (C) propranolol
   (D) sumatriptan

7. In administering the Phalen test in a primary care office, the clinician is evaluating:

   (A) stereognosis.
   (B) CN II impingement.
   (C) median nerve inflammation
   (D) CN V impingement.

8. A 75-year-old male presents to the clinic with concerns of changes in the vision of his left eye. Symptoms started this morning after showering. He denies any injury or changes in his current medications. During assessment, vitals and neurologic exams are normal except profound vision loss in the left eye. The patient also indicates that he is experiencing some unexplained pressure on the left side of his temple. Which of the following is most likely the cause of his symptoms?

    (A) a cluster headache
    (B) a migraine with auras
    (C) a migraine without aura
    (D) giant cell arteritis

9. A patient who has experienced a cerebrovascular accident (CVA) may have residual deficits affecting the neurologic system. One complication following CVA is aphasia. Aphasia refers to:

    (A) the loss of one's voice.
    (B) an inability to produce or understand speech.
    (C) a muscular derangement controlling oral movement.
    (D) decreased level of consciousness.

10. During an adult wellness check for a 56-year-old man, you learn that your patient has a history of having a transient ischemic attack (TIA) one year ago and rheumatoid arthritis. His current daily medications are amlodipine, spironolactone, and metformin. As part of the medication reconciliation process, what other intervention would you initiate for the patient based on his history of TIA?

    (A) daily baby aspirin (81 mg)
    (B) daily multivitamins
    (C) daily non-steroidal anti-inflammatory drugs
    (D) daily calcium (1,000 mg)

11. A 13-year-old teenage boy presents with unresolved neck pain, headache, and fever. He was last treated at another clinic two days ago for a migraine. His vital signs are as follows: heart rate = 89, respiration = 19, blood pressure = 140/90, and temperature = 103.2°F. During the assessment, both Brudzinski's and Kernig's signs are positive. What is the possible diagnosis for this patient?

    (A) cervicitis
    (B) bacterial meningitis
    (C) cervical sprain
    (D) chronic migraine

12. Trigeminal neuralgia is a chronic pain condition that affects which of the following cranial nerves?

    (A) CN V
    (B) CN IX
    (C) CN X
    (D) CN XII

13. A patient with a diagnosis of trigeminal neuralgia would likely avoid all the following activities, EXCEPT:

    (A) closing both eyes.
    (B) washing the face.
    (C) applying makeup.
    (D) brushing teeth.

14. A 31-year-old patient recently returned from a hunting trip and presents with lethargy, mild fever, and paralysis of CN VII. What is the appropriate diagnostic test to order?

    (A) complete blood count (CBC)
    (B) erythrocyte sedimentation rate (ESR)
    (C) liver function tests
    (D) Lyme disease antibody titer

15. A 35-year-old male presents with nasal stuffiness and a constant stabbing pain behind his left eye for the past four days. Vital signs are stable. He denies a fever, lethargy, or pharyngitis. An assessment reveals clear nasal discharge, with no sinus tenderness. Which of the following conditions is this patient most likely experiencing?

    (A) migraine headache with aura
    (B) cluster headache
    (C) tic douloureux
    (D) cranial neuralgia

Answer Explanations

1. **(C)** The Weber test and the Rinne test may be used to assess cranial nerve (CN) VIII. These tests are used to evaluate hearing via air conduction compared with bone conduction. During a Rinne test, normal hearing will show an air conduction time that is twice as long as bone conduction (air conduction time 2 > bone conduction 1). During a Weber test, normal hearing should produce equal sound in both ears. Conductive hearing loss will cause abnormalities on the affected side. Likewise, sensorineural loss will cause the sound to be heard in the normal ear and diminished or absent in the affected ear. CN III is the oculomotor nerve, which innervates the superior rectus, inferior rectus, and medial rectus, as well as the inferior oblique muscles of the eye (choice (A)). Extraocular muscle function may be assessed using the corneal light reflex test (Hirschberg test) and the diagnostic positions test. CN V is the trigeminal nerve, which innervates the facial and jaw area (choice (B)). This nerve has three branches and may be assessed by looking for symmetry of jaw movement and equal bilateral jaw strength and by evaluating for pain occurring when teeth are clenched. The sensory function of CN V may be tested by using a cotton ball against the cheek to assess for symmetric response. CN X is the vagus nerve, which may be evaluated by eliciting a gag reflex (choice (D)).

2. **(D)** The sternocleidomastoid and trapezius muscles are supported by cranial nerve (CN) XI (the spinal accessory nerve). The sternocleidomastoid muscle enables the head to tilt and rotate. Trapezius muscles are connected to the scapula and act to assist with shrugging shoulders. CN II is the optic nerve, which is evaluated by testing visual acuity and visual fields (choice (A)). CN III is the oculomotor nerve, which innervates the extraocular eye muscles (choice (B)). This nerve may be tested by using the corneal light reflex test (Hirschberg test) and the diagnostic positions test. CN IX is the glossopharyngeal nerve, which controls the movement of the uvula and soft palate (choice (C)). This nerve may be assessed by having the patient say "aaaahhhh."

3. **(A)** A Mini-Mental State Exam should be administered as a baseline assessment when dementia is suspected. A score of 23 or lower on the MMSE is indicative of cognitive impairment. A CT scan of the brain emits radiation and is not indicated for an initial screen (choice (B)). A PHQ-9 is used to assess depression (choice (C)). EEG is used to evaluate the activity of the brain waves (seizure, epilepsy, sleep disorder, or stroke) (choice (D)).

4. **(D)** The Romberg test requires the patient to stand with eyes closed. It is used to evaluate gait and balance. It can also be used to detect imbalance, which may be the result of alcohol intoxication. Tandem gait is used to help diagnose ataxia (where the toes of the back foot touch the heel of the front foot at each step) (choice (A)). Rapid alternating movements test is used to check for dysdiadochokinesia (choice (B)). The heel-to-shin test is a measure of coordination and may be abnormal if there is loss of motor strength, proprioception, or a cerebellar lesion (choice (C)).

5. **(A)** Foods with aspartame (NutraSweet and Equal) can trigger migraines and should be avoided. Foods and beverages that contain aspartame include diet beverages, light yogurts, sugar-free candies, and low-calorie desserts. Caffeine (choice (D)) and foods rich in magnesium (choice (B)), calcium, complex carbohydrates (choice (C)), and fiber may relieve the symptoms of migraines.

6. **(C)** Propranolol (Inderal) is a beta blocker and may be used as prophylactic treatment for migraines. Other prophylactic treatments for migraines include anticonvulsants (such as topiramate) and antidepressants (such as amitriptyline). Prochlorperazine is used to treat severe migraines that are associated with nausea; however, this medication often causes drowsiness (choice (A)). Because the patient is a commercial pilot, it is important to consider this when prescribing medications. Naproxen sodium (choice (B)) and sumatriptan (choice (D)) are medications used to treat migraines.

7. **(C)** The Phalen test assesses median nerve inflammation or impingement. The test is performed by instructing the patient to hold both hands back-to-back while flexing the wrists to a 90-degree angle. This position is maintained for 60 seconds. Acute flexion of the wrist should produce no symptoms unless there is impingement or inflammation of the median nerve. A positive Phalen's is consistent with a diagnosis of carpal tunnel syndrome. Stereognosis is the ability to perceive and understand the form and nature of objects through touch (choice (A)). Cranial nerve (CN) II is the optic nerve, which may be assessed by checking visual acuity (choice (B)). CN V is the trigeminal nerve, which controls facial sensations (choice (D)). The sensory functions of CN V may be tested by using a cotton ball against the cheek to assess for symmetric response.

8. **(D)** Giant cell arteritis involves the ophthalmic, temporal, and carotid vessels. Symptoms include acute onset of unilateral headache around the temple region, fever, fatigue, and tongue claudication. Cluster headaches present with abrupt onset of excruciating pain behind one or both eyes and are associated with increased lacrimation and rhinorrhea (choice (A)). Migraines present as unilateral throbbing pain in the head often associated with nausea and vomiting and may or may not be accompanied by aura (choice (C)). Aura is a prodromal characteristic symptom that occurs prior to the development of headache (choice (B)).

9. **(B)** Aphasia is a neurological term for the inability to produce or understand speech/language. Loss of voice is called aphonia and may be seen with dysfunction of the larynx or its innervating nerve network (choice (A)). Dysarthria is defined as a defect in the muscles assisting in speech and controlling oral movement (choice (C)). A decreased level of consciousness is a more generalized dysfunction of the neurologic system that does not specifically affect speech (choice (D)).

10. **(A)** A patient with a history of TIA should incorporate a daily baby aspirin into his or her medication regimen. Aspirin inhibits the enzyme cyclooxygenase and reduces thromboxane A2 production, which stimulates platelet aggregation. Lower doses of aspirin (baby aspirin) have fewer GI-related side effects than full adult doses. The U.S. Preventive Services Task Force recommends daily aspirin therapy for patients between 50 and 59 years of age, who have no increased bleeding risk, and who have an increased risk of heart attack or stroke of 10% or greater over the next 10 years. Chronic use of NSAIDs increases the risk of gastritis (choice (C)). Targets for daily calcium intake are 1,000 mg per day for men and women between 25 and 65 years of age and 1,500 mg per day for postmenopausal women (choice (D)). However, the question is focused on stroke prevention due to a history of TIA. A daily multivitamin is not appropriate treatment for this patient (choice (B)).

11. **(B)** Acute onset symptoms of bacterial meningitis include a fever, headache, nuchal rigidity, and rapid changes in mental status. Brudzinski and Kernig tests can be used to evaluate nuchal rigidity. Cervicitis is the inflammation or infection of the cervix (choice (A)). Cervical (neck) sprain (choice (C)) and migraine (choice (D)) do not result in nuchal rigidity.

12. **(A)** Trigeminal neuralgia (also known as tic douloureux) is a chronic pain condition associated with nerve injury or a nerve lesion that affects the trigeminal nerve (CN V).

13. **(A)** Activities that could potentially trigger or increase trigeminal neuralgia-related pain include vibration or contact with the cheek, such as when shaving, washing the face (choice (B)), applying makeup (choice (C)), brushing teeth (choice (D)), eating, drinking, talking, or being exposed to the wind. Opening and closing the eyes is an activity not controlled by the trigeminal nerve and should remain painless.

14. **(D)** Because Bell's palsy (paralysis of CN VII) is frequently associated with Lyme disease, a Lyme disease titer should be ordered based on the patient's history and possible tick exposure. Bell's palsy is also associated with other disorders, many of which are viral, such as herpes simplex virus and herpes zoster. A stroke or brain tumor may also cause facial paralysis. The CDC currently recommends a two-step process when testing blood for evidence of antibodies against Lyme disease bacteria. Both steps can be done using the same blood sample. The first step is the enzyme immunoassay (EIA), and, if negative, no further testing is required. However, if the EIA is positive, the second step is a western blot test. CBC (choice (A)), ESR (choice (B)), and liver function tests (choice (C)) are not needed in this situation, unless the diagnosis remains uncertain.

15. **(B)** Symptoms of cluster headaches include excruciating, constant pain behind the eye, with nasal congestion and rhinorrhea. Migraine headaches with aura include trigger signs (such as visual changes, blind spots, or the appearance of flashing lights) that occur prior to the onset of headache (choice (A)). Tic douloureux (or trigeminal neuralgia) is a chronic pain condition associated with nerve injury or nerve lesion that affects the trigeminal nerve (CN V) (choice (C)). Cranial neuralgia is a generalized term that refers to dysfunction in one or more cranial nerves (choice (D)).

8

Disorders of the Musculoskeletal System

Musculoskeletal disorders are responsible for a large percentage of patient visits to urgent care as well as primary care offices. These disorders and dysfunctions present in many different ways, making diagnosis challenging. Knowledge of anatomy and physiology is key to effectively identifying and managing these disorders. Musculoskeletal disorders are the leading cause of disability in the United States, and these conditions often negatively impact quality of life. One important aspect of providing efficacious care to patients with musculoskeletal complaints is knowing which physical examination tests should be administered to narrow down the list of differential diagnoses. A common way of classifying musculoskeletal disorders is by noting whether the problem is acute (lasting six weeks or less) or chronic (lasting more than six weeks). This chapter will discuss some of the most common musculoskeletal disorders seen in primary care.

Acute Musculoskeletal Injuries

The term *acute musculoskeletal injury* describes a number of common musculoskeletal conditions associated with acute pain and/or muscle spasm. Since these injuries are acute, symptoms have been occurring for less than six weeks. Symptoms may be associated with other conditions, such as chronic spinal stenosis, arthritis, or tendonitis. Most injuries seen in primary care are caused by musculoskeletal trauma resulting in a derangement in function and subsequent pain, limitations of movement, and a decreased ability to use the involved extremity.

Sprains and Strains

The most frequently encountered acute musculoskeletal injuries that are seen in family practice are sprains. A sprain is the result of twisting or stretching the ligaments in a joint beyond its normal range of motion. A strain, on the other hand, is associated with microscopic tears or stretching of muscle tissue. Often, a sprain and a strain appear the same on physical examination. One way to differentiate between these two types of injuries is to recognize that strains are frequently the result of overuse or unusual force applied to a joint. Sprains usually involve joints and are associated with falls, twisting, and hyperextension of a joint. A patient's ability to place weight on the injured extremity immediately after the injury is a guide to the severity of the injury. Evaluate joint stability with all sprains. Diagnostic evaluation should include X-ray of the affected area.

Ankle sprains specifically are classified by their degree of injury. These classifications include Grade 1, Grade 2, and Grade 3, as outlined in Table 8.1.

Table 8.1. Grades of Ankle Sprains

Grade	Ligament's Condition	Assessment Findings
1 (Mild)	Slight stretching and microscopic tearing	Mild tenderness Swelling on the ankle
2 (Moderate)	Partial tearing	Moderate tenderness Swelling around the ankle Some abnormal looseness of the ankle joint
3 (Severe)	Complete tearing	Significant tenderness (even without palpation) Substantial instability noted on pushing on the joint

Symptoms

Patients are usually aware they have injured their joint and should be asked to describe the mechanism of injury. Patients may report excruciating, abrupt pain, the presence of swelling immediately after the injury, and that the joint "gave way" and the patient was unable to place weight on the area of injury. Edema may be present immediately following the injury or may develop hours later.

Management

Management of most acute musculoskeletal injuries includes RICE (rest, ice, compression, elevation). Injuries that do not improve and resolve with conservative therapy should be referred for orthopedic evaluation.

Fractures

A fracture represents a break in the bone and is usually associated with a blunt force injury. Fractures may be open or closed, depending on overlying tissue derangement associated with the injury. Open fractures carry increased risk for infection and must be evaluated and managed aggressively. Fractures may involve the entire circumference of the bone (complete) or just a portion of the bone structure (partial). Complete fractures are unstable injuries and urgent management is required. Assessment should include asking about the mechanism of injury and consideration that fractures may occur at sites away from the primary site.

Symptoms

Patients report an injury and are usually aware that a fracture has occurred, especially if the bone is out of alignment or displaced. Reports of associated bleeding, swelling, numbness, or tingling are important components to incorporate into the management plan. Suspected fractures in pediatric patients should include evaluation for a Salter-Harris fracture. These fractures occur within the growth plate area of the long bones and are more commonly found in boys than in girls.

Salter-Harris Classification

Classification	Description
Salter I (Slipped)	Fracture extends through the physis of the bone.
Salter II (Above)	Most common: Fracture extends through the physis and the metaphysis.
Salter III (Lower)	Intra-articular fracture extending from the physis into the epiphysis.
Salter IV (Through/Transverse)	Intra-articular fracture extending through the epiphysis, physis, and metaphysis.
Salter V (Rammed/Ruined)	Rare: Occurs with severe crushing or compression injury extending through the epiphysis and physis.

Management

Fractures should be stabilized in primary care, usually with a temporary cast or splint, and referred for orthopedic evaluation.

Osteoarthritis (OA)

Osteoarthritis is a degenerative joint disease that is related to "wear and tear" stress on the joints of the body. It is the most common joint disease in adults 45 years and older. OA is a significant cause of chronic pain, disability, and diminished quality of life for many older adults and is a frequent cause for acute care health care visits. OA is a disease that presents and progresses gradually, with symptoms usually beginning in middle age. Risk factors for the development of OA include a positive family history, past injury or trauma to a joint, obesity, and advanced age. This disease occurs in men and women equally; however, women usually become symptomatic at an earlier age than men.

Symptoms

Patients will usually report a gradual progression of joint stiffness and pain. Several joints may be involved when the patient seeks care, or only one joint may be the focus of evaluation. OA joint pain typically worsens as the day progresses. Joint deformities seen in OA include Heberden's nodes (nodules/deformities affecting the DIP joints of the hands) and Bouchard's nodes (nodules/deformities affecting the PIP joints of the hands).

Management

Nonpharmacological measures include the use of heat or cold to the affected area, splints as needed, and gentle range of motion exercises to maintain joint function. Pharmacological management includes NSAID therapy for pain management. Intra-articular corticosteroid injections and topical analgesics are also used in the management of OA. For severe disease, surgical arthroscopic surgery and joint replacement may improve patient mobility and quality of life.

Gouty Arthritis

Gouty arthritis, often called simply *gout*, is a monoarticular acute condition that commonly affects the first metatarsophalangeal (MTP) joint of the great toe. The disorder may also be chronic and affect other joints of the body such as the elbow, knee, and ankle. Gout is associated with elevated levels of uric acid in the serum with deposition of urate crystals in joint fluid. Tophi are hardened growths composed of urate crystals that may develop on the feet, ears, hands, and prepatellar and olecranon bursae. There is a genetic component associated with development of gout involving genes that handle urate. There is often a family history of the disorder. Secondary gout may be caused by medications (especially diuretics, niacin, cyclosporine, low-dose aspirin), chronic kidney disease, and myeloproliferative disorders.

As the patient ages, and with repeated episodes of gout inflammation, other joints may become involved. Men are affected more often than women and the age is usually over 30 years of age. Alcohol consumption decreases renal excretion of gout, leading to hyperuricemia and may trigger painful episodes. Other triggers include fasting prior to medical procedures and changes in medications. Gold-standard diagnostic test for diagnosis is aspiration and presence of sodium urate crystals in joint fluid or tophus.

Symptoms

Gout produces severe pain in the affected joint that often begins during the night or when the patient wakes up in the morning. The pain is described as excruciating and is made worse by walking, movement, or even slight pressure over the area.

Management

Management of exacerbations includes the early initiation of NSAID therapy. Gout is exquisitely responsive to NSAID therapy and offers fairly rapid relief of acute pain. Oral colchicine may also be used for episodes lasting less than 36 hours. Other measures include oral corticosteroids for alleviation of symptoms and avoidance of all trigger foods and beverages, such as alcohol and foods high in purine content, such as meats, seafood, and purine-rich vegetables. Patients who experience recurrent episodes of gout should be considered for chronic pharmacological management with allopurinol. Allopurinol is a xanthine oxidase inhibitor that blocks the final enzymatic step in the production of uric acid. Because this medication may actually worsen a gouty attack, it should not be used during an acute episode. Patients should receive prophylactic doses of colchicine when initiating allopurinol therapy.

Rheumatoid Arthritis (RA)

Rheumatoid arthritis is a chronic, systemic, inflammatory disease which causes a progressive synovitis of multiple joints, usually the wrists, elbows, knees, and ankles. RA also affects many other organ systems of the body, including the heart, lungs, viscera, and eyes. The disease is more common in women than men and has a population prevalence of 1% in the United States. Peak onset of RA symptoms occurs between ages 40 and 60 years, with actual disease onset between ages 20 and 40 years. Patients with a positive family history of RA are at higher risk for development of the disease, but the exact cause is unknown. Untreated RA causes joint destruction with disability and is associated with a shortened life expectancy. Other nonarticular complications of this systemic disease include keratoconjunctivitis (dry eye), which may lead to blindness, pericardial effusion, pleural effusion, and bronchiolitis obliterans with organizing pneumonia (BOOP). Splenomegaly and neutropenia occur in a condition called Felty's syndrome.

Diagnostics include the presence of rheumatoid factor (RF) in the serum, which is suggestive of RA. However, other conditions can contribute to the presence of rheumatoid factors, such as other autoimmune disorders and chronic infections. Serum testing for anti-CCP auto-antibodies is the most specific blood test to detect RA and can be used for early diagnosis of disease. The ESR and CRP levels are elevated during acute episodes. Patients may develop superimposed septic arthritis, and arthrocentesis is used to capture this diagnosis.

Symptoms

Early in the disease, patients may develop vague systemic symptoms such as weight loss, low-grade fever, and malaise. During acute episodes, the presentation is usually symmetrical involving numerous joints. Characteristically, deformities occur in the proximal interphalangeal (PIP) and metacarpophalangeal (MCP) joints in the hands. In the later stages of disease, boutonniere deformity develops in which the PIP joint is in a nonreducible flexed position and occurs with distal interphalangeal (DIP) hyperextension of the same digit. Another joint deformity seen with advanced disease is the Swan neck deformity, characterized by PIP hyperextension and DIP flexion.

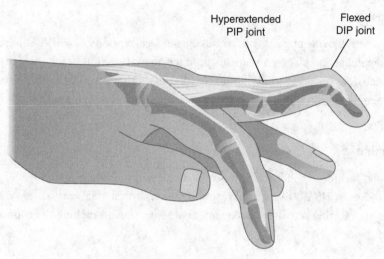

Figure 8.1. DIP vs. PIP

Management

Goals of management are to decrease inflammation and pain, preserve function, and prevent deformity of affected joints. These patients should also be screened for the presence of hepatitis B. Pharmacological therapy for RA includes the use of low-dose corticosteroids for acute flares, which provides a rapid anti-inflammatory effect. Intra-articular injections may be performed if only one or two joints are primarily affected. Updated guidelines recommend initiation of disease-modifying antirheumatic drugs (DMARDs) when the diagnosis is confirmed to suppress disease activity. Synthetic DMARDs used in the treatment of RA include methotrexate, sulfasalazine, and leflunomide. Biological DMARDs include tumor necrosis factor inhibitors such as etanercept, infliximab, and adalimumab. DMARD agents work by inhibiting structural damage to cartilage and bone, thereby slowing disease progression. Because the mechanism of action of DMARDs is to decrease inflammatory response, use of these medications predisposes individuals to development of infection and disease. Patients are instructed to recognize and quickly report signs of infection, such as sore throat or productive cough. Early aggressive management of these illnesses is crucial.

Bursitis

Bursitis is inflammation affecting the bursae, which are the synovium-like membranes that overlay bony processes and act as shock absorbers. Bursae are located between bony prominences, tendons, and muscles and are sacs filled with synovial fluid. They may be located superficially or within deeper tissue. In addition to shock absorption, bursae provide lubrication within joints promoting smooth function. These structures can be damaged by trauma, disease, infection, as well as inflammation. The two most common sites of involvement are the olecranon and the prepatellar bursae; however, other areas may be affected, including subdeltoid, ischial, and trochanteric. Baker's cyst is bursitis affecting the posterior aspect of the knee. Septic bursitis is a more serious form that results from bacterial infection of the bursa. Bursitis may be associated with systemic disease, but more often presents to primary care from overuse and aging.

Symptoms

Individuals with bursitis present with complaints of focal tenderness and swelling of the involved bursae. Prepatellar and olecranon bursitis produce an oval swelling at the tip of the knee or elbow, which does not affect joint motion. Tenderness with warmth, cellulitis, history of trauma, or fever are indicative of septic bursitis. However, one-third of patients with septic bursitis do not have fever.

Management

Management includes application of moist heat or ice, immobilization of the affected joint during acute episodes, NSAID therapy, ultrasound therapy, intrabursal corticosteroid injections, and avoidance of triggering activities. Management of septic bursitis includes incision and drainage with IV antibiotics.

Osteoporosis

Osteoporosis is a skeletal disorder characterized by normal mineralization of bone but with damage to the microarchitecture of the bone tissue. Because the bony architecture of the skeleton is weakened, there is significantly increased risk for fractures and disability. Osteopenia is a less severe form of the disease with less decrease in bone density. Osteomalacia is a disorder of bone mineralization itself, causing skeletal weakness and instability. The disease is seen in both sexes but is more common in women after menopause. Menopause is the trigger for a change in bone turnover. Osteoclastic mechanisms, which break down bone, predominate over osteoblastic activity, which creates new bone. Nonmodifiable risk factors include age, ethnicity, postmenopausal status, family history, predisposition, and autoimmune disease. Modifiable risk factors include low body weight, smoking, excessive alcohol use, low dietary calcium and vitamin D, and long-term use of medications such as phenytoin.

Screening for osteoporosis via dual-energy X-ray absorptiometry (DXA) scan is recommended for all postmenopausal women aged 65 and older and all men aged 70 and older. Other groups for which screening may be indicated include younger postmenopausal women with higher risk (family history, early menopause). Younger individuals with pathologic fractures should also be screened. Bone mineral density (BMD) is expressed as g/cm^2, and normal varies by bone and machine used. The T-score is a reporting tool for screening. This score compares patient bone density measures with mean density of younger women. The World Health Organization Criteria for diagnosis of osteoporosis is provided in Table 8.2.

Table 8.2. T-Score Classification

T-score	Interpretation
≥ -1.0	Normal
-1.0 to -2.5	Osteopenia (low bone density)
< -2.5	Osteoporosis
< -2.5 (with fracture)	Severe osteoporosis

The DXA measures bone density at two or three areas, including lumbar spine and total hip. Frequency of DXA screening is based on T-score.

Symptoms

Patients with osteoporosis are often asymptomatic until a fracture occurs, most commonly an acute vertebral compression fracture.

Management

Prevention and management goals include stabilization of bone mass, prevention of fractures, symptom relief, and maximizing function. Pharmacological management includes calcium and vitamin D supplementation with adequate dietary intake, estrogen replacement therapy, selective estrogen-receptor modulators (SERM), bisphosphonates, calcitonin, and androgen supplementation for men.

Carpal Tunnel Syndrome (CTS)

Carpal tunnel syndrome is an entrapment neuropathy and the most common cause of peripheral nerve compression. CTS is seen more commonly in adults between the ages of 40 and 60 years. Females are affected more frequently than males. Middle-aged and pregnant women are most commonly affected. Patients with CTS are often engaged in repetitive motion activities, such as computer work. Testing for CTS should include Phalen's maneuver, which is accomplished by having the patient acutely flex the wrists and press the backs of both hands together for 60 seconds. A positive Phalen's is recorded when the patient complains of numbness and tingling of the thumb or first two digits. Another test is Tinel's sign, which is done by light percussion of the palmar surface of the wrist with a percussion hammer. If the patient reports a shock-like or tingling sensation, the test is positive and is suggestive of CTS.

Symptoms

Classic presentation is burning, tingling paresthesias of one or both hands that is worse during the night and often wakes the patient from sleep.

Management

Conservative management is recommended with wrist splinting with free movement of thumb and fingers. NSAID therapy for analgesia and anti-inflammatory properties. CTS occurring during pregnancy usually resolves with delivery of the baby. For severe CTS, surgery may be required.

Knee Injuries

Knee injuries are commonly occurring events that are seen primarily in the family practice or urgent care setting. The knee is a complex modified hinge joint with a constellation of three bones, five major tendons, four large ligaments, and two menisci. These structures all play a role in maintaining stability of the knee. Derangement of any of these structures may cause limited mobility and decreased joint range of motion. Fractures of the bony architecture of the knee are also possible and may cause significant disruption of all articulations in this joint.

Collateral Ligament Injuries

The two collateral ligaments of the knee are the medial collateral ligament (MCL) and the lateral collateral ligament (LCL). These two strong ligaments provide lateral stability to the knee. Injuries may include strains, sprains, or tears. Most injuries to these ligaments are sports-related involving an injury occurring when the foot is planted and the knee pivots and twists.

CLINICAL PEARL

Vitamin D should always be recommended with calcium supplementation because vitamin D is better at absorbing calcium.

Symptoms

Patient presents with a painful, swollen knee and a feeling of joint instability. Swelling usually begins within 20–30 minutes of the injury, and the greater the amount of swelling, the more severe the injury.

Management

In the primary care setting, injury to collateral ligaments may be assessed by placing varus and valgus stress on the knee. Laxity in either direction indicates joint instability. Obtain an X-ray initially to rule out fracture. First- and second-degree sprains may be managed with RICE (rest, ice, compression, elevation). More severe presentations should be referred to orthopedics for evaluation.

Cruciate Ligament Injuries

There are two cruciate ligaments in the knee, and these structures provide rotational stability to the knee. The anterior cruciate ligament (ACL) attaches to the anterior part of the tibia and the lateral condyle of the femur. The posterior collateral ligament (PCL) attaches to the posterior part of the tibia and attaches to the anterior portion of the femur. The ACL is involved in the majority of knee injuries and often occurs along with MCL and lateral meniscus ruptures. Injury to these ligaments causes profound instability to the joint. Most of these injuries occur during athletics.

Symptoms

The patient often reports hearing a "pop" and feeling the knee "give way." Pain from this type of injury is so severe that the athlete is unable to return to the game. On examination, the patient is unable to fully extend the leg.

Management

Four standard tests to perform include the valgus stress test, varus stress test, Lachman test, and thumb sign. Each test evaluates a specific ligamentous area. All injuries of the cruciate ligaments should be referred to orthopedics.

Meniscal Injuries

The menisci are crescent-shaped structures composed of cartilage and fiber that serve as shock absorbers for the knee. The two menisci are positioned medially and laterally within and surrounding the knee joint acting to maintain buffer space between bone surfaces. The medial meniscus is injured more frequently than the lateral meniscus, because it is in an inherently more vulnerable position and is more rigid. Meniscal injuries may occur alone or in combination with ligamentous injuries. Knee function is disrupted by meniscal tears, and the knee is then susceptible to the development of osteoarthritis. There are two groups of individuals who are more susceptible to meniscal injury; these are young adults who are athletic and older individuals who have osteoarthritis. Sports most likely to produce meniscal injuries include football, basketball, and soccer. Degenerative tears, which are seen in older individuals, occur as a result of normal wear and tear of the joint over time and in association with arthritic changes in the knee. With these tears, traumatic injury is often not involved.

Symptoms

The patient will usually complain of pain, stiffness, locking, or weakness of the knee. This is representative of degenerative tears seen with aging. With traumatic tears, there is usually a history of a "twisting injury" to the knee with an acute onset of pain. On exam, there will be tenderness over the lateral or medial joint line and effusion with traumatic injury. A positive McMurray test is indicative of a tear.

Management

Meniscal injuries may heal spontaneously (in younger individuals) but should be evaluated by an orthopedic clinician. The following table shows common orthopedic maneuvers.

Table 8.3. Common Orthopedic Maneuvers

Ligament/Test	Evaluates	How to Perform
Medial collateral ligament/ valgus stress test	Stability of ligament	While supporting the thigh, apply stress with the knee extended and then flexed 25 degrees. Place one hand on the lateral side of the knee and grasp the medial tibia with the other hand and abduct the knee. If knee opens up in a valgus (knock-kneed) direction more than the unaffected knee, test is positive for partial or complete tear of MCL.
Lateral collateral ligament/ varus stress test	Stability of ligament	With knee in extension and 25-degree flexion, reverse the stress pattern used in the valgus stress test. If the knee opens up more than the opposite knee in a varus (bow-legged) direction, there is a partial or complete tear of the LCL.
Anterior cruciate ligament/ Lachman test	Ligament injury	With patient supine and knee flexed 15–20 degrees, wrap hand around leg with thumb on tibial tubercle. With the other hand, stabilize distal femur pressing thumb through quadricep tendon with rest of hand encircling the thigh above the knee. The knee should be relaxed, with you supporting the weight. Simultaneously apply pressure to tibia posteriorly, attempting to push it forward while pushing backward on the femur. Feel for any forward movement of the tibia. Any forward movement of the tibia indicates an ACL tear.
Posterior cruciate ligament/ thumb sign	PCL tear	With patient supine, flex the knee to 90 degrees and support the foot. Normally you should be able to place your thumbs on the medial and lateral tibial plateaus. With PCL injury, the proximal tibial moves backward and there is a smaller area for the thumb. When the tibial plateaus are at the same level of the femoral condyles, this indicates a complete PCL tear.
Meniscus/ McMurray test	Tear of meniscus	Flex knee to maximum pain-free degree and hold position while externally rotating the foot. Gradually extend the knee while maintaining the foot rotation. A click or pain indicates a posterior tear. When rotating the foot internally, pain or click indicates a lateral meniscus tear.
Patella/ apprehension sign	Joint instability	Patient is seated with quadriceps flexed. Extend the knee to 30 degrees. With instability, this will displace the patella to an abnormal position. This elicits pain and thus causes apprehension about further movement.
Patella/ bulge sign	Joint effusion	Apply pressure to the lateral area of the knee. A medial bulge will appear if there is fluid in the joint.

Lumbar Stenosis

Lumbar stenosis refers to a narrowed lumbar spinal canal and compression of nerve roots. The most frequently affected areas are from L4 to L5, L3 to L4, and L1 to L2. The condition may be congenital or acquired and most frequently occurs as a result of large osteophytes at facet joints, ligamentous hypertrophy, or bulging intervertebral discs. Osteoarthritis in the lumbar spine can cause narrowing. Compression of nerve structures may result in "claudication" symptoms with walking or movement. Obesity and osteoporosis are predisposing factors for the development of lumbar stenosis.

Symptoms

Individuals with lumbar stenosis seek care for progressive, chronic lumbar back pain. These patients obtain short-term relief of pain by "stooping" forward and often adopt this position.

Management

Management includes physical therapy, prescribed exercise, and reduction of abdominal fat. A decompression laminectomy may be done if there is no response to conservative measures.

CLINICAL PEARL

Always evaluate for neurologic deficit such as bowel and bladder incontinence or gait problems. This could indicate cauda equina syndrome and requires emergency referral!

Low Back Pain (LBP)

Low back pain is extremely common and is the leading cause of disability for individuals below the age of 45 years. The cause of LBP is often multifactorial and difficult to determine. Degenerative changes in the lumbar spine are found in most patients with LBP. Risk factors for LBP include long-term corticosteroid use, back trauma, osteoporosis, presence of contusion, and age over 70 years. The majority of cases of LBP resolve spontaneously within six weeks.

Symptoms

Individuals with LBP seek care for chronic lower back discomfort that is causing disruption of daily activities, may be made worse by sitting or standing, may radiate down the legs, and may be unresponsive to NSAIDs.

CLINICAL PEARL

Suspect nerve root impingement when pain is leg-dominant rather than back-dominant.

Management

Examination should include assessment for symmetrical movement, range of motion, motor strength, reflexes, and sensation. The hip should be evaluated with the patient supine, and assessment of range of motion and the straight leg raise test should be used to evaluate for lower lumbar nerve root compression. Alarming symptoms include LBP accompanied by unexplained weight loss, pain unresolved with management, and pain at night or at rest. This presentation may indicate a malignancy. Alarm symptoms for infection include rest pain, fever, recent infection (urinary tract, pneumonia, cellulitis), immunocompromise, or injection drug use.

Paget's Disease of the Bone (Osteitis Deformans)

Paget's disease is a condition of disordered remodeling of bone. There is excessive osteoclast bone resorption. This process leads to structurally unsound bone structure. There may be one or more bony lesions present, and the resultant damage leads to bones that are enlarged and demonstrate skeletal deformity. The disease is fairly common and has a striking geographic prevalence. Paget's disease is seen most often in the United Kingdom, New Zealand, Australia, the United States, and Brazil. In the United States, around 2–3% of individuals over age 55 years are affected, and this prevalence increases with aging. It is often identified incidentally on plain film radiographs.

The cause is unknown but a familial, genetic tendency has been identified. Patients with Paget's disease of the bone may exhibit bowed extremities and enlargement of the skull. The most commonly involved areas include the sacrum, pelvis, and lumbar spine.

Symptoms

This disease may be asymptomatic or bone pain may be the first symptom. Patients will have a large head, deafness, kyphosis, bowed tibias, and frequent fractures. Serum calcium and phosphate are normal, but alkaline phosphatase is elevated. On X-ray, bones appear dense and expanded.

Management

Management may be conservative and aimed at managing symptoms. Physical therapy may improve muscle strength and tone. Bisphosphonates or calcium may be prescribed to improve bone strength and analgesia for any associated pain. Patients often report an increase in pain at involved sites with the initiation of bisphosphonate therapy. This is a "first-dose effect," which usually resolves with continued administration. IV zoledronate is superior to oral bisphosphonates and is the treatment of choice in the management of Paget's disease. Patients may experience flu-like symptoms, fever, myalgia, and fatigue following administration of this agent. Prompt bisphosphonate treatment decreases disease activity and may prevent complications.

Practice Questions

1. A modifiable risk factor for the development of osteoporosis is:

   (A) gender.
   (B) genetics.
   (C) smoking.
   (D) race.

2. Your patient is a 17-year-old male with an injury to his left knee during lacrosse practice. On examination, you note a positive anterior drawer sign. This finding is indicative of injury to the:

   (A) collateral ligament.
   (B) anterior cruciate ligament.
   (C) medial meniscus.
   (D) lateral meniscus.

3. Postmenopausal women are advised to take daily calcium (1,500 mg) along with vitamin D. The vitamin D is needed because:

   (A) it increases intestinal absorption of calcium and helps to mobilize calcium from the bone itself.
   (B) it binds with the calcium to assist in active transport into tissue cells.
   (C) deficiency of vitamin D causes irreversible bone loss.
   (D) it replaces all dietary vitamin D requirements.

4. Lumbar radiculopathy may produce early neurological changes such as:

   (A) reduced muscle strength in the legs.
   (B) inability to flex the foot.
   (C) loss of discriminatory sensation of the extremities.
   (D) loss of deep tendon reflexes.

5. Your patient is a 16-year-old female with an acute knee injury incurred during a soccer game. Based on the history and physical exam, you suspect a complete medial meniscus tear. Which of the following findings would help confirm this diagnosis?

   (A) loss of joint movement
   (B) joint effusion
   (C) inability to squat
   (D) warmth over the knee

6. First-line pharmacological therapy for management of acute lower back pain includes:

   (A) NSAIDs.
   (B) muscle relaxers.
   (C) topical lidocaine.
   (D) opioid pain relievers.

7. Your patient is a 65-year-old female with a diagnosis of osteoarthritis. On a routine follow up exam you note swelling over the proximal interphalangeal joints of the hands. These findings are documented as:

   (A) Heberden's nodes.
   (B) Bouchard's nodes.
   (C) Murphy's sign.
   (D) Osler's nodes.

8. Stiffness or fixation of a joint is called:

   (A) contracture.
   (B) ankylosis.
   (C) subluxation.
   (D) dislocation.

9. A 76-year-old male is seen with complaints of progressively increasing right hip pain. He is an active, older gentleman who continues to live independently. Following a physical examination, the FNP orders radiographs of the right hip. The film demonstrates that there is significant "bone on bone" involvement of the hip joint. Which of the following courses of action would be most efficacious for this patient?

   (A) recommend physical therapy and analgesic control with acetaminophen
   (B) recommend NSAID therapy for pain control
   (C) prescribe physical therapy and follow-up exercises at home
   (D) prescribe acetaminophen for pain and initiate an orthopedic referral

10. A 60-year-old female presents to the office with a history of lower back pain. Her chief complaint today, however, is that she is suddenly having difficulty walking and cannot control her bladder or bowels. Based on this history, which of the following is the best response by the nurse practitioner?

    (A) initiate a referral to a neurologist
    (B) refer to the emergency department for immediate evaluation
    (C) order non-weight-bearing status until diagnostic imaging is complete
    (D) initiate a referral to physical therapy for strengthening exercises

11. Jake is a 45-year-old male presents for care with a chief complaint of pain in his left foot. He reports he fell off a 4-foot stepladder and injured his foot. On physical examination, the FNP notes point tenderness over the lateral malleolus. Edema is present at the site of injury; however, the patient is able to ambulate. What is the appropriate plan for management in this scenario?

    (A) RICE therapy
    (B) elevation of foot with ACE wrap
    (C) X-ray of left foot and ankle
    (D) recommend non-weight-bearing for seven days

12. A male patient is seen in the clinic with complaints of lower back pain following a lifting injury at work one day ago. Based on patient history and the physical examination, the nurse practitioner diagnosed lumbar sprain. The patient requests a note for his employer saying he needs to be off work and to rest for seven days. Which of the following statements would be appropriate based on this diagnosis?

   (A) Stop doing any activity that causes pain in your back.
   (B) You can continue your regular activities, with limited walking.
   (C) Bed rest for several days will help alleviate your pain.
   (D) Continue your daily activities, including walking.

13. The nurse practitioner is examining a patient's feet during an office visit. She notes a dusky-red-colored area of swelling that extends beyond the margin of the metatarsophalangeal joint of the right great toe. It is warm to palpation and exquisitely tender. These findings are suggestive of:

   (A) acute cellulitis.
   (B) acute gouty arthritis.
   (C) acute tenosynovitis.
   (D) acute epicondylitis.

14. A 35-year-old female is seen with a chief complaint of burning, aching pain in her hands that wakes her up from sleep. She works in an office and has no other medical problems. The nurse practitioner wants to rule out carpal tunnel syndrome as a diagnosis. The nurse practitioner instructs the patient to hold her wrists in flexion with the backs of the hands pressed together. She is to hold this position for 60 seconds. If positive, this could be an indicator of carpal tunnel syndrome. The name of this test is:

   (A) Finkelstein's test.
   (B) Allen's test.
   (C) Phalen's test.
   (D) thumb abduction.

15. The Lachman test is used in the clinical setting to assess instability of the:

   (A) medial collateral ligament (MCL).
   (B) lateral collateral ligament (LCL).
   (C) anterior cruciate ligament (ACL).
   (D) posterior cruciate ligament (PCL).

Answer Explanations

1. **(C)** Risk for development of osteoporosis includes modifiable and nonmodifiable factors. Nonmodifiable risk factors include gender (choice (A)), genetics (choice (B)), and race (choice (D)). Modifiable risk factors include smoking, high alcohol intake, sedentary lifestyle, calcium deficiency, and menopause. Menopause causes a state of relative estrogen deficiency, which is a significant risk factor for the development of osteoporosis, particularly when combined with other risk factors. This explains the disease prevalence in older women.

2. **(B)** The anterior drawer sign is a test used to assess for rupture of the anterior cruciate ligament. The test is considered positive if there is increased forward (anterior) movement of the tibia when the knee is in 90-degree flexion. To assess stability of the collateral ligaments, varus and valgus stress tests are performed (choice (A)). The McMurray test is used to evaluate for meniscal injury (choices (C) and (D)). This test is positive when flexion-circumduction movement is associated with a positive audible click.

3. **(A)** Postmenopausal women are advised to take 1,500 mg of calcium daily, along with vitamin D. Research has demonstrated the efficacy of this regimen in preventing osteoporosis in this population. A patient who is deficient in vitamin D is unable to fully absorb calcium, thus supplementation is advised. The other responses are incorrect.

4. **(D)** Low back pain is technically an injury to the paravertebral spinal muscles. The hallmark presentation of chronic low back pain is recurrent pain that may radiate to one or both buttocks. Loss of deep tendon reflexes may be an early sign of neurologic involvement in the pathology. Discriminatory sensation of the legs is preserved (choice (C)). The other two options, reduced muscle strength in the legs (choice (A)) and the inability to flex the foot (choice (B)) indicate muscular, rather than neurologic, pathology and are not usual components of chronic low back pain pathology.

5. **(C)** A patient presenting with a suspected medial meniscus tear usually has preserved ability to move the joint. There may be effusion and warmth of the knee; however, this is not a specific finding related to meniscus rupture. Usually, with a complete rupture, the patient is unable to obtain a squatting position because of knee instability and pain. The other choices are incorrect.

6. **(A)** Acute low back pain is a commonly occurring problem and usually involves strain or sprain of the muscles of the lower back. The resultant tissue inflammation causes pain; therefore, first-line treatment should include NSAIDs because of their anti-inflammatory and analgesic properties. Muscle relaxer (choice (B)) and topical lidocaine (choice (C)) are sometimes used for persistent pain that does not respond to NSAID therapy. However, these are used judiciously and are not first-line. Opioid therapy is not recommended for acute low back pain (choice (D)).

7. **(B)** Bouchard's nodes are bony deformities of the proximal interphalangeal (PIP) joints of the hands and are associated with osteoarthritis. Heberden's nodes are also seen with osteoarthritis but affect the distal interphalangeal joints (DIP) of the hands (choice (A)). These findings, too, are bony deformities that occur with advanced osteoarthritis. Osler's nodes are tender reddish subcutaneous nodules on the ends of fingers or toes that are seen with bacterial endocarditis (choice (D)). Murphy's sign is an abdominal exam technique to assess for gallbladder disease (choice (C)).

8. **(B)** Ankylosis is a term used to describe stiffness or fixation of a joint or multiple joints. A contracture is an abnormal, usually permanent derangement of a joint or multiple joints, which are in a position of flexion and fixated in place (choice (A)). Atrophy and shortening of the muscles occur. Subluxation is a term referring to an incomplete dislocation of a joint (choice (C)). Dislocation is the movement or displacement of a bone or bones from their normal anatomical positions (choice (D)). This displacement occurs within joint structures, negatively impacting joint function and mobility.

9. **(D)** Radiographic results of "bone on bone" evidence of the joint space indicates severe degenerative osteoarthritis of the hip. Initial analgesic therapy is acetaminophen as needed. Because of the joint derangement evident on the film, physical therapy and follow-up exercises will not be of great benefit at this time (choices (A) and (C)). NSAID therapy may be prescribed if adequate pain relief is not obtained with acetaminophen (choice (B)). A referral to an orthopedic specialist would be appropriate as this patient may be a good candidate for surgical repair/replacement of the right hip.

10. **(B)** Based on this patient presentation, she may have cauda equina syndrome, which is a medical emergency. This syndrome indicates severe spinal nerve root impingement requiring rapid evaluation and management. Other signs of cauda equina syndrome include bilateral leg weakness, saddle anesthesia, and bilateral sciatic pain extending to both legs. Although a neurologist will likely be involved in her care, this patient should be evaluated emergently and this can be facilitated in the emergency department. The other answer choices would be incorrect in this situation.

11. **(C)** This patient suffered a traumatic injury to his left foot. Sprains and strains are the most commonly seen injuries of this type; however, a fracture must be ruled out before proceeding to other treatment recommendations. Recommended management for a sprain includes rest, ice, compression, and elevation (RICE) (choice (A)). An order for an ACE wrap and rest is not detailed enough to provide safe care for this patient (choice (B)). Non-weight-bearing status will be determined based on findings of diagnostic studies (choice (D)).

12. **(D)** Research on management of low back sprain demonstrates that early and continued activity promotes resolution of symptoms faster than bed rest, which is no longer recommended. Patients are often reluctant to continue movement because they will continue to experience some pain following a lumbar strain. Acetaminophen or short-term NSAID therapy may be appropriate, but the patient should continue to move around normally. The other choices would not be appropriate.

13. **(B)** Acute gouty arthritis is a disorder that is often related to hyperuricemia. The body is overproducing uric acid or under-excreting uric acid. This excess of uric acid produces crystals that precipitate out of the serum in areas of the body that are cooler, such as the toes. The metatarsophalangeal joint of the great toe is the most frequently affected joint in an episode of acute gout. The presentation of a painful, dusky-red, swollen joint is pathognomonic for gout. Uric acid levels may or may not be elevated during an acute attack. Cellulitis presents as an edematous, expanding, warm indurated area most often on the lower leg (choice (A)). The patient may have systemic symptoms of infection such as fever, chills, and malaise. Cellulitis is caused most commonly by a Gram-positive bacteria and involves the dermis and subcutaneous tissue of the limb as opposed to focal joint involvement. Tenosynovitis is inflammation involving a joint tendon sheath and the synovium within the joint itself (choice (C)). There are many causes of tenosynovitis including calcium deposits, repeated trauma, high cholesterol, and gonorrhea. Tenosynovitis may be a component of gouty arthritis; however, the description given is not indicative of this disorder.

14. **(C)** Phalen's test is performed by asking the patient to hold both wrists in flexion for 60 seconds while keeping the backs of the hands pressed together. If the patient experiences numbness and tingling of the hands with this test, it is considered positive and is one indicator of possible carpal tunnel syndrome. Finkelstein's test is used to assess for de Quervain's disease (choice (A)). The patient is instructed to touch the thumb to the palm of the hand and make a fist. The test is positive if moving the wrist into ulnar deviation causes pain. Allen's test or Allen's sign is used to assess patency of the radial and ulnar arteries into the hand (choice (B)). To perform this test, the clinician compresses the radial artery at the wrist and has the patient rapidly open and close the hand several times. The patient then opens the hand, which should be pale in color or white. When the clinician relieves the pressure on the artery, the hand should flush, which indicates the artery is patent. To perform thumb abduction, the patient is asked to point the thumb upward against downward applied resistance (choice (D)).

15. **(C)** The Lachman test is used clinically to evaluate stability or instability of the ACL. To perform this test, the knee is passively held in 30 degrees of flexion and the patient is asked to relax. With one hand, the clinician stabilizes the distal femur, and with the other hand, a gentle anterior force on the proximal tibia is applied. It is important to test both knees to interpret findings. To assess the posterior cruciate ligament, the patient is asked to lie supine and the knee is flexed to 90 degrees with support (choice (D)). Normally, the anterior tibial plateau is 1 cm anterior (in front of) the femoral condyles. The clinician is able to place their thumb on top of the medial and lateral tibial plateaus. If the PCL is injured, the proximal tibia falls back and the area available to the thumb decreases. When the tibial plateaus are flush with the femoral condyles, there is 10 mm or more of posterior laxity, indicating a complete tear of the PCL. To assess stability of the LCL, the varus stress test is performed (choice (B)). With this test, the knee is in extension and 25-degree flexion, which reverses the stress pattern used for the MCL. If the knee opens up more than the opposite knee in a varus direction (outward), the patient has either a partial or complete tear of the LCL. The valgus stress test is used to assess the stability of the MCL (choice (A)). To perform this test, the clinician should support the thigh area to relax the quadriceps muscle. Stress is applied initially with the knee extended and then flexed to 25 degrees. With the thigh supported and knee extended, place one hand on the lateral area of the knee, grasp the distal tibia with the other hand, and abduct the knee. If the knee opens up in a valgus direction more than the opposite knee, the patient has either a partial or complete tear of the MCL.

9

Disorders of the Hematologic and Immunologic Systems

Hematologic disorders affect every organ system in the body. Many common complaints associated with hematologic disorders include fatigue, bruising, fever, and lymphadenopathy. These complaints are signs of another pathologic condition occurring in the body. Because oxygen delivery via red blood cells is so critical, it is important for the FNP to be familiar with the different types and functions of blood components. Because anemia is the most common hematologic condition seen in family practice, understanding the components of the complete blood count (CBC) and peripheral smear is critical to being able to piece together patient history, physical examination findings, and laboratory studies. This chapter will discuss and highlight some of the most common hematologic conditions seen in primary care. Along with hematologic disorders, the discussion will include descriptions of immunologically driven conditions.

Anemia

Anemia is a disorder caused by another pathologic process in the body. The World Health Organization identifies anemia as a hemoglobin level less than 13.0 g/dL in men and less than 12.0 g/dL in women. The estimated level of hematocrit is three times that of hemoglobin, thus a hemoglobin of 12.0 would correspond to a hematocrit of 36%. Classifying anemia according to blood components, such as size, shape, and color of red blood cell, may assist in diagnosis. RBC size is captured by the mean corpuscular volume (MCV) on the CBC. RBCs with a MCV less than 80 fL are considered smaller than normal, or microcytic. RBCs with a MCV of equal to or greater than 100 fL are larger than normal and are termed macrocytic. Normocytic RBCs have a MCV between 80 fL and 100 fL. Shape of the RBC is important as well. Normal RBCs have a biconcave shape, which facilitates hemoglobin attachment to the cell. Hemoglobin represents the oxygen-carrying capacity of the cell. Certain disease states, such as sickle cell disease, produce RBCs that are shaped like sickles and are unable to carry hemoglobin. Color of the RBC is described using the suffix "chromic." RBCs that are pale are described as hypochromic, which compares with normochromic cells. Red blood cells are not considered to be hyperchromic. Color of the cell is derived from oxygen, thus hypochromic cells are carrying little oxygen. Another parameter of the RBC captured on the CBC is the red cell distribution width (RDW). This value indicates how much variation exists between RBCs. An elevated RDW means that circulating RBCs have a wide range of size. This type of abnormality occurs when anemia is severe or prolonged and the body is producing and releasing RBCs before they are mature in order to meet oxygen demand of the body. Reticulocytes are baby RBCs, and production and release into the bloodstream indicate normal bone marrow function. With a diagnosis of anemia, this relative lack of oxygen in the body produces corresponding changes in other systems, such as the cardiovascular and pulmonary. When a patient presents with anemia, always look for and treat the underlying cause.

Iron Deficiency Anemia (IDA)

Iron deficiency anemia is the most common anemia worldwide and continues to affect millions across the globe each year. This type of anemia is occasionally seen in infants as they expend maternal stores of iron they had at birth, and it is often related to diet. Adults with anemia require a high index of suspicion for bleeding as the cause. The most common cause of IDA globally is lack of dietary iron. However, in the United States, gastrointestinal bleeding is the primary cause in adults. There is an increased need for iron during pregnancy, lactation, and in premature infants. Iron is required for hemoglobin production, thus IDA will demonstrate a hemoglobin level of < 13.5 g/dL in males; and < 12 g/dL in females. IDA is a hypochromic (pale RBCs), microcytic (small RBCs) anemia.

Symptoms

Patients with IDA will complain of fatigue, fast heart rate, and dyspnea with any exertion. Mucous membranes may be pale. Many females with IDA develop pica, which is a craving for a nonfood item, such as ice. Lab evaluation includes: serum ferritin (stored iron) is decreased, total iron binding capacity (TIBC) is increased, H&H is decreased, mean corpuscular volume (MCV) is decreased, and reticulocyte count is decreased.

Management

Management includes identification and treatment of underlying causes. IDA itself is treated with supplemental iron; oral ferrous sulfate at 325 mg daily; parenteral iron only if PO is not tolerated. Iron should be taken with citrus juice (vitamin C improves absorption) on an empty stomach. Treatment should last at least three to six months. Patients with suspected gastrointestinal bleeding should be referred for further evaluation.

Vitamin B12 Deficiency

Vitamin B12 deficiency causes macrocytic anemia. Pernicious anemia (a malabsorption problem) results from autoimmune destruction of intrinsic factor, which normally binds with B12 and is critical for DNA production and RBC development. Conditions associated with decreased gastric acid production also add to vitamin B12 deficiency because of decreased protein carriers available for binding. The body needs only 10 mcg/day of vitamin B12. Because most individuals ingest more than enough B12 in their diet, the liver usually stores up to 5,000 mcg/day. This means that several years may elapse before vitamin B12 deficiency is identified.

Symptoms

Patients will often present with stomatitis, glossitis, diarrhea, peripheral neuropathy, nausea, and anorexia. Lab findings include an elevated MCV, normal MCHC (normochromic), low or normal reticulocytes, serum B12 levels less than 0.1 mcg/mL with hypersegmented neutrophils.

Management

Management is based on treating the cause of the anemia if possible and replacing vitamin B12. Oral supplementation of true B12 deficiency is recommended with 1,000 mcg/day of cobalamin until normal serum B12 levels are reached. For pernicious anemia, treatment is undertaken with IM administration of B12 daily, weekly, then monthly for life. Neurologic symptoms associated with B12 deficiency, such as peripheral tingling, numbness, memory loss, personality changes, and ataxia may resolve or may be permanent.

Folic Acid Deficiency

Deficiency of folic acid leads to a normochromic, macrocytic, megaloblastic anemia that results in impaired DNA synthesis and red blood cell production. Folic acid deficiency in pregnant

---

CLINICAL PEARL

An increase in reticulocyte count should occur within a week of beginning iron therapy. This confirms diagnosis of iron deficiency anemia and response to therapy.

women is associated with fetal neural tube defects. Risk factors for this type of anemia include pregnancy, alcoholism, aging, and medications such as trimethoprim-sulfamethoxazole, phenytoin, oral contraceptives, and phenobarbital. These agents interfere with folic acid absorption.

Symptoms

Patients will often report a history of indigestion, anorexia, fatigue, and diarrhea. Findings upon physical exam include pallor, glossitis, stomatitis, tachycardia, murmur, and mental status changes. Lab findings: serum folate < 3 ngm/mL, < HCT, normal Hgb, RDW elevated, TIBC normal. MCV elevated. This type of deficiency is often seen with vitamin B12 deficiency.

Management

Management includes identification and treatment of underlying cause. Folic acid replacement at 400 mcg/day for pregnant women; 200 mcg/day for all others. Treatment should continue for two months or until folate level normalizes. Encourage a folate-rich diet, which includes green leafy vegetables, red beans, asparagus, fish, bananas, and wheat bran.

Sickle Cell Disease (SCD)

Sickle cell disease is an autosomal recessive disorder that presents with abnormal hemoglobin production leading to a chronic hemolytic anemia. SCD is characterized by production of hemoglobin S. The most commonly seen problem in SSD is sickle cell anemia (HbSS). Abnormal hemoglobin S causes widespread vasoconstriction and tissue ischemia throughout the body. Hemolysis occurs as these abnormal cells travel through the spleen, precipitating a hemolytic anemia.

Symptoms

SCD presents within the first 6 to 12 months of life with recurrent pain episodes. Initial symptoms may be irritability and swelling of hands and feet. On peripheral blood smear, Hgb S is seen. The diagnostic gold standard is the presence of irreversibly sickled cells on electrophoresis. Strokes are common, even in childhood.

Management

Management includes prevention of crises through adequate hydration and avoiding situations causing hypoxia, fever, infection, or cold temperatures. Prompt management of infection, fever, and pain is critical. These children should receive appropriate immunizations. For outpatient management of crises that are mild in nature, supplemental oxygen and nonnarcotic analgesics are recommended. Supportive care within the primary care office includes administration of immunizations and early recognition and treatment of infections. Refer these patients to a hematologist for evaluation. An allogeneic hematopoietic stem cell transplant can cure 80% of children with the disorder if performed early in the disease process.

Polycythemia Vera

Polycythemia vera is an acquired myeloproliferative disorder that causes overproduction of all hematopoietic cell lines. The most prominent pathology is overproduction of red blood cells. The disorder is more common in men over the age of 40 years.

Symptoms

Patients present with headaches, tinnitus, fatigue, dizziness, and blurred vision due to increased viscosity of blood and expanded volume. On a physical exam, a palpable spleen and evidence of thrombosis or retinal vein engorgement may be noted.

Management

Management involves regular phlebotomy to maintain hematocrit below 45%. Patients are advised to remain well hydrated and avoid risk factors for thrombosis. Hydroxyurea is given as myelosuppressive therapy.

Glucose-6-Phosphate Dehydrogenase (G6PD) Deficiency

Glucose-6-phosphate dehydrogenase deficiency is an x-linked recessive disorder that is seen in American Black males. This hematologic disorder decreases the red blood cells' ability to handle oxidative stress in the body. GSPD deficiency causes episodic hemolysis when the patient is exposed to oxidant drugs or infection is present.

Symptoms

These patients are usually healthy with no chronic organomegaly or anemia identified. With exposure to oxidative stress, hemolysis occurs, which is usually self-limiting.

Management

Management includes avoidance of oxidant medications: dapsone, phenazopyridine, methylene blue, quinolone antibiotics, nitrofurantoin, and trimethoprim-sulfamethoxazole.

Coagulation Disorders

The body's process of coagulation is a seemingly precarious balance moving between prothrombotic and antithrombotic activity involving coagulation factors, the vascular endothelium, and platelets. A dysfunction or deficiency of one of the elements results in hemorrhagic or thrombotic disease. Disorders may be inherited or acquired, with acquired disorders being more common. Examples of inherited disorders include hemophilia A/B, von Willebrand disease, and Factor XI deficiency. Acquired clotting disorders have variable causes such as vitamin K deficiency, hepatic disease, anticoagulant medications, massive blood loss, as well as transfusion and platelet disorders. Patients with liver disease are at high risk for clotting disorders because of defective or deficient synthesis of coagulation factors and natural anticoagulants, including protein C and S.

Symptoms

Inherited clotting disorders present early in life with episodes of massive bleeding associated with minor injury. Individuals with acquired clotting disorders may present to primary care with complaints of excessive bruising, bleeding gums, and frequent nosebleeds. Patients may appear pale, and there may be physical evidence, such as ecchymosis, hemarthrosis, or petechiae.

Management

Individuals with known clotting disorders should receive education related to decreasing risk for bleeding as well as emergency management of bleeding episodes. Overall management will be pursued in specialty care.

Table 9.1. Antithrombotic Therapy

Classes of Anticoagulants	Description	Uses/Dosing/Comments
Unfractionated heparin & LMWHs	Heparin is derived from porcine intestinal tissue and is a biologic product with wide variation in chemical structure, making it poorly predictable with respect to response. LMWHs have more predictable pharmacokinetics (than unfractionated heparin) and allow for weight-based dosing.	
Fondaparinux	Chemically related to LMWHs and exerts almost no thrombin inhibition. Works directly to inhibit factor Xa by binding to antithrombin. Predictable pharmacokinetics allow for weight-based dosing.	Metabolized by kidneys and is contraindicated with a creatinine clearance less than 30 mL/min. Has a long half-life (17–21 hours) and may be dose once-daily via subcutaneous injection. Unlike heparin, no neutralizing agent exists to address bleeding events.
Vitamin K antagonist	Warfarin inhibits activity of vitamin K dependent carboxylase important for coagulation factor production.	May be taken orally; however, individual response varies based on nutritional status, comorbid conditions, concomitant medications, and genetic polymorphisms. Patients must undergo periodic monitoring to verify intensity of anticoagulant effect. This is reported as the INR, which corrects for differences in product potency.
Direct-acting oral anticoagulants (DOACs)	Have a predictable dose effect and do not require lab monitoring. Anticoagulant effect is independent of vitamin K, thus diet does not alter patient response. Are renally metabolized to varying degrees, thus renal function must be monitored during therapy.	Products include: - dabigatran etexilate - Rivaroxaban - Apixaban - Edoxaban Indications and dosing for each agent are individualized. Many drug interactions exist with these agents.

Leukemias

The leukemias represent a group of malignant blood disorders in which normal bone marrow is replaced by abnormal, dysfunctional lymphocytes called blast cells. Unregulated proliferation of abnormal cells produces symptoms and diagnostic findings associated with these disorders.

Chronic Myeloid Leukemia (CML)

Chronic myeloid leukemia results from an overproduction of myeloid (bone marrow) cells. Because this is a myeloproliferative disorder, myeloid cells continue to differentiate and circulate in the peripheral blood. CML is characterized by a specific chromosomal abnormality, identified as the Philadelphia chromosome. CML occurs during middle age, and early disease is basically a chronic disorder. The bone marrow continues to function as normal, and neutrophils are able to fight infection normally. Diagnosis is confirmed via bone marrow biopsy.

Symptoms

Patients usually present with complaints of fatigue, night sweats, and low-grade fever. Overproduction of white blood cells triggers a hypermetabolic state. Individuals may also report abdominal discomfort, and splenomegaly may be identified on exam. CML is characterized by an elevated white blood cell count, usually greater than 100,000/mcL but less than 500,000/mcL.

Management

During the long chronic phase of CML, the goal of therapy is to normalize hematologic abnormalities, and treatment includes the use of a tyrosine kinase inhibitor (e.g., imatinib, dasatinib, nilotinib). These medications achieve hematologic control of the disease in almost 98% of patients. Introduction of these medications has greatly expanded life expectancy with 80% of patients alive at nine years post diagnosis.

Acute Nonlymphocytic Leukemia (ANLL)

Acute nonlymphocytic leukemia affects adults, and approximately 80% of adults with leukemia have ANLL. This disorder usually presents after age 40, and incidence increases with age. Chromosomal and molecular abnormalities have been identified that assist in determining overall prognosis for this disease.

Symptoms

Patients often present with bone and joint pain along with fever and chills. Shortness of breath, palpitations, and signs of infection are common. Bleeding of the gums is frequently present at diagnosis and may be the reason for seeking care.

Management

ANLL will be managed by oncology.

Chronic Lymphocytic Leukemia (CLL)

Chronic lymphocytic leukemia is the most common leukemia occurring in adults over age 60 years.

Symptoms

Because CLL is a chronic form of leukemia, patients often present with fatigue, low-grade fever, and night sweats. Lymphocytosis with a white blood cell count greater than 500,000 cells/mcL may be present on diagnosis.

Management

Patients with a diagnosis of CLL should be referred to an oncologist.

Acute Lymphoblastic Leukemia (ALL)

Acute lymphoblastic leukemia (ALL) is the predominant form of leukemia seen in children between ages 2 and 15 years. At the present time, approximately 90% of children diagnosed with ALL may be cured. Management is strongly guided by genetic features individual to each child.

Symptoms

Individuals present with fatigue, bruising, pallor, shortness of breath, and constitutional symptoms such as fever and weight loss.

Management

Children with ALL should be referred to pediatric oncology for care.

Immune Disorders

Allergic Reactions

Allergic reactions occur due to hypersensitive, immune system-related responses to common substances, or antigens. Many of these antigens are found in the environment and usually do not cause illness. Allergic response may remain localized at the site of inoculation or may become widespread and systematic with potentially lethal consequences. Allergens are substances that are "nonself" and thus foreign to the body. Immune response at the cellular and humoral level to these substances initiate a cascade of immunological events that produce the symptoms associated with the allergy.

- **Type 1:** Allergic responses are IgE-mediated hypersensitivity reactions to a previously encountered antigen. Symptoms include nasal congestion, mucus production, and eye irritation all occurring within seconds to minutes of exposure.
- **Type 2:** Responses are antibody-mediated cellular responses that involve activation of IgM and IgG molecules causing a cytotoxic reaction to an antigen. An example of this type of reaction is Rh-incompatibility hemolysis in neonates.
- **Type 3:** Responses also involve IgM and IgG activation that form complexes directly with the allergen. These complexes become deposited in various parts of the body leading to a delayed onset of symptoms, sometimes weeks after exposure. Rashes that occur in response to medications are an example of this type of reaction.
- **Type 4:** Responses are delayed reactions to antigen exposure, such as development of a dermatologic reaction with repeated exposure to nickel.

Symptoms

Patient presentation is variable depending on the type of allergic response. Type 1 reactions usually present with immediate symptoms of tearing, increased nasal mucosa, and itchy eyes when exposed to the allergen. Type 2 reactions present fairly rapidly but not as quickly as type 1. Infants exposed to maternal antibodies during birth develop signs of hemolysis within hours. Type 3 reactions present within hours to days after exposure to allergen. Type 4 reactions may present until days to weeks after exposure.

Management

Management is based on the type of reaction with allergen avoidance first-line intervention. Type 1 reactions are immediate and require immediate administration of IM or subQ epinephrine. Other classes of medications include antihistamines, histamine-2 receptor antagonists, and corticosteroids.

Chronic Fatigue Syndrome (CFS) and Fibromyalgia Syndrome (FMS)

Chronic fatigue and fibromyalgia syndromes, although separate diagnoses, have significant overlap in symptom presentation. These illnesses affect women three times as often as men and usually present between the ages of 20 and 55 years. CFS and FMS are associated with other autoimmune disorders such as systemic lupus erythematosus (SLE) and rheumatoid arthritis (RA).

Symptoms

Altered pain perception is considered a central factor of both disorders along with much symptomatic overlap such as fatigue, pain in multiple joints, headaches, mood and memory changes, depression, sore throat, post-exercise malaise, sleep problems, and generalized muscle pain. A diagnosis of FMS requires a report of widespread muscle pain for at least three months and pain elicitation with pressure on at least 11 of 18 trigger points. Please refer to Table 9.2 and Figure 9.1 reference tender points in the diagnosing of fibromyalgia.

Management

Goal of management of these disorders is to improve and maintain a good quality of life in the setting of chronic pain. Cognitive behavioral therapy (CBT) and graded exercise both have demonstrated efficacy in achieving management goals.

Table 9.2. Tender Points in Fibromyalgia

Front	Back
▪ Neck (under the lower sternomastoid muscle) ▪ Chest (near the second costochondral junction) ▪ Elbow (distal to the lateral epicondyle) ▪ Waist (at the prominence of the greater trochanter) ▪ Knee (at the medial fat pad of the knee)	▪ Head (insertion of the suboccipital muscle) ▪ Shoulders (mid upper trapezius muscle) ▪ Mid upper back (origin of the supraspinatus muscle) ▪ Hip (upper outer quadrant of the buttock)

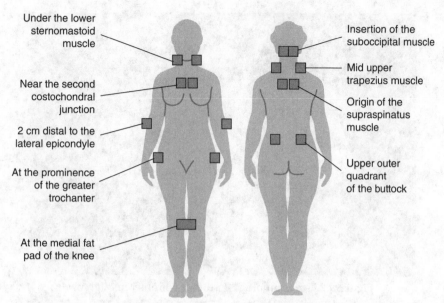

Under the lower sternomastoid muscle

Near the second costochondral junction

2 cm distal to the lateral epicondyle

At the prominence of the greater trochanter

At the medial fat pad of the knee

Insertion of the suboccipital muscle

Mid upper trapezius muscle

Origin of the supraspinatus muscle

Upper outer quadrant of the buttock

Figure 9.1. The 18 Tender Points Important for Diagnosing Fibromyalgia

Lyme Disease

Lyme disease is the most common tick-borne illness in the United States and is included in this chapter because untreated disease triggers autoimmune illness. Lyme disease is caused by the spirochete *B. burgdorferi* and transmitted to humans via a tick bite that must be attached for at least 24 to 48 hours. The disease has three stages and may lead to a chronic, disabling condition with severe neurologic and musculoskeletal sequelae.

Symptoms

Erythema migrans is characteristic of stage 1 disease. The patient may report flu-like symptoms such as headache, myalgias, and fatigue. Without treatment, the rash clears in three to four weeks. Stage 2 is early disseminated infection with bacteremia occurring in 50–60% of untreated individuals within days to weeks of infection. During this stage, the organism may lodge in certain areas causing focal symptoms, such as in the heart (myopericarditis) and the neurologic system (aseptic meningitis). Stage 3 is a late persistent infection that may last for years after the initial illness and affects the musculoskeletal, dermatologic, and neurologic systems. Arthritis of one joint or several is a classic presentation of late disease.

Management

Management is based on the stage of disease and manifestation. A patient with a tick bite only requires observation. If erythema migrans develops, treat with doxycycline, amoxicillin, or cefuroxime axetil for two weeks. Patients with stage 2 or stage 3 disease with cardiac or neurologic system involvement should be referred to an infectious disease specialist.

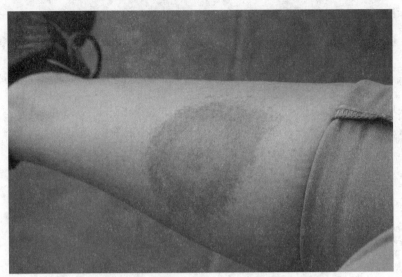

Figure 9.2. An Example of Erythema Chronicum Migrans

Sjogren's Syndrome (SS)

Sjogren's syndrome is a chronic systemic autoimmune, inflammatory disorder caused by dysfunction of exocrine glands. Clinical presentation usually includes dry eyes and mouth caused by abnormal function of the lacrimal and salivary glands. This disorder is primarily seen in women, usually between the ages of 40 and 60 years. Sjogren's syndrome may be seen alone, but the disorder often accompanies other autoimmune disorders such as rheumatoid arthritis.

Symptoms

Individuals with Sjogren's syndrome present with complaints of very dry eyes and dry mouth (sicca components). Patients may complain of burning, itching, or foreign-body sensation of the eyes. Photophobia, if present, may indicate corneal ulceration as a result of severe dryness.

Management

Management is symptom-based and includes artificial tears to relieve ocular symptoms, improved oral hygiene, and oral lubrication. Patients with systemic or resistant symptoms should be referred to a rheumatologist.

Systemic Lupus Erythematosus (SLE)

Systemic lupus erythematosus is an inflammatory autoimmune disorder that affects multiple organ systems. Antigen-antibody complexes become trapped in capillaries of visceral structures and cause many of the symptoms associated with the disease. SLE occurs mainly in young women and has a clinical course characterized by periods of spontaneous remission and relapses. Triggers for disease flares include exposure to sunlight, stress, microbial infection, pregnancy, postpartum state, and surgery. Lab diagnostics should include CBC, direct Coombs, urinalysis, and ANA.

Symptoms

Classic presentation includes a malar (butterfly) rash over cheeks and nose, anorexia, malaise, fever, and weight loss. Joint symptoms are common and may be the first manifestation of SLE. Symptoms often wax and wane, and medication management should be tailored based on disease activity.

Management

Goal of therapy is symptom control. Fatigue, which is the most disabling symptom, may be managed with the use of hydroxychloroquine, corticosteroids, or DHEA. Antimalarial medications, such as hydroxychloroquine, may be effective in managing rashes and joint symptoms. Regular use of this drug has also been associated with decreased disease flares. Referral to a rheumatologist is indicated for overall disease management.

Human Immunodeficiency Virus (HIV) Disease

Human immunodeficiency virus disease is the initial stage of eventual destruction of immune function if untreated. HIV affects men and women of all races as well as infants, children, and adolescents. At the present time, two-thirds of people with HIV live in sub-Saharan Africa and most of them are women. Recent data related to HIV in the United States indicates that the population groups with the highest incidence of HIV include African American men and women as well as Asian and Latino individuals. Transmission occurs through mucous membrane inoculation of the virus via saliva, blood, semen, and breast milk. HIV may also be transmitted from mother to unborn child via the placenta. Other sources of transmission include needle-stick injuries and needle-sharing.

Symptoms

Presentation may consist of acute infection: fever, sore throat, myalgias, headaches, cervical lymphadenopathy, and night sweats; many patients are asymptomatic. Physical exam findings include persistent generalized lymphadenopathy, cough, dyspnea, shortness of breath, localized Candida infections, sexually transmitted infections, and weight loss.

Management

Management involves initial disclosure of HIV status, initiation of viral suppressive drug therapy, and monitoring of viral activity throughout treatment. Prevention of transmission, preservation of immune function, prophylaxis for opportunistic infections, and optimization of quality of life are treatment goals. With overall management by a specialist in HIV care and current regimens of antiretroviral therapy (ART), this disease has become a chronic condition and individuals often live a normal life span.

Acquired immune deficiency syndrome is a result of untreated HIV infection. When the CD4 T-cell count drops below 200 cells/mcL, opportunistic infections become more frequent and more devastating. When the CD4 T-cell level is below 200 cells/mcL or the patient develops an AIDS-defining illness, AIDS is diagnosed. Patients with AIDS will be managed by a specialist in AIDS care.

Practice Questions

1. A 36-year-old female has a chief complaint of progressive fatigue and anorexia. With a diagnosis of pernicious anemia, which of the following sets of symptoms would the FNP also expect in this patient?

   (A) hypertension, chest pain, peripheral edema
   (B) blurred vision, double vision, decreased vibratory sensation in the feet and hands
   (C) peripheral neuropathy, lethargy, fatigue, ataxia
   (D) jaundice, hepatomegaly, right upper quadrant pain

2. A young patient is seen in the clinic with a history and presentation suggestive of sickle cell anemia. The FNP should order which of the following studies?

   (A) CBC with peripheral smear
   (B) hemoglobin electrophoresis
   (C) bone marrow biopsy
   (D) hemoglobin and hematocrit

3. Which laboratory test is most useful in diagnosing iron deficiency anemia?

   (A) direct Coombs
   (B) serum ferritin level
   (C) serum folate level
   (D) RBC count

4. A 45-year-old Black male presents with a two-day history of illness. He has a medical history significant for erythrocytosis. He is otherwise healthy. Which of the following represents the most serious concern for complications based on the patient's history?

   (A) a two-inch laceration on his left ankle
   (B) vomiting and diarrhea
   (C) productive cough
   (D) fatigue

5. What type of leukemia is most commonly seen in older adults and is usually asymptomatic with a median survival of 10 years?

   (A) chronic myelogenous
   (B) acute lymphoblastic
   (C) acute myelogenous
   (D) chronic lymphocytic

6. At what age should infants be screened for anemia?

   (A) birth
   (B) six months
   (C) nine months
   (D) no screening recommended

7. The erythrocyte sedimentation rate (ESR) may be used as a screening test to detect presence of a systemic disease. Which of the following is true regarding the ESR?

   (A) An elevated ESR is diagnostic for rheumatoid arthritis.
   (B) The ESR is a very specific indicator of inflammation.
   (C) The ESR is useful in detecting pancreatic cancer.
   (D) An elevated ESR is a normal part of the aging process.

8. A 70-year-old male is being seen for an annual physical examination and labs. His CBC indicates iron deficiency anemia (IDA). The patient is currently being treated for several chronic conditions. Treatment for which of the diseases below is most likely the cause of his IDA?

   (A) osteoarthritis
   (B) hyperlipidemia
   (C) diabetes mellitus
   (D) hypertension

9. An adolescent is seen in an urgent care clinic for an illness. His CBC demonstrates leukocytosis. What does this indicate?

   (A) The patient has a viral infection.
   (B) The patient has a bacterial infection.
   (C) The patient has an infection of unknown origin.
   (D) The patient does not have an infection.

10. A 32-year-old female has a history of gastric bypass surgery. She is diagnosed with pernicious anemia. Which of the following findings would be an expected finding with this type of anemia?

    (A) glossitis
    (B) severe headaches
    (C) nausea and vomiting
    (D) thrombocytopenia

11. Your patient is a six-year-old female with sickle cell anemia. She underwent a splenectomy six months ago. Which of the following is true regarding patients who have had a splenectomy?

    (A) They are at high risk for bleeding disorders.
    (B) They are more likely to demonstrate worsening anemia.
    (C) They are at increased risk of hepatomegaly.
    (D) They are more susceptible to infection.

12. Which of the following disorders is considered to be a macrocytic anemia?

    (A) thalassemia
    (B) iron deficiency
    (C) sickle cell
    (D) folic acid deficiency

13. A 40-year-old male has a new diagnosis of glucose-6-phosphate dehydrogenase (G6PD) deficiency. Which of the following should be done to prevent red blood cell lysis?

    (A) maintain adequate hydration
    (B) avoid aspirin and sulfa medications
    (C) minimize consumption of iron-containing foods
    (D) receive all recommended immunizations

14. A 15-year-old thin female presents to the clinic for care. Her weight is 10% the ideal body weight. She reports that she becomes dizzy when she stands up. Laboratory testing was performed. Besides malnutrition, which of the following findings could account for the patient's dizziness?

    (A) mildly elevated blood urea nitrogen (BUN)
    (B) hemoglobin 9.6 mg/dL
    (C) glucose 90 mg/dL
    (D) potassium 3.5 mEq/L

15. A patient presents to the clinic with a history of thalassemia minor. Which of the following should be limited in the diet to avoid hepatotoxicity?

    (A) multivitamin with iron
    (B) vitamin B12
    (C) folic acid supplementation
    (D) vitamin C

Answer Explanations

1. **(C)** Pernicious anemia is an autoimmune disorder that causes macrocytic anemia. Patients often present with peripheral neuropathy, lethargy, fatigue, and ataxia. With this disorder, autoantibodies destroy gastric parietal cells, which produce intrinsic factors. Atrophic gastritis results with further binding to or neutralizing of intrinsic factors. Intrinsic factor is required for digestion and absorption of nutrients, DNA synthesis, and maturation of red blood cells. This type of anemia is a macrocytic anemia. Research has found that prolonged use of medications that decrease gastric acid production, such as histamine-2 blockers and proton pump inhibitors, also decrease nutrient absorption and use. Metformin, which is a medication commonly used in the treatment of diabetes mellitus, can decrease vitamin B12 absorption in up to one-third of patients. Hypertension, chest pain, and peripheral edema reflect abnormality or dysfunction of the cardiovascular system and are not normally seen with pernicious anemia (choice (A)). Blurred vision, double vision, and decreased vibratory sensation are neurologic signs that are not usually found in individuals with pernicious anemia (choice (B)). Jaundice, hepatomegaly, and right upper quadrant abdominal pain are findings consistent with a liver or gastrointestinal system abnormality (choice (D)).

2. **(B)** Hemoglobin electrophoresis is the most sensitive method for diagnosing sickle cell disease/anemia. CBC with peripheral smear will identify anemia based on hemoglobin and hematocrit levels, but is unable to differentiate the type of hemoglobin present (choice (A)). Bone marrow biopsy is indicated if presentation is suggestive of myelodysplastic disorder such as anemia (choice (C)). Hemoglobin and hematocrit will indicate serum percentage/levels of these two components of the blood, but will not identify hemoglobin S (choice (D)).

3. **(B)** Ferritin is the storage form of iron and reflects total body iron stores. This blood component will be depleted before signs/symptoms of anemia are present. The direct Coombs test is used to detect IgG antibodies or components of the complement cascade on the surface of the red blood cell membrane (choice (A)). The direct Coombs is useful in identifying hemolytic anemia. Serum folate level reflects folic acid level present in the body and is helpful in identifying folic acid deficiency (choice (C)). The red blood cell count is the total number of red blood cells in the body and may indicate anemia, but will not differentiate the type of anemia present (choice (D)).

4. **(B)** Erythrocytosis is polycythemia vera, a condition in which all blood cell lines are overproduced, most notably red blood cells. The blood in these individuals is thick and viscous because of too many blood cells. Vomiting and diarrhea represent a risk for dehydration, which would markedly exacerbate the viscosity of the blood, leading to hypoxia of tissues. Although otherwise healthy, illnesses that could lead to dehydration should be addressed quickly. A laceration would not be cause for concern unless there were signs of infection (choice (A)). A productive cough would be indicative of a respiratory tract infection, which poses no increased risks for this patient (choice (C)). Fatigue is a generalized symptom associated with almost every illness (choice (D)). In this patient, fatigue would not be of increased concern based on his medical history.

5. **(D)** Chronic lymphocytic leukemia (CLL) is a progressive condition characterized by accumulation of mature but functionally incompetent lymphocytes. Lymphocytes are non-phagocytic white blood cells that circulate throughout the blood, lymph system, and peripheral lymphatic tissues. These cells are categorized as B and T lymphocytes and are responsible for tumor surveillance and cellular immunity. CLL occurs in older individuals and has an insidi-

ous onset with localized or generalized lymphadenopathy, splenomegaly, hepatomegaly, petechiae, and pallor. Most patients are asymptomatic and do not require treatment. The median survival time after diagnosis is 10 years; however, some patients live much longer. Chronic myelogenous leukemia (CML) has a hallmark Philadelphia chromosome, which aids in diagnosis (choice (A)). There are three clinical phases: chronic, accelerated, and blast phase. Most patients present in the chronic phase with fatigue, weight loss, night sweats, and abdominal fullness. This type of leukemia accounts for around 10–15% of adult leukemia. Acute lymphoblastic leukemia (ALL) is a malignant proliferation of immature lymphocytes and is the most common malignancy in children (choice (B)).

6. **(C)** Infants should be screened for anemia at nine months of age. This is accomplished by obtaining blood for a hemoglobin and hematocrit level. A diagnosis of anemia is considered with a hemoglobin below 11 g/dL or a hematocrit below 33%. Children who live in high altitudes have lower cutoff points for anemia. Many children are rescreened around three to four years of age.

7. **(D)** As a person ages, their normal ESR rises to a new normal. The ESR is an indicator of inflammation but is not very specific because many conditions cause an elevation (choice (B)). Inflammatory musculoskeletal conditions may cause an elevated ESR, but this is not specific for rheumatoid arthritis (choice (A)). Anemia may cause an elevated ESR. A useful test to detect pancreatic cancer (choice (C)) is the CA 19-9 blood marker, not the ESR.

8. **(A)** Medical management of osteoarthritis frequently includes the use of NSAIDs for pain control. NSAIDs may cause gastric erosions and occult gastrointestinal bleeding. This etiology should be considered for this patient. Pharmacologic therapy for hyperlipidemia (choice (B)), diabetes mellitus (choice (C)), and hypertension (choice (D)) does not carry this same risk.

9. **(C)** Leukocytosis indicates an elevated number of white blood cells are identified on the peripheral blood smear/CBC. These white blood cells become elevated with infections that are either viral or bacterial in origin, thus it is not helpful in differentiating the pathogen, making choices (A), (B), and (D) incorrect. The lymphocyte and neutrophil counts may be helpful in distinguishing the type of infection.

10. **(A)** Glossitis is an inflammation of the tongue that is often seen with pernicious anemia. With glossitis, the tongue appears beefy-red in color and often has a smooth or shiny appearance. This is not a universal finding with pernicious anemia, but if present, should raise the suspicion of the diagnosis. The other findings are not consistent with pernicious anemia.

11. **(D)** The spleen plays an active part in removing bacteria and aging RBCs from the bloodstream. A patient who has had a splenectomy will, therefore, have a higher risk for serious infection without this line of defense in place. *Streptococcus pneumoniae* is a serious pathogen that is seen in patients who are asplenic. These patients should receive the pneumococcal vaccine. Removal of the spleen is not associated with enlargement of the liver (choice (C)), hepatomegaly), does not increase bleeding risk (choice (A)), and does not contribute to more pronounced expression of anemia (choice (B)).

12. **(D)** Folic acid deficiency and B12 deficiency anemias both present with macrocytic (large) red blood cells. Thalassemia (choice (A)) and iron deficiency (choice (B)) are both microcytic (small RBC) anemias. Sickle cell anemia is diagnosed based on sickle-shaped RBCs during hypoxic crises (choice (C)).

13. **(B)** G6PD deficiency is an x-linked disorder that decreases the red blood cell's ability to neutralize oxidative stressors in the body. Foods or medications that have significant oxidative properties may initiate lysis of red blood cells in patients with this deficiency. Substances to avoid include aspirin, sulfa medications, and fava beans. Immunizations (choice (D)) and adequate hydration (choice (A)) are important but do not impact RBC lysis. There is no reason for this patient to limit consumption of iron-containing foods (choice (C)).

14. **(B)** A low hemoglobin is indicative of anemia and could cause dizziness when standing up. This patient may have an eating disorder, and this should be explored. However, the low hemoglobin should be addressed with iron supplementation if the serum ferritin level is low. A glucose of 90 (choice (C)) is normal, and a mildly elevated BUN (choice (A)) could be caused by mild dehydration. The potassium level is normal (choice (D)).

15. **(A)** Thalassemia minor is characterized by overproduction of one chain of the hemoglobin molecule. Patients with beta thalassemia usually require no specific treatment. Patients with thalassemia minor are asymptomatic and may have a mild anemia. Unless they have a coexistent IDA, they should avoid iron supplements to avoid hepatotoxicity.

10

Disorders of the Dermatologic System

The skin is the largest organ of the body, and disruption of this protective barrier can predispose the individual to more serious problems that may become systemic. Diagnosis of dermatologic disorders begins with describing the type of lesion. Morphology is an important clue to etiology; therefore, being able to correctly identify and document the presenting problem is important. Obtaining a thorough history, performing a focused physical examination, and ordering correct laboratory studies are crucial in moving from differential diagnoses to a final diagnosis and treatment plan. Nurse practitioners who work in family practice will care for individuals with dermatologic conditions on a daily basis and must become familiar with the common presentation of the most frequently encountered problems. This chapter will discuss the most common conditions presenting to primary care.

Atopic Dermatitis (AD)

Atopic dermatitis, also called eczema, is an extremely common disorder worldwide, with increasing incidence and prevalence. Onset is usually between two and six months of age (infantile eczema), and there is often a positive family history of the disorder. AD is a pruritic, xerotic (dry), or lichenified condition of the skin that occurs on the face, trunk, arms, legs, neck, antecubital fossa, and popliteal folds. Age is a consideration for affected areas. Infants will likely have involvement of the cheeks, face, upper extremities, trunk, and extensor surfaces, as well as the scalp. Presentation in adults involves lesions on the trunk and extremities. AD is part of a trio of conditions known as the "atopic triad." The other two conditions in this triad are allergic rhinitis and asthma.

Symptoms

Dry skin is often the only initial sign of eczema in infants, and more than one-third will present before three months. Infants with eczema may present with acute symptoms of intense redness and itching, with vesicles, papules, serous discharge, and crusting of affected areas. Skin will demonstrate generalized xerosis (dryness), with sparing of the diaper area. Infants and children with chronic AD will have scratch marks, flaky, rough skin, and lichenification. For adults, the presenting symptom is severe pruritus, which often develops before the rash. As with infants and children, chronic AD leads to lichenification of the skin.

Management

Management includes maintenance of skin hydration through use of emollients and avoidance of triggers. Parents are instructed to avoid daily bathing of infants with AD. Topical agents such as corticosteroids are first-line recommendations for AD management. Topical corticosteroid medications are available in different delivery vehicles (cream, ointment, gel) and potency. Low-potency medications include triamcinolone acetonide 0.025% and alclometasone 0.05%. Most patients will require management with an intermediate potency agent, such as betamethasone valerate 0.05%, 0.12%. Super high-potency topical corticosteroids include augmented betamethasone dipropionate 0.05% and clobetasol propionate 0.05%. All topical corticosteroids should be used sparingly as long-term, indiscriminate use will cause atrophy and hypopigmentation of the skin. Use of super high-potency medications in primary care should be avoided; refer patients with resistant AD to dermatology. Topical calcineurin inhibitors, tacrolimus, and pimecrolimus, used twice a day, may also be effective. Other therapies for AD include UVB light exposure and psoralen plus ultraviolet A (PUVA).

CLINICAL PEARL

Infants and children with AD are more likely to have asthma and allergic rhinitis.

Acne Vulgaris

Acne vulgaris is a common skin disorder that affects approximately 85% of the population between the ages of 10 and 25 years. Onset often coincides with or shortly follows onset of puberty. The disease ranges from very mild to severe nodulocystic acne and can greatly impact patient self-esteem.

Symptoms

Characteristic acne lesions are open and closed comedones. There may be mild tenderness, pain, or itching of lesions, which occur mainly over face, neck, upper chest, upper back, and shoulders.

Management

Management includes patient education about skin hygiene and cosmetic use. Topical retinoids (Tretinoin) are effective but may cause irritation. First-line treatment is benzoyl peroxide, which is often used in combination with other products. Moderate acne may require systemic antibiotics such as doxycycline, minocycline, trimethoprim-sulfamethoxazole, or cephalosporin until clear, and then tapering. For severe acne, referral to a dermatologist is needed. Dermatologists may prescribe isotretinoin (Accutane), which is a potentially toxic medication with teratogenic properties; pregnancy category X.

Impetigo Contagiosa

Impetigo is a common contagious, autoinoculable bacterial infection of the skin that affects infants and children. It is transmitted via direct and indirect contact and is more common in the summer and with crowded living conditions. There are two forms: bullous and nonbullous impetigo.

Symptoms

Bullous impetigo is caused by *Staphylococcus aureus* and presents with superficial blisters that coalesce to form bullae. These bullae rupture with resultant moist, inflamed, honey-colored crusts. The nonbullous form is caused by *Staph aureus*, *Streptococcus pyogenes*, or a combination of both pathogens. Lesions begin as small vesicles with honey-colored serum. Yellow-brown crusts form when vesicles rupture and a honey-colored crust is present.

Management

Management includes topical mupirocin, topical fusidic acid, or oral antibiotics for more severe cases.

Candidiasis

Candida albicans is a ubiquitous organism normally present on the skin. Candidiasis represents an overgrowth of this fungal organism, causing pathology. Candidiasis may affect the skin and/or mucosa of the body. Conditions that impair the body's natural immune system predispose individuals to the development of candidiasis. Other conditions in which candidiasis is seen more frequently include pregnancy, diabetes mellitus, and obesity, and it is also frequently seen in individuals who are taking systemic corticosteroids. Severe candidiasis is often the presenting illness in HIV infection.

Symptoms

Candidiasis often presents with intense itching and an erythematous rash in body folds such as the groin, gluteal cleft, beneath the breasts, in vulvar and anal areas and the umbilicus. The rash is beefy red with denuded areas and satellite lesions; mucous membrane involvement appears as white, curd-like patches on mucosa. Lab findings: clusters of budding yeast and hyphae seen under microscope with 10% KOH solution. Systemic disease may occur in individuals who are immunocompromised.

Management

Keep affected areas dry with exposure to air as much as possible. Nystatin or clotrimazole topical agents are usually first-line agents. Gentian violet solution or oral nystatin is used for mucocutaneous areas. Severe, widespread disease may require oral fluconazole. Patients with widespread disease should be referred.

Tinea

Dermatophytosis, or tinea, causes superficial skin infections. Three fungal infections are primarily responsible: *Trichophyton*, *Epidermophyton*, and *Microsporum*. The organism is transmitted through contact with an infected person or animal (dog or cat). Fungal spores in soil may also cause a tinea infection if the individual comes into contact. Tineas affect most parts of the body and are classified according to location. Tinea capitis affects the scalp and may become serious in children. Tinea corporis, or ringworm, affects the body. Tinea cruris is ringworm of the groin area and is often called "jock itch." Tinea pedis affects the feet, while tinea versicolor is development of hypopigmented or hyperpigmented areas and occurs most often in the summer. Tinea unguium is also called onychomycosis and affects the nails.

Symptoms

Tinea capitis is usually found in a toddler or school-age child. The parent usually reports a bald spot on the scalp. If the condition is severe, a kerion may develop, which is an inflamed, boggy infected lesion, which may involve a large portion of the scalp. This area is tender and requires treatment with griseofulvin for eradication. The patient with tinea corporis will present with an area of redness and induration, often in a circular pattern with central clearing (ringworm). Tinea cruris presents as a red, pruritic rash in the groin area and occurs most commonly on individuals who are obese. Tinea pedis (athlete's foot) usually affects males in their teen years. There will be a strong foot odor and reddened macerated areas between the toes. Tinea versicolor is completely painless and is often found incidentally as a hypopigmented or hyperpigmented area of skin.

Management

Management of most types of tinea begins with topical treatment with an "azole" type medication. Miconazole 2% cream is used for tinea pedis, cruris, and corporis. Clotrimazole 1% is effective for tinea pedis, cruris, and corporis. Treatment is often for four weeks. Development of a kerion requires oral griseofulvin, although many tinea strains are becoming resistant. Liver function and renal function studies should be performed prior to starting griseofulvin.

Scabies

Scabies is a highly contagious skin infection caused by *Sarcoptes scabiei* itch mites and is usually seen in individuals with crowded living conditions, in long-term care facilities, or in hospitals. Facility-associated disease is increasing in incidence. Index patients are usually immunosuppressed and/or elderly. Scabies is transmitted through close physical contact and through shared bedding and linens.

Symptoms

Patients with scabies present with severe, generalized itching. Vesicles, burrows, and pustules may be seen within finger web spaces and wrist creases. The head, neck, and face are usually spared. Red papules or nodules present on the scrotum and penis are pathognomonic.

Management

Management is with permethrin 5% cream applied from the neck down and left on for 8–12 hours before showering. Repeat treatment in one week. Bedding and clothing should be laundered or cleaned and placed in a plastic bag for 14 days. All household members should be treated at the same time. Triamcinolone cream 1% may be used for persistent itching.

Pediculosis (Lice)

Pediculosis is a parasitic infection of the scalp, trunk, or pubic areas. There are three different varieties of lice that cause infestation: *Pediculosis pubis* (genital area), *Pediculosis corporis* (body), and *Pediculosis capitis* (head lice).

Symptoms

Patients present with severe itching and multiple excoriated areas from scratching. Nits may be seen on the hair shaft, with actual lice seen on the scalp, skin, or clothes.

Management

Dispose of infested clothing or launder in very hot water.

Pubic lice: Treated with permethrin 1% rinse applied for 10 minutes and permethrin cream 5% left on for eight hours.
Scalp: Permethrin 1% cream rinse (Nix) application applied to scalp and left on for eight hours. Resistance to permethrin is increasing. Malathion lotion 1% (Ovide) is another treatment option; however, the product is highly flammable and application must be done in a well-ventilated area.

Rosacea

Rosacea is a chronic dermatologic condition that is characterized by facial erythema and maculopapular lesions. The cause is unknown; however, the underlying pathophysiology is one of inflammation instead of infection. There are three components to the disorder: a vascular component, which causes persistent erythema of affected areas; a recurrent acneiform component, promoting development of acneiform erythematous papules and pustules around the central facial area; and a connective tissue hyperplasia component, which causes sebaceous gland hyperplasia, especially of the nose (rhinophyma). Women are affected more frequently than men; however, men have more severe symptoms. Peak incidence of rosacea is from the fourth to the seventh decade of life. The disease is characterized by exacerbations and periods of inactivity. Risk factors include family history, temperature extremes, sunburn, stress, alcohol, caffeine intake, foods high in histamine (red wine, aged cheese, beer), and medications such as tretinoin and isotretinoin.

Symptoms

Rosacea typically begins as redness of the forehead, cheeks, nose, or chin. It also occasionally affects the ears, neck, chest area, or scalp. Patients usually do not seek care because they believe the lesions are acne. Characterized by papules, pustules, telangiectasia, rhinophyma (thickened skin of the nose), and red, irritated eyes. Ocular rosacea may cause watery, irritated, red eyes.

Management

Moderate to severe cases should be treated with antibiotic therapy, such as oral tetracycline and topic metronidazole. Lifelong treatment is required.

Cellulitis/Erysipelas

Cellulitis and erysipelas are skin infections affecting deeper skin tissues. Bacterial pathogens invade the skin or are transmitted from localized infections within the body. Erysipelas affects upper dermatologic skin layers and superficial lymph nodes. Cellulitis causes infection within deeper skin layers and subcutaneous fat. Cellulitis is seen more frequently in adults, whereas erysipelas commonly affects children and older adults from 60 to 80 years of age. Risk factors include immunosuppression, diabetes mellitus, insect bites, tattoos, piercings, eczema, psoriasis, obesity, edema, chemotherapy, pregnancy, and recent Strep pharyngitis.

Symptoms

Erysipelas often affects the face, whereas cellulitis is seen as an area of bright red, shiny skin that is warm to the touch and is edematous and often involves the lower legs. There is no clear line of demarcation within the affected area. Patients will complain of malaise and fatigue. Presentation of erysipelas involves acute onset of fever, chills, nausea, and vomiting within the first 48 hours of pathogen invasion, and the rash will have a clear line of demarcation. Cellulitis has a slower onset of symptoms with a more localized area of involvement. Lymphadenopathy is seen with both disorders. Desquamation of skin occurs in the resolving stages of both disorders. Cellulitis and erysipelas may spread rapidly to deeper tissues and enter the lymphatic system. This may lead to septicemia with a high mortality rate.

Management

Management includes oral or IV antibiotics and hospitalization for severe illness. Penicillin is the first-line agent of choice, although erythromycin or clindamycin are acceptable if the patient is unable to take penicillin.

Contact Dermatitis

Contact dermatitis represents an inflammatory response of the skin in response to antigen exposure systemically or via the skin. If this is a second or subsequent exposure to the allergen, the illness is called allergic contact dermatitis (ACD). If there is an immediate response to an initial exposure to an allergen, the condition is called irritant contact dermatitis (ICD).

Symptoms

ACD presents as a pruritic rash at the site of exposure with erythema, papules, vesicles, and bullae. Lesions appear one to two days after exposure and may last for up to one month. ICD presents as a dry, red, rough area of skin. Lesions may look like a burn injury and the area is more irritated than pruritic.

Management

Management involves identification of the trigger/allergen and avoidance. For mild to moderate presentation, topical corticosteroids are first-line, and cool compresses and oral

CLINICAL PEARL

Butterfly rash over the cheeks or ears seen with erysipelas is called the Milian's ear sign.

CLINICAL PEARL

Patients with erysipelas should be referred to the ED immediately for management. Rapid progression may lead to death!

diphenhydramine are recommended for itching at night. Severe reaction requires systemic corticosteroid along with a topical steroid. Tacrolimus or pimecrolimus may be added on if needed.

Psoriasis

Psoriasis is a chronic skin condition that is immune-mediated and characterized by erythematous areas with silvery scales, patches, and plaques. These lesions are often painful and pruritic. Psoriasis commonly presents between the ages of 15 and 25 years but affects all age groups. The hallmark of psoriasis is accelerated skin turnover with plaque accumulation on the skin surface. Risk factors include ulcerative colitis, Crohn's disease, family history, alcohol use, stress, and medications such as NSAIDs, beta blockers, and lithium.

Symptoms

Patients with psoriasis vulgaris present with silvery plaques on elbows, knees, back, and scalp. Pustular psoriasis presents with raised, pustular lesions. Psoriatic erythroderma involves plaque formation over much of the body, usually an exacerbation of psoriasis vulgaris. Psoriasis, although a skin condition, also causes psoriatic arthritis with painful joint inflammation. Approximately 30% of individuals with psoriasis vulgaris will develop psoriatic arthritis.

Management

Management includes moisturizers that are scale-lifting agents containing salicylic acid, as well as calamine and corticosteroid lotions/creams to reduce itching. Severe psoriasis should be referred to dermatology.

Herpes Simplex Virus (HSV)

Herpes simplex infections are caused by two different viruses: HSV1 and HSV2. Historically, HSV1 has been associated with oral infections, whereas HSV2 causes genital infections. HSV1 genital infections are becoming more common, and HSV2 oral lesions are also becoming more common, most likely based on changing sexual practices.

Symptoms

Oral-labial herpes presents as herpetic gingivostomatitis in children and young adults with fever, sore throat, and painful vesicles on tongue, palate, gingiva, buccal mucosa, and lips. Lesions of HSV are typically vesicular clusters with an erythematous base; as vesicles rupture, scabbing occurs. No cure exists for HSV; recurrences are usually milder than initial episodes.

CLINICAL PEARL

Vesicular lesions on the face or near the eyes (herpetic conjunctivitis) requires an emergent referral for ophthalmologic evaluation as blindness may result from ocular involvement.

Management

Therapy is supportive and symptom driven. Goal is to reduce or eliminate pain, decrease viral shedding, heal affected lesions, and prevent complications. Oral antiviral medications are first-line therapy. Valacyclovir and famciclovir require less frequent dosing and have better bioavailability than other antivirals. Treatment may be episodic or suppressive.

Herpes Zoster Virus (HZV): Shingles

Varicella zoster (herpes zoster) viral infection is a reactivation of latent varicella zoster virus in the dorsal root ganglia. This viral reactivation produces a painful vesicular rash along one dermatome of the body. Shingles mainly affects older adults who have had chickenpox as a child. Risk factors include immunosuppression, physical trauma, and increasing age.

Symptoms

Shingles presents with a prodrome of pain, burning, tingling, or numbness of a focal area of skin. Rash appears days to weeks after pain begins. Rash is unilateral consisting of vesicular lesions that coalesce. Clear fluid in vesicles becomes cloudy after several days, and vesicles rupture and crust over. Rash causes severe, sharp, stinging pain that resolves in two to four weeks.

Management

The zoster vaccine is considered the first line of defense. Shingrix vaccinations after age 50 are available for all adults. Antiviral medications are given to reduce severity and duration of illness. They are given for 7–10 days and should be started within 72 hours of symptom onset.

Actinic Keratosis

Actinic keratosis is a common premalignant skin lesion that is found in persons with light complexions. These lesions are also known as solar lentigines or solar keratoses. Actinic keratosis occurs on sun-exposed areas of the body and, if left untreated, can progress to squamous cell carcinoma.

Symptoms

Patients will often complain of a scaly rash or irritated area of skin. Pruritus, tenderness, or stinging may be present. Most lesions are asymptomatic. Lesions appear as scaly, reddened papules approximately 0.2–5 mm in diameter with a rough, uneven surface (sandpaper texture). Most common sites are the face, ears, neck, neckline, backs of arms, and backs of legs (in women).

Management

Removal is controversial as a means to prevent cancer. Refer to dermatology for evaluation.

Skin Cancer

Basal Cell Carcinoma (BCC)

Basal cell carcinoma is the most common skin cancer in the United States with over two million individuals diagnosed annually. Basal cell carcinomas have the propensity to invade deeper tissues, causing significant tissue destruction if untreated.

Symptoms

These lesions are slow-growing papules with a pearly, nodular appearance with telangiectasias. Eighty percent are found on the head and neck and often look like ulcerated lesions that do not heal.

Management

Refer to dermatology for management. Mohs surgery, which is the removal of the tumor followed by immediate frozen section with evaluation of tissue margins and subsequent re-excision if indicated, has cure rates of around 98%.

> **CLINICAL PEARL**
>
> Herpes zoster ophthalmicus, lesions around or near the eye, requires emergency referral!

Squamous Cell Carcinoma (SCC)

Squamous cell carcinoma occurs in areas of prolonged sun exposure and appears as rough, pink patches of skin that may appear suddenly or develop from actinic keratoses. SCC of the ear, lip, temple, oral cavity, and genitalia have a higher rate of metastasis.

Symptoms

May appear as an ulcerated lesion that may bleed. These lesions have a significant risk of metastasis if not removed.

Management

Management is referral to dermatology for evaluation and treatment. Because of the propensity for metastasis, patients with SCC should be seen regularly in follow-up with examination and evaluation for lymphadenopathy.

Malignant Melanoma

Malignant melanoma is the most lethal of all skin cancers. Malignant cells arise from epidermal melanocytes, which produce melanin. Most melanomas develop from the skin; however, a few develop in the eye and rarely do not have a primary site identified. Prognostic factors for melanoma include age and gender, tumor location, and tumor thickness.

Symptoms

Patients usually report the presence of a large mole with a changing appearance. Lesions appear most often on sun-exposed areas of skin. The neck and back are common sites in men, with the legs commonly involved in women. For Asian and Black individuals, the fingers, nail beds, feet, mucous membranes, and eyes are common sites for melanoma. Lesions appear as symmetrical areas with irregular borders and color variation and a diameter of more than 6 mm. The lesion is usually elevated. Figure 10.1 and Figure 10.2 shows ABCDEs of Malignant Melanoma and examples of lesions.

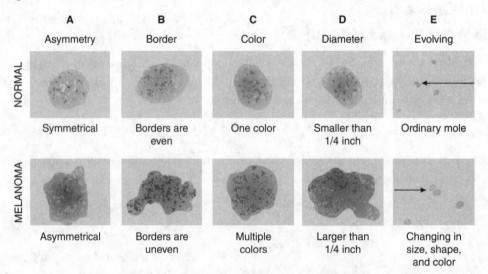

Figure 10.1. ABCDEs of Malignant Melanoma

Primary Lesions	Definition	Morphology	Examples
Macule	Flat (nonpalpable) circumscribed skin discoloration	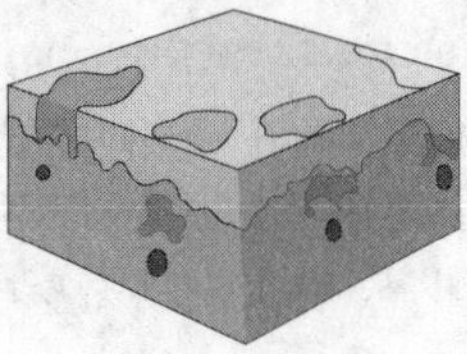	Café au lait Vitiligo Freckle Junctional nevi Ink tattoo Tinea versicolor Melasma
Patch	Large macule, ≥1 cm	Same as above	Vitiligo Nevus flammeus
Papule	Solid elevation, < 0.5 cm in diameter	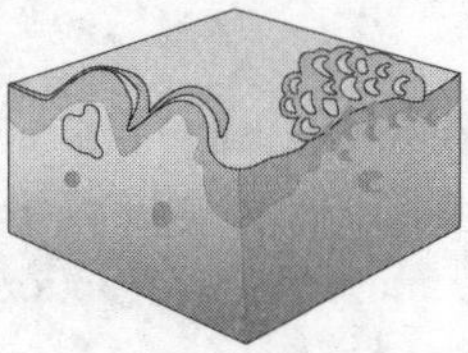	Acrochordan (skin tag) Acne Nevus Melanoma Molluscum contagiosum
Plaques	Broad papule or confluence of papules, >0.5 cm, no deep component	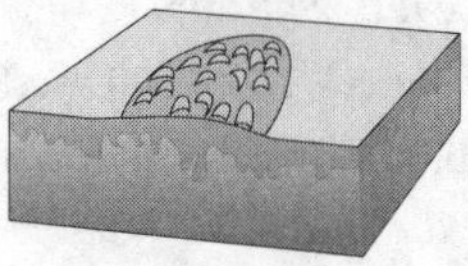	Psoriasis Eczema Tinea corporis Mycosis fungoides
Nodules	Solid elevation, >0.5 cm in diameter, larger deeper papule	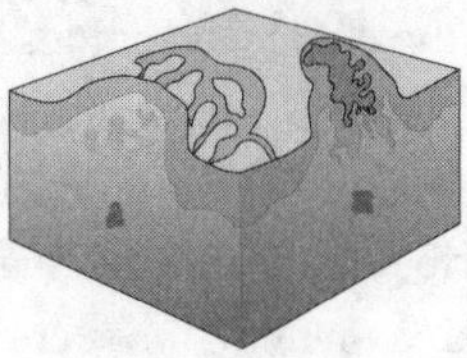	Rheumatoid nodule Xanthoma Lipoma Metastatic carcinoma Erythema nodosum
Tumors	Large nodule	Same as above	Lipomas, Melanoma, TB
Wheals	Evanescent, pruritic edematous, plaque (a hive)	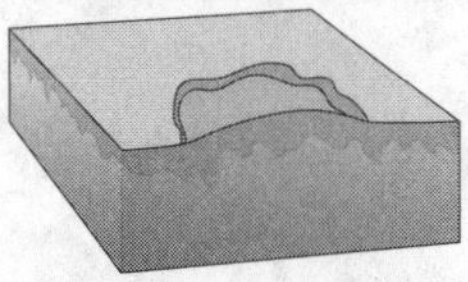	Urticaria Dermographism Urticaria Pigmentosum
Vesicle	Papule that contains clear fluid (a blister), epidermal, may be unilocular or multilocular	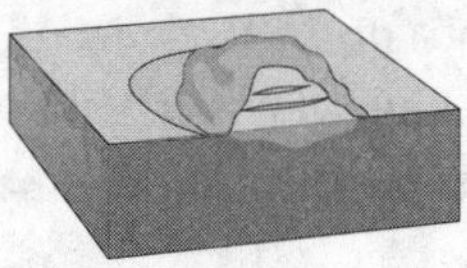	Herpes simplex Herpes Zoster Contact Dermatitis Poison Ivy Dermatitis

Figure 10.2. Examples of Lesions

Management

Referral to dermatology for evaluation, biopsy, and staging.

Practice Questions

1. Your patient is a 36-year-old male with a chief complaint of pain and swelling of his left leg. He reports that he cut his left lower leg three days ago while roofing a house. On examination, you note swelling, warmth, erythema, and tenderness over his left lower leg. The area is reddened, but there is no sharply defined border. Based on this presentation, which of the following is the likely diagnosis?

   (A) erysipelas
   (B) cellulitis
   (C) abscess
   (D) tetanus

2. A patient is brought into the urgent care clinic after being stung by a bee. The patient's mother tells you the patient is allergic to bees. The patient is wheezing slightly. What is the drug of choice for an acute anaphylactic reaction?

   (A) prednisone by mouth every 24 hours
   (B) diphenhydramine (Benadryl) 50 to 100 mg PO
   (C) epinephrine 1:10,000 0.1 mg/mL Injection, 0.3 to 0.5 mg subcutaneously
   (D) topical hydrocortisone cream

3. You are seeing a patient in the clinic who comes in with a complaint of "skin problems." The patient is a 32-year-old female who reports she has had this problem with her skin for several years, but she feels it is getting worse. On examination, you note areas of reddened papules and plaques in a circumscribed pattern. The area is slightly raised, feels rough, and has a powdery, white scale over the area on her elbows and knees. This presentation is consistent with:

   (A) eczema.
   (B) actinic keratosis.
   (C) seborrheic dermatitis.
   (D) psoriasis.

4. A female, aged 30, presents to the office with several problems. She reports fatigue for several weeks with development of a distinctive rash on her face, covering her nose and cheeks. She also reports joint pain and blurred vision. Based on her presenting history, the FNP should consider which of the following in the differential diagnosis list?

   (A) lymphoma
   (B) leukemia
   (C) rheumatoid arthritis
   (D) systemic lupus erythematosus

5. The patient is a 19-year-old male with a large carbuncle on the back of his neck. After incision and drainage of the lesion, the FNP prescribes an antibiotic. The agent should cover the most common organism associated with carbuncle development, which is:

   (A) *Staphylococcus aureus.*
   (B) *Klebsiella sp.*
   (C) actinomycosis.
   (D) *Moraxella catarrhalis.*

6. A patient presents to the clinic with concerns about a recent tick bite. He tells the FNP that he noticed a tick crawling up his leg while he was hiking in the woods yesterday. He does not know if the tick bit him, but he is worried about Lyme disease. In order for a tick to transmit Lyme disease (*Borrelia burgdorferi*), it must be attached for at least:

   (A) 8–10 hours.
   (B) 12–16 hours.
   (C) 24–48 hours.
   (D) 72 hours.

7. Rosacea is a chronic skin disorder that can significantly impact the quality of life for patients with the diagnosis. Oral antibiotic treatment has proven to be effective in reducing symptoms in some patients. All of the following agents have proven efficacy in the treatment of rosacea, EXCEPT:

   (A) levofloxacin.
   (B) metronidazole.
   (C) tetracycline.
   (D) amoxicillin.

8. Transmission of the human papilloma virus (HPV) that is responsible for nongenital warts commonly occurs via:

   (A) exposure to bodily fluids such as saliva and semen.
   (B) person-to-person contact.
   (C) respiratory droplet.
   (D) contact with contaminated surfaces.

9. Type I hypersensitivity/allergic reactions are mediated through which of the following pathways?

   (A) interleukin (IL)-10 binding to T-cells
   (B) tumor necrosis factor (TNF) alpha binding to T-cells
   (C) IgG antibodies binding to basophils
   (D) IgE antibodies binding to mast cells

10. A patient presents to the clinic with concern about a skin lesion. The patient is a 60-year-old female who reports a "bump" on the back of her leg that is slightly itchy. On examination, the FNP discovers a lesion consistent with an actinic keratosis. Which of the following descriptions is consistent with this diagnosis?

   (A) a warty-appearing growth
   (B) an asymmetrical lesion on a sun-exposed area
   (C) a reddened, scaly, rough-appearing lesion with an uneven surface
   (D) an elevated papule with crusting and a pearly appearance

11. An 11-year-old child is brought into the clinic by his dad, who reports concern about a lesion on the child's stomach. On examination of the area, the FNP finds an annular lesion with central clearing and a slightly scaly border. The patient reports the area does not itch. This finding is consistent with:

   (A) tinea corporis.
   (B) contact dermatitis.
   (C) eczema.
   (D) impetigo.

12. The topical agent permethrin (Elimite) is used in the treatment of which of the following disorders?

   (A) psoriasis
   (B) eczema
   (C) scabies
   (D) herpes simplex virus

13. The most common trigger for rosacea is:

   (A) cold weather.
   (B) perfumed lotions.
   (C) caffeine intake.
   (D) sun exposure.

14. The underlying etiology of seborrheic keratosis is likely:

   (A) dermal hyperplasia.
   (B) benign proliferation of immature keratinocytes.
   (C) nevus transformation.
   (D) lichenification of epidermal tissue.

15. Your patient is a 15-year-old female with a chief complaint of "itchy" lesions that come and go on her upper thighs. She reports that when she gets cold or goes swimming, they get worse. Based on this history, the FNP gives a diagnosis of benign urticaria. Which class of medications would be appropriate for this patient?

   (A) NSAIDs
   (B) benzodiazepines
   (C) topical metronidazole
   (D) oral antihistamines

Answer Explanations

1. **(B)** Cellulitis presents as an infection of the epidermis and subcutaneous tissue as a result of bacterial invasion, usually through a break in the skin. Characteristically, cellulitis presents as a painful, swollen, warm, reddened area without sharp borders indicating where the infection stops. Erysipelas is also a dermatologic infection; however, the patient often has signs of systemic toxicity, and the involved area is red, raised, swollen, and hot to the touch (choice (A)). The borders are circumscribed, meaning they clearly define the involved area of infection. An abscess (furuncle or boil) is a localized inflammatory area that is the result of a more deep-seated infection, usually by *Staphylococcus aureus* (choice (C)). These lesions drain pus and are autoinoculable, meaning the patient can spread the infection to other areas. A carbuncle is an area consisting of several abscesses that have merged together. Tetanus is a systemic infection caused by neurotoxin *C. tetani* (choice (D)). There is a history of a wound and possible contamination of the wound by the organism. Signs of tetanus include stiffness of the jaw with muscle spasms and convulsions. This is a fatal illness and can be prevented by immunization with tetanus toxoid.

2. **(C)** Treatment for an acute anaphylactic reaction is epinephrine administered subcutaneously. Anaphylaxis is a rapidly lethal allergic reaction requiring emergent management. A patient who presents to an outpatient clinic with developing anaphylaxis should be given epinephrine and immediately transported to an emergency department. Prednisone is a medication that modulates immune response but does not prevent anaphylaxis from progressing (choice (A)). An oral dose would not be appropriate for any medication in this situation. Diphenhydramine IV is a second-line drug for anaphylaxis management (choice (B)). The PO form works well as an antihistamine but should not be used in this scenario. Topical hydrocortisone cream works well for mild dermatologic reactions and rashes (choice (D)). This medication works well to decrease pruritus and promote resolution but is not applicable during an anaphylactic reaction.

3. **(D)** Psoriasis is a chronic, recurring skin disorder that is characterized by the presence of silvery scales on bright red, well-circumscribed plaques and occurs often on the knees and elbows. Psoriasis is made worse by obesity, and individuals with psoriasis who lose weight may see a significant clearing in the disease. Eczema is also called atopic dermatitis and presents as an itchy, dry eruption that occurs on the face, neck, trunk, hands and wrists, and in the antecubital and popliteal folds (choice (A)). Eczema usually has its onset in childhood and may improve as the patient becomes an adult. A family history of atopic (or allergic) disorders is common. Actinic keratoses are small papules or macules that are usually flesh-colored or pale pink and occur on parts of the body that have had extensive sun exposure (choice (B)). These lesions feel rough, like sandpaper, to palpation and are considered premalignant. Therefore, they are usually ablated with liquid nitrogen or excised. Seborrheic dermatitis is a disorder that may be acute or chronic and presents with dry scales with underlying redness (choice (C)). Seborrheic dermatitis usually occurs on the scalp, central facial area, umbilicus, body folds, presternal area, and behind the ears.

4. **(D)** Systemic lupus erythematosus (SLE) presents predominantly in young adult women. Findings of a butterfly (malar) rash over the nose and cheeks along with joint pain is characteristic of SLE. The rash is composed of red papules and plaques with a fine scale overlying the area. In the acute phase of the disease, the patient often reports a fever and feeling ill. Other symptoms that are pathognomonic for SLE include transient or permanent episodes of monocular blindness and a rash over sun-exposed areas. SLE is an inflammatory autoim-

mune disorder in which autoantibodies attack nuclear antigens, causing widespread pathology affecting many body systems, including the central nervous system, renal system, and hematologic system. Lymphoma is a cancer affecting the lymphocytes and may progress rapidly or slowly (choice (A)). The patient with lymphoma often presents with painless lymphadenopathy, and the diagnosis is confirmed through tissue biopsy. The leukemias are a group of cancers that affect the leukocytes (white blood cells) and may present with fever, fatigue, and bleeding abnormalities (choice (B)). These cancers affect the bone marrow production of cell lines and have varied presentation based on the type of leukemia. Rheumatoid arthritis is a chronic, systemic, inflammatory disorder that manifests as synovitis of multiple joints (choice (C)). Presentation is usually insidious with prolonged morning stiffness and symmetric polyarthritis. Rheumatoid factor (RF) and antibodies to cyclic citrullinated peptides (anti-CCP) are present in the majority of patients with rheumatoid arthritis.

5. **(A)** The most common organism responsible for the development of dermatologic infections, such as furuncles and carbuncles, is *Staphylococcus aureus*. Other common organisms associated with these types of lesions are *Escherichia coli*, *Pseudomonas aeruginosa*, and *Streptococcus faecalis*. Systemic antibiotic therapy is indicated in the setting of carbuncles, which are a large collection of furuncles. *Klebsiella* is a Gram-negative diplococcus that is responsible for several respiratory infections, including pneumonia (choice (B)). Actinomycosis is a chronic bacterial disorder that affects the jaw, thorax, or abdomen (choice (C)). This disease causes the formation of deep, lumpy abscesses that develop numerous sinus tracts. *Moraxella catarrhalis* is an aerobic bacterium that is present in the nasopharynx (choice (D)). *Moraxella* is a major cause of ear infections in infants and children and is also associated with respiratory illnesses.

6. **(C)** Lyme disease is a tick-borne illness caused by the spirochete *B. burgdorferi*. There is a geographic distribution for the disease; however, this seems to be expanding in recent years as the disease has been identified in new areas of the country. Research has demonstrated that in order to transmit the infection to a human, the tick needs to be attached for at least 24 to 48 hours. Lyme disease is characterized by the development of erythema migrans, a bulls-eye rash occurring within days to weeks of the bite. The transmitting tick is very small, and a bite may go unnoticed, thus history of activities is an important component of assessment for Lyme disease. The disease has three stages: early localized, early disseminated, and late persistent infection.

7. **(A)** Rosacea is a common dermatologic disorder presenting in adults that affects the face. The characteristic appearance of erythema, telangiectasia, and an acneiform rash is a classic presentation. Patients with rosacea often report flushing, and worsening of the rash is triggered by exposure to sunlight, heat, spicy foods or drink, exercise, and alcohol. Treatment includes consistent use of sunscreen, avoidance of triggers, and metronidazole gel (choice (B)) applied topically. Oral antibiotics are used when topical therapy is ineffective. Antibiotics with proven efficacy in the treatment of rosacea include tetracycline (choice (C)), metronidazole (choice (B)), amoxicillin (choice (D)), or rifaximin. Levofloxacin is a fluoroquinolone agent used in the treatment of acute sinusitis, community-acquired pneumonia, complicated urinary tract infections, and acute pyelonephritis.

8. **(B)** Transmission of the HPVs responsible for nongenital warts (HPV types 1, 2, and 4) occurs mainly through person-to-person contact. These HPV types are not spread via contact with body fluids (choice (A)), respiratory droplets (choice (C)), or contaminated surfaces (choice (D)). The HPV types associated with anogenital warts include 6, 11, 16, 18, 31, 33, 45,

52, and 58. Vaccines are available to prevent infection with HPV types associated with the development of anogenital disease and are recommended for boys and girls.

9. **(D)** Type I hypersensitivity reactions occur within minutes of exposure to an antigen. The antigen links adjacent IgE molecules together, which activates and degranulates mast cells. Clinical manifestations of this type of reaction are a result of this mast cell degranulation. Type 2 reactions involve the activation of antigen-specific IgM and IgG immunoglobulins, which bind to foreign antigens and activate serum immune complements, which destroy cells with the antibody-antigen complex. Type 2 reactions are, thus, cytotoxic. Type 3 reactions also require activation of IgM and IgG gamma globulins. Complexes form between the gamma globulin and the antigen, and these complexes are deposited into various tissues of the body. This deposition triggers an inflammatory mediator response, which affects many organs and tissues throughout the body. Type 4 reactions are delayed responses that are T-cell dependent and begin in the skin. An example of a Type 4 reaction is dermatitis associated with poison ivy exposure. Choices (A), (B), and (C) are not the correct pathways.

10. **(C)** Actinic keratosis is the most common premalignant lesion found in light-skinned individuals. These lesions appear as reddened, scaly, and rough, with an uneven appearance. When palpated, they often have a sandpaper-like texture. A warty-appearing growth is characteristic of seborrheic keratosis (choice (A)). An asymmetrical lesion on a sun-exposed area is typical of a malignant melanoma (choice (B)). An elevated papule with a crusty, pearly-appearing surface is a basal cell carcinoma (choice (D)).

11. **(A)** A finding of an annular lesion with central clearing and a scaly border describes tinea corporis, which is caused by a *Microsporum* infection, usually *Trichophyton rubrum*. This benign skin infection is often transmitted by a pet. Diagnosis can be made clinically and by examining a scraping of skin under a microscope using a KOH preparation. Contact dermatitis may be irritant or allergic and is an acute or chronic skin condition resulting from direct contact with an irritant or an allergen (choice (B)). The lesions are erythematous with vesicles, bullae, and weeping or crusting. These areas are usually pruritic, and the patient often has a history of previous contact with the antigen. Eczema is an atopic skin condition with distinct presentations in individuals of different ages and races (choice (C)). Diagnostic criteria for atopic dermatitis (eczema) include pruritus, typical lesion morphology and distribution, onset in childhood, and chronicity. Poorly defined scaly, red plaques are seen on the face, neck, and flexural surfaces and upper trunk areas. In chronic cases, the skin becomes lichenified from persistent scratching and irritation. Impetigo is a contagious infection of the skin caused by *Staphylococcus* and/or *Streptococcus* found mainly in young children (choice (D)). The lesions appear as superficial blisters filled with purulent material. The blisters break and a classic "honey-colored" scab forms.

12. **(C)** Permethrin is a topical medication used in the treatment of scabies. Scabies is caused by the *Sarcoptes scabiei* mite and is transmitted from person to person through close physical contact with an infected person. Scabies may also be acquired by sharing bedding, linens, etc., with an infected individual. This disorder causes intense itching and causes generalized excoriations with small vesicles or "burrows" on the skin. Treatment goals are to kill all mites and control the dermatitis. Permethrin 5% cream is very effective and is applied from the neck down and left on for 8–12 hours, then showered off. Treatment often needs to be repeated in one week, and all linens, etc., must be treated as well. All household members should be treated. Permethrin is not used in the treatment of psoriasis (choice (A)), eczema (choice (B)), or herpes simplex virus infection (choice (D)).

13. **(D)** The most common trigger for rosacea is sun exposure. Other common triggers include spicy or hot foods, alcohol intake, and hot weather. Identifying and avoiding triggers is an important component of disease management. Choices (A), (B), and (C) are not triggering factors for rosacea.

14. **(B)** Seborrheic keratoses are benign growths with a warty appearance occurring on the trunk as well as the face and hands. They are seen commonly in older adults. Seborrheic lesions develop from the horny layer of the epidermis and result from proliferation of immature keratinocytes. These lesions are not considered premalignant but have some association with the presence of skin cancer, such as basal cell carcinomas occurring at other sites.

15. **(D)** Urticaria is characterized by eruptions of wheals or hives in response to various stimuli. Intense pruritus is usually a component of the condition but, in rare cases, may be absent. Special forms of urticaria have unique characteristics, such as dermatographism, cholinergic urticaria, solar urticaria, and cold urticaria. Treatment of choice for urticaria is antihistamines. Identification of triggers is an important part of management of the disorder. The other choices are not medications that would be used to treat benign urticaria.

PART II
Reproduction

11

Men's Health Issues

The average life expectancy of a man has increased due to the advancement of medical knowledge, the advent of health care screening and treatment technology, and the increasing emphasis on preventative care in our society. When discussing men's health issues, male patients may prefer to seek male family nurse practitioners (FNPs) to address any concerns they may have. Unfortunately, the preferred provider may not be an option. Therefore, all FNPs should be comfortable and competent in addressing men's health issues.

Impotence

Impotence is the inability of an adult male to achieve or sustain an erection and may be caused by psychological factors (functional) or vascular, neuro, endocrine, or anatomical abnormalities (organic). Impotence can be caused by a variety of issues. It could be due to the presence of chronic diseases, injury, drug side effects, lack of sexual desire, lack of orgasms, issues involving problems with ejaculation, and the impairment of blood flow within the penile organ nerves. Loss of libido could be due to an androgen deficiency from either dysfunction of the pituitary gland or testicular disease. The condition may be verified via serum testosterone level, gonadotropin levels, and thyroid-stimulating hormone (TSH) testing. Testosterone level testing should be performed in the early morning.

Erectile Dysfunction (ED)

Erectile dysfunction is the inability to maintain an erection sufficient for sexual intercourse. Incidence of ED increases with age: At 40 years old, the rate is 5%; at 65 years old, the rate is 15–25%. Other risk factors include diabetes mellitus, hypertension, chronic alcohol and tobacco use, and neuropathy. Patients with ED may be reluctant to discuss the problem with the FNP. However, most men eventually verbalize their problem, and the FNP should routinely ask patients about this common problem.

Symptoms

The main symptom is a man's inability to get or keep an erection firm enough for sexual intercourse.

Management

Management of ED begins with treating or minimizing underlying causes such as uncontrolled blood sugar or hypertension, and it often includes pharmacologic agents. Different classifications of ED drugs are widely available, although there is little difference in the efficacy of the medications. However, some may have a longer duration of action (half-life). For example: tadalafil (Cialis) has a longer half-life than sildenafil (Viagra). One common side effect associated with both medications is hypotension, and a longer half-life could result in longer side effects of hypotension. These medications are taken as needed prior to sexual activity.

Testicular Torsion

Testicular torsion is a twisting or rotation of the testes within the scrotum and is a urological emergency. The condition occurs most often in school-age males, and the left testicle is affected more than the right.

Symptoms

Assessment may reveal unilateral pain in the scrotum, swelling in the testicles, and the lack of cremasteric reflex. Elevation of the scrotum does not relieve the pain.

Management

Patients suspected for testicular torsion require an **immediate testicular ultrasound**. If an ultrasound cannot be obtained, the FNP should immediately **refer the patient to the emergency department**.

Hydrocele

Hydrocele is a swelling in the scrotum or inguinal canal and is usually painless. A transilluminated assessment with a pen light in a dark room may reveal trapped fluid that appears pink, yellow, or red in the scrotum area. Hydrocele is a benign, self-limiting condition that resolves on its own and is not an emergency.

Varicocele

Varicocele is a painful condition involving the scrotal vessels. A varicocele occurs when blood backs up in the main veins that drain the scrotum. The condition is most noticeable when the patient is standing. A dilated spermatic vein is noted within the scrotum. Obesity predisposes an individual for the development of a varicocele.

Symptoms

Assessment findings may include soft and movable blood vessels that feel like a "bag of worms" under the scrotal skin.

Management

Treatment is symptomatic, such as scrotal support. Although varicocele is a non-emergent condition, prolonged edema may decrease sperm count.

Benign Prostatic Hyperplasia (BPH)

Benign prostatic hyperplasia is a condition in which there is a nonmalignant enlargement of the prostate gland. Incidence of BPH increases with age: At 50 years old, the rate is 50%; at 70 years old and older, the rate is 80%.

Symptoms

Presenting symptoms include increased frequency of voiding due to feeling of constriction, incomplete emptying, and post void dribbling of urine. Medications and substances that may exacerbate symptoms include over-the-counter cold and allergy medications and antihistamines, as well as caffeine. On examination, the prostate will feel firm and will be uniformly enlarged. Serum prostate-specific antigen (PSA) is commonly used to evaluate for the presence of BPH. A PSA elevation of less than 10 ng/mL is indicative of BPH. An elevation of greater than 10 ng/mL requires urology evaluation to rule out prostate cancer.

Management

Treatment includes tamsulosin (Flomax), finasteride (Proscar), dutasteride (Avodart), and tadalafil (Cialis).

CLINICAL PEARL

Urologist detorsion of the organ and the restoration of testicular blood flow is crucial within the first six hours or testicle loss will occur.

CLINICAL PEARL

Tadalafil (Cialis) is approved for benign BPH, but it is also commonly prescribed for treating erectile dysfunction. Do not prescribe tadalafil for patients taking nitrates or a combination of other alpha blocker medications.

Bacterial Prostatitis

In general, acute bacterial prostatitis is caused by Gram-negative bacteria (*E. coli, Pseudomonas*). It is prevalent among elderly men. In populations 35 years and under, it is usually caused by sexually transmitted infections such as gonorrhea or chlamydia. For age groups over 35 years and older, including men who have sex with men, Gram-negative *Enterobacteriaceae* is a more common etiology. Risk factors include a history of prostatitis, use of urinary catheter, a history of urethral or bladder infections, and dehydration.

Symptoms

Symptoms include difficulty in starting the urine stream, inability to empty the bladder (resulting in frequent bathroom visits), weak urine stream, the urge to frequently stop and restart the stream, and episodes of urine leakage.

Management

Treatment for acute bacterial prostatitis is similar to treatment for acute pyelonephritis. Treatment for men younger than 35 is single dose intramuscular (IM) ceftriaxone followed by oral doxycycline. When treating men 35 and older, a higher dose ciprofloxacin or levofloxacin.

Prostate Cancer

Prostate cancer is the most commonly reported cancer in American men, second in the number of cancer deaths. Risk factors include an age greater than 50, a positive family history, obesity, African American ethnicity, and avid long-hour cycling. The prostate is palpable via digital rectal examination (DRE). The prostate gland is 2–3 cm across, soft, smooth, and symmetrical. Findings of a painless hard nodule require further evaluation. A prostate-specific antigen (PSA) level greater than 4.0 ng/mL requires consultation with a urologist. Routine DRE and PSA testing for patients with limited life span (ten years or less) is not recommended by the United States Preventative Task Force (USPTF).

Priapism

Priapism is a prolonged (ranges from two to four hours or more) and painful erection of the penis due to adverse effects from medication (or intentional overdoses on phosphodiesterase-5 inhibitors: sildenafil, vardenafil, avanafil, and tadalafil), illicit drug use, or sickle cell disease. Do not initiate any treatment for priapism in primary care. **Refer the patient to the emergency department as soon as possible.**

Epididymitis

Epididymitis is an inflammation of the epididymis that often results from bacterial pathogens moving up from the urethra or from the prostate gland. In children, this condition often results from direct trauma to the scrotum, torsion of the appendix epididymis, or reflux of urine into the epididymis. In individuals younger than 35 years, the most common pathogens are *Chlamydia trachomatis* or *Neisseria gonorrhoeae*. For men older than 35 years, the inflammation is usually the result of infiltration by *E. coli* or *Enterococcus*. For all men who practice anal intercourse, the most common organisms are enteric pathogens such as *E. coli*. The presence of a urinary tract infection (UTI) may also lead to epididymitis through migration of bacteria from the bladder.

CLINICAL PEARL

The use of fluoroquinolone has been linked to tendon disorders especially in patients over the age of 60 who are concurrently taking steroids (corticosteroids) or in those who have undergone a kidney, heart, or lung transplant.

CLINICAL PEARL

Prostate-specific antigen, or PSA, is a protein produced by normal, as well as malignant, cells of the prostate gland. A PSA value should serve as a historical note for baseline comparison and should not be used to rule out prostate cancer.

Symptoms

Symptoms of epididymitis include fever, dysuria, and swelling of the epididymis or scrotum. When elevation of the scrotum relieves the pain, this indicates a positive Prehn's sign. Other symptoms include gradual development of scrotal pain, painful urination, fever, chills, and a positive cremasteric reflex. Younger sexually active men and older patients may be diagnosed with epididymitis caused by a sexually transmitted disease (*Chlamydia* or *Neisseria gonorrhoeae*). When this is the cause, other symptoms may include penile discharge or the presence of a lesion on the penis.

Management

Supportive management for epididymitis begins with NSAIDs for pain and discomfort. For men who practice insertive anal sex, epididymitis is often the result of infection with chlamydia or gonorrhea. In this situation, treatment includes a single dose of azithromycin (Zithromax) 1 g orally plus a single dose of ceftriaxone (Rocephin) 250 mg IM. Quinolones such as ciprofloxacin (Cipro), ofloxacin (Floxin), or levofloxacin (Levaquin) are no longer recommended for chlamydial or gonorrheal infections because of drug resistance.

For men with epididymitis resulting from a urinary tract infection, treatment options are trimethoprim-sulfamethoxazole (Bactrim or Bactrim DS) orally for 10 days, ciprofloxacin (Cipro) 500 mg twice daily for 10 days, or ofloxacin (Floxin) 300 mg twice daily for 10 days. In men 35 years old and older, acute epididymitis could be a result of secondary prostatitis caused by *Enterobacteriaceae*, such as *Salmonella, E. coli, Yersinia pestis, Klebsiella,* and *Shigella.* In this situation, treatment includes levofloxacin 500 mg once a day for 10 days or ofloxacin 300 mg twice a day for 10 days.

Chlamydia Trachomatis

CLINICAL PEARL
Patients treated for chlamydia should abstain from sexual activity for seven days after a single dose of antibiotics or until completion of a seven-day course of antibiotics to prevent spreading the infection to partners.

Chlamydia is a **reportable** sexually transmitted infection (STI) and the most prevalent sexually transmitted disease (STD) in the United States. Risk factors for males include sex with other men, multiple sex partners, and inconsistent use of condoms.

Symptoms

Symptoms include lymphadenopathy, dysuria, proctitis, epididymitis, prostatitis, and penile discharge. Differential diagnoses include gonorrhea, urinary tract infection, and trichomonas. The diagnostic gold standard is the nucleic acid amplification test (NAAT).

Management

Treatment includes azithromycin 1,000 mg orally in a single dose or doxycycline 100 mg orally twice a day for seven days. The CDC recommends annual chlamydia and gonorrhea testing in all sexually active women younger than 25 years and in older women at increased risk of infection.

Neisseria Gonorrhoeae

Gonorrhea is a **reportable** disease caused by intracellular, Gram-negative bacteria. Risk factors include unprotected sexual exposure to an infected sexual partner (vaginal/anal) and recent gonococcal infection (due to reinfection from an untreated partner).

Symptoms

Symptoms include purulent urethral discharge, penile edema, acute epididymitis, prostatitis, painful ejaculation, rectal infection (discharge), tenesmus, and rectal burning or itching.

Management

Treatment includes ceftriaxone 250 mg IM in a single dose and azithromycin 1,000 mg orally in a single dose.

Genital Herpes (HSV-2)

Approximately 15% of the adult population in the United States are seropositive for genital herpes. Less than 20% of the seropositive population have clinical signs of genital herpes. Risk factors include unprotected sex, contact with herpetic lesions, genital/mucosal secretions, the use of immunosuppressive medication, and HIV infection.

Symptoms

Symptoms include painful ulcerated genital lesions with possible inguinal lymphadenopathy, lethargy, myalgia, headache, dysuria, localized pruritus, and a burning sensation in the infected site.

Management

Treatment for genital herpes includes acyclovir 400 mg orally three times a day for 7–10 days (first clinical episode of genital herpes), acyclovir 400 mg orally three times a day for 5 days (episodic therapy for recurrent genital herpes), and 400 mg twice daily (suppressive therapy for recurrent genital herpes).

Syphilis

Syphilis is a complex **reportable** disease that often includes the involvement of multiple organ systems. The disorder is caused by infection with the spirochete *Treponema pallidum*. This organism can penetrate intact skin and mucous membranes during sexual activity. The organism then enters the bloodstream, where it is transported to other organ systems. Infection of the cerebrospinal fluid is associated with the development of neurosyphilis, which is a complication of syphilis that is often fatal. The disease is diagnosed according to organ involvement and presentation. Stages include primary, secondary, latent, and tertiary.

Symptoms

Symptoms for primary syphilis include a painless genital ulcer with a clean base, indurated margins, and localized lymphadenopathy. Symptoms for secondary syphilis include a diffuse maculopapular rash on the torso and upper and lower extremities, lethargy, and flu-like symptoms. Symptoms for late or tertiary syphilis include aortic insufficiency, seizures, mental status changes, and granulomatous lesions. Those most at risk for syphilis include men who have unprotected sex, men who use IV drugs, men who have multiple sexual partners, men who have sex with men, and men who have HIV infection or another sexually transmitted disease caused by the spirochete *Treponema pallidum*. Examples of lab testing include the rapid plasma reagin (RPR) test, venereal disease research laboratory (VDRL) test, and treponemal test.

Management

Treatment for all individuals diagnosed with syphilis includes benzathine penicillin G 2.4 million units IM in a single dose. All sexual partners should also be treated.

CLINICAL PEARL

Any child with confirmed syphilis should be reported to child protective services (CPS) for possible sexual abuse.

Human Immunodeficiency Virus (HIV) Screening/Prevention

PrEP (pre-exposure prophylaxis) is a current HIV prevention treatment via once-a-day pill regimen. This treatment is recommended for uninfected people who engage in behaviors that place them at risk for HIV exposure. However, the medication does not prevent any other STDs, and patients still need to use condoms. The standard daily dosage is Truvada, one tablet (emtricitabine 200 mg and tenofovir DF 300 mg orally once a day).

In May 2018, the Food and Drug Administration (FDA) approved Truvada PrEP for adolescents weighing more than 35 kg (the average weight of an 11-year-old).

Human immunodeficiency virus is a retrovirus that invades human CD4-T lymphocytes, causing cell death and profound immunodeficiency. Infection with HIV predisposes an individual to many opportunistic infections as well as cancer. Possible HIV symptoms include fever, chills, fatigue, mouth ulcers, rashes, Kaposi sarcoma, night sweats, myalgia, sore throat, swollen lymph nodes, and frequent oral thrush. HIV infection is the precursor to the development of acquired immunodeficiency syndrome (AIDS). HIV is a **reportable** disease. The current recommendation for HIV screening is for all patients aged 13–64 years in any health care setting. Repeat screening should be initiated for high-risk individuals (sex workers, men having sex with men, and individuals having sex with multiple partners) at least once a year.

A preferred method of HIV screening for asymptomatic patients is the fourth-generation combination HIV-1/2 immunoassay. The fourth-generation test will detect both HIV-1 and HIV-2 antibodies, as well as HIV P24 antigen. If the fourth-generation combination assay is negative, the person is considered HIV-uninfected, and no further testing is needed. However, if the fourth-generation combination assay is positive, an HIV-1/HIV-2 antibody differentiation immunoassay is performed, such as the Bio-Rad Geenius HIV 1/2 confirmatory assay or the Bio-Rad Multispot HIV-1/HIV-2 rapid test.

Chancroid

Chancroid is a sexually transmitted condition. The causative organism for chancroid is the Gram-negative bacillus *Haemophilus ducreyi*.

Symptoms

Clinical presentation for chancroid includes single or multiple painful vesicular(s) and pustular lesion(s) with a necrotic base. Inguinal lymphadenitis is also common.

Management

Treatment for chancroid is a single dose of azithromycin 1 g orally or a single dose of ceftriaxone 250 mg IM. Another treatment alternative for patients unable to take azithromycin is ciprofloxacin 500 mg twice a day for three days or erythromycin 500 mg three times a day for one week.

Patients who present with chancroid should also be tested for other STIs such as HIV, syphilis, gonorrhea, chlamydia, and hepatitis B and C.

Practice Questions

1. All of the following statements are true concerning erectile dysfunction (ED) in elderly adults, EXCEPT:

    (A) Erectile dysfunction is very common after age 70.

    (B) Tadalafil (Cialis) is significantly more effective than sildenafil (Viagra).

    (C) Erectile dysfunction may be caused by concurrent medical disorders.

    (D) Frail, elderly persons are still interested in sex.

2. All of the following are common risk factors for ED, EXCEPT:

    (A) testosterone deficiency.

    (B) a history of radical prostatectomy.

    (C) long-term tobacco use.

    (D) chronic alcohol use.

3. A 17-year-old teenager presents in the office experiencing severe scrotal pain following a direct kick in his groin area during a school fight. What is your next action?

    (A) order a STAT urine specimen

    (B) order a STAT scrotal ultrasound

    (C) encourage the patient to apply ice and elevate the affected area

    (D) refer the patient to the emergency department

4. Which of the following procedures is a common, noninvasive method to evaluate a patient with possible hydrocele?

    (A) transillumination

    (B) ultrasound

    (C) check for cremasteric reflex

    (D) palpate for tenderness

5. While teaching a 16-year-old boy how to perform a testicular self-exam, upon palpation of the scrotum you note soft and movable blood vessels similar to a "bag of worms" under the scrotal skin. There is no other sign of scrotal abnormality. What is the probable diagnosis?

    (A) hydrocele

    (B) testicular torsion

    (C) varicocele

    (D) epididymitis

6. You are reviewing a PSA report on a 64-year-old patient who had a firm, non-tender, symmetrical enlarged prostate during his wellness physical one week ago. The urinalysis is normal. His PSA is 3.9 ng/mL. What is your conclusion?

    (A) The patient may have prostate cancer.

    (B) The patient may have prostate infection.

    (C) The patient may have benign prostatic hypertrophy (BPH).

    (D) The patient is experiencing a normal aging process.

7. All of the following options are risk factors for prostate cancer EXCEPT:

    (A) aging.

    (B) having a positive family history of prostate cancer.

    (C) being obese.

    (D) occupation as a long-haul truck driver.

8. What is an appropriate treatment for a 25-year-old commercial truck driver with a diagnosis of acute bacterial prostatitis?

    (A) levofloxacin

    (B) IM ceftriaxone followed by oral doxycycline

    (C) clear fluids

    (D) cranberry juice

9. A five-year-old boy presents with his father at the clinic with complaints of scrotal pain. The family has recently returned from a camping trip. The patient's vital signs are stable, and he was able to void without any concerns. Physical examination shows a mild swollen lump noted on his left scrotum, mild tenderness on palpation, and no sign of injury or infection. An in-house urinalysis is normal. What is your diagnosis?

    (A) acute bacterial prostatitis

    (B) chronic prostatitis

    (C) epididymitis

    (D) asymptomatic bacteriuria

10. What is the preferred treatment for uncomplicated gonococcal infection for a 16-year-old male with no drug-allergy history?

    (A) amoxicillin

    (B) TMP-SMX

    (C) metronidazole

    (D) ceftriaxone IM plus azithromycin

11. Which of the following is a recommended treatment for acute epididymitis most likely caused by sexually transmitted gonorrheal and chlamydial infection in men who practice insertive anal sex?

    (A) oral azithromycin (Zithromax) and IM ceftriaxone (Rocephin)

    (B) topical clindamycin and oral tinidazole

    (C) topical metronidazole gel 0.75% and IM ceftriaxone (Rocephin)

    (D) oral doxycycline and IM penicillin

12. Which of the following is a recommended treatment for an initial genital herpes (HSV-2) episode?

    (A) abacavir (Ziagen)

    (B) acyclovir (Zovirax)

    (C) raltegravir (Isentress)

    (D) darunavir (Prezista)

13. The differential diagnosis for a 27-year-old male sex worker who presents with genital ulceration should include all of the following, EXCEPT:

    (A) syphilis.
    (B) genital herpes.
    (C) hemangioma.
    (D) chancroid.

14. A 19-year-old male who is homeless presents at your clinic inquiring about pre-exposure prophylaxis (PrEP) treatment. He is sexually active and has sex with multiple partners. The patient is tested for HIV, syphilis, gonorrhea, chlamydia, and hepatitis A, B, and C. All test results are negative. What is the appropriate next step?

    (A) prescribe dolutegravir (Tivicay) and administer a purified protein derivative (PPD) test for tuberculosis
    (B) prescribe Truvada (emtricitabine 200 mg and tenofovir DF 300 mg), with a written recommendation for condom use
    (C) refer the patient to an infectious disease specialist for evaluation
    (D) explain to the patient that he is not a candidate for pre-exposure prophylaxis (PrEP) treatment because he is homeless

15. Which of the following options is the correct causative organism for chancroid lesions?

    (A) *Haemophilus ducreyi*
    (B) *Treponema pallidum*
    (C) *Neisseria gonorrhoeae*
    (D) *Mycoplasma genitalium*

Answer Explanations

1. **(B)** Tadalafil and sildenafil are both prescribed for treatment of erectile dysfunction. Both medications are equally effective, making choice (B) false and therefore the correct answer. The major difference between the two medications is that tadalafil has a longer half-life than sildenafil. A common side effect associated with both medications is hypotension. This effect may last longer with tadalafil than with sildenafil. Contraindications for this class of medications include the concomitant administration of nitrates or alpha blockers, as these drugs may potentiate the hypotensive effect. By age 70, around 80% of men experience some degree of erectile dysfunction, so choice (A) is true. Chronic, concurrent medical conditions such as diabetes mellitus, hypertension, and cardiovascular disease may cause erectile dysfunction, so choice (C) is true as well. Older adults continue to have an interest in sexual activity, thus choice (D) is also a true statement.

2. **(A)** Testosterone deficiency may pose a significant risk for ED, but it is not a common risk factor for ED. Diabetes mellitus, hypertension, a history of a radical prostatectomy (choice (B)), chronic tobacco and alcohol use (choices (C) and (D)), neuropathy, and other urological surgery represent 70% of cases possibly responsible for ED.

3. **(D)** Due to the history and location of the trauma, the patient should be referred to the emergency department as soon as possible to rule out testicular torsion. Ordering any other labs (choices (A) and (B)) will only delay the treatment for the patient. Applying ice to the area along with elevation (choice (C)) may further compromise blood flow to the testes and should be avoided until a complete evaluation has been done.

4. **(A)** Transillumination is a technique used with a light source to visualize fluid below the skin surface. It is simple and poses no risk or additional cost. It may be used to evaluate possible sinusitis, hydrocephalus in newborns or infants, hydrocele in males, and breast lesions or cysts in females prior to any further testing such as X-ray, CT scan, or ultrasound (choice (B)). The purpose of checking for cremasteric reflexes (choice (C)) is to evaluate the elevation of the testicle in response to stroking the upper inner thigh. This test is useful in diagnosing testicular torsion. Normally, hydrocele is painless; thus, palpation of the scrotum (choice (D)) should not elicit discomfort and would not help in the diagnosis of hydrocele.

5. **(C)** A varicocele occurs when blood backs up in the main veins that drain the scrotum. No treatment is indicated. However, some studies have reported a possible association between varicocele and infertility. Hydrocele, choice (A) is fluid buildup around the testicle(s). Choice (B), testicular torsion, happens when the testicle is twisted around the spermatic cord. Symptoms of testicular torsion include severe unilateral scrotal pain. This condition is a urological emergency and the patient should be referred to the emergency department. Epididymitis (choice (D)) is an inflammatory and infectious process affecting the epididymis. Patients usually report gradual development of scrotal pain, and the epididymis is tender to palpation.

6. **(C)** There is a probable case for benign prostatic hypertrophy based on the physical findings and prostate-specific antigen (PSA) value. A PSA level of less than 10 ng/mL is indicative of BPH. A PSA of 10 ng/mL or greater requires urologist consultation and may indicate possible cancer (choice (A)). The PSA value should serve as a historical note for baseline comparison and should not be used to rule out prostate cancer. The PSA value is normally not affected by prostate infection (choice (B)). An elevated PSA level is not considered to be a normal part of aging (choice (D)).

7. **(D)** Commercial long-distance truck drivers may be prone to prostatitis, not prostate cancer, due to limited bathroom breaks during the long-distance drives. Risk factors for prostate cancer include an age greater than 50 years old (choice (A)), avid long-hour cycling, a positive family history (choice (B)), obesity (choice (C)), and African American ethnicity.

8. **(B)** The treatment for acute bacterial prostatitis is similar to the treatment for acute pyelonephritis. For men younger than 35 years, the treatment is single dose IM ceftriaxone followed by oral doxycycline. For men 35 years old and older, a higher dose of ciprofloxacin or levofloxacin (choice (A)) is recommended. Levofloxacin is a quinolone antibiotic that is effective in treating acute bacterial prostatitis but is no longer used first line because of increasing rates of drug resistance and adverse effects, such as tendinitis. Clear fluids (choice (C)) and cranberry juice (choice (D)) may relieve some of the symptoms of acute bacterial prostatitis; however, they do not have the mechanism to treat the infections.

9. **(C)** In most cases, epididymitis will get better on its own over time. In children, the condition may develop due to inflammation from direct trauma to the scrotum, torsion of the appendix epididymis, or reflux of urine into the epididymis, however it may develop with no known trauma or injury to the area. Rest and ibuprofen can help decrease the inflammation and improve the pain. Acute bacterial prostatitis (choice (A)) is seen in adult men and often results from a sexually transmitted infection. Chronic prostatitis (choice (B)) is also a condition seen in adults. The prostate gland in children is underdeveloped until puberty and rarely causes problems. Asymptomatic bacteriuria (choice (D)) is the incidental finding of bacteria on urinalysis. This condition is common and, if no symptoms are present, no treatment is required in young children.

10. **(D)** Ceftriaxone 250 mg IM as a single dose plus a single dose of oral azithromycin 1 g is the preferred treatment for uncomplicated gonococcal infection for a 16-year-old. The treatment regimen is simple, with IM given at the clinic, and the patient only needs to take one pill at home. Thus, medication adherence is higher. The other options, (choice (A)) amoxicillin, (choice (B)) TMP-SMX, and (choice (C)) metronidazole, are not the recommended treatment for uncomplicated gonococcal infection.

11. **(A)** According to the 2015 CDC STD treatment guidelines, oral azithromycin 500 mg once per day for 10 days and ceftriaxone 250 mg IM as a single dose is the recommended treatment for an acute epididymitis case most likely caused by sexually transmitted gonorrheal and chlamydial infection in men who practice insertive anal sex. Topical clindamycin and oral tinidazole (choice (B)) and metronidazole gel 0.75% (choice (C)) are recommended for bacterial vaginosis. Doxycycline (mono therapy) (choice (D)) is not recommended for gonorrhea and chlamydia infection.

12. **(B)** Acyclovir (Zovirax) is the current medication used to treat genital herpes. However, the dosage varies based on the acuity of the infections (primary, recurrent, and suppression treatment). Abacavir (choice (A)), raltegravir (choice (C)), and darunavir (choice (D)) are antiretroviral medications used to prevent and treat HIV/AIDS.

13. **(C)** Hemangioma is not part of the differential diagnosis for genital ulceration. A hemangioma forms on top of the skin or in the subcutaneous layer. It usually appears as a red mark (burgundy-colored birthmark) occurring in the head and neck area. Syphilis (choice (A)) is a chronic, systemic infectious disease caused by the pathogen *Treponema pallidum*. Syphilis is a sexually transmitted infection that may affect every organ system. An ulceration at the site of inoculation may be seen. Genital herpes (choice (B)) is a viral infection caused by

herpes virus. Presentation often includes the development of an ulcerated area on the penis (in men) along with burning pain and dysuria. This ulcerated area often evolves into a vesicular lesion, which may secrete fluid containing the virus. Chancroid (choice (D)) is a sexually transmitted infection presenting with single or multiple vesicular and/or pustular lesions on genital tissue.

14. **(B)** Emtricitabine (Truvada) is recommended as pre-exposure prevention for uninfected people who engage in behaviors that place them at risk for HIV exposure. However, the medication does not prevent any other STDs, and patients still need to use condoms. Truvada is approved as an HIV medication for people 12 and older, but only as PrEP for people 11 and older. Dolutegravir (choice (A)) is an antiretroviral medication used in the treatment of HIV/AIDS. A referral to an infectious disease specialist (choice (C)) is not indicated at this time. Choice (D) is incorrect because the patient is a good candidate for PrEP, based on his social history and lab screening. PrEP is offered in primary care and community health clinics, among others.

15. **(A)** The Gram-negative bacillus *Haemophilus ducreyi* causes chancroid, which presents as a painful vesicular, pustular ulcer with a necrotic base. Chancroid is commonly contracted sexually. *Treponema pallidum* (choice (B)) is associated with the development of the sexually transmitted infection syphilis. *Neisseria gonorrhoeae* (choice (C)) is the causative organism in gonorrheal infections. *Mycoplasma genitalium* (choice (D)) is an uncommon condition associated with immunocompromised conditions.

12

Women's Health Issues

Women's health encompasses a wide range of conditions occurring throughout the life span of a woman. Many conditions, such as menstruation, pregnancy, and menopause, represent stages of life and are not pathological in nature. The family nurse practitioner should be aware of normal as well as abnormal processes associated with women's health and be prepared to provide holistic patient-centered guidance, support, and health care. This chapter will highlight important topics specific to the care of women throughout the life span.

Contraception

Contraception is an important consideration for the majority of women during reproductive years. Currently, women have a wide range of choices relating to contraception and almost every woman should be able to find and comfortably use a method of her choice. Despite availability of contraception in the United States, the majority of pregnancies are unintended. Although contraception is primarily used for pregnancy planning, the use of some forms of contraception may provide protection against sexually transmitted infections, may improve dermatologic and menstrual disorders, and may allow women to control menstruation.

CONTRACEPTIVE METHODS

- Barrier: male and female condom, diaphragm, cervical cap.

- Spermicidal: vaginal contraceptive sponge, contraceptive jelly, foam, cream, and suppository.

- Hormonal (may be a combination of estrogen and progestin, or progestin only): oral contraceptives, patch, implantable device, injection, and certain intrauterine devices. Absolute contraindications for hormonal contraception include a history of smoking, breast cancer, and/or thromboembolic disease, and women over age 35 years who present with any of these conditions. The effectiveness of hormonal contraception is directly related to patient adherence.

- Intrauterine device: Paraguard, a copper "T" that provides contraception for up to 10 years; Mirena provides pregnancy protection for about 5 years.

- Regulated abstinence: Patient monitors fertile periods and abstains from intercourse during those times.

- Postcoital controls: withdrawal, postcoitus douche, and emergency contraception.

- Sterilization: permanent method of birth control; vasectomy for males; tubal ligation for females.

Disorders of Menstruation

Amenorrhea

Amenorrhea is the absence of menses. Normally, menarche (the onset of menses) occurs between the ages of 11 and 15 years old. Primary amenorrhea is defined as no menses by the age of 14 in girls who have not developed any secondary sexual characteristics (breast buds), or by age 16 in girls who may or may not have developed secondary sexual characteristics. Secondary amenorrhea may be associated with polycystic ovarian syndrome (PCOS), disorders of the hypothalamic system, hyperprolactinemia, ovarian failure, and excessive exercise (low BMI). The most common causes of amenorrhea are pregnancy, hypothalamic disorders, and PCOS. Women who are amenorrheic should be evaluated if there is no menses by age 14 without a growth delay disorder, if there is no menses by age 16 even with a growth delay disorder, or if they have had menstruated previously and then stopped having menstrual cycles for at least the past three consecutive months.

Symptoms

The patient presents with concern about absence of menses. The FNP should determine if this is primary or secondary.

Management

> **CLINICAL PEARL**
>
> Women who are very athletic and those with eating disorders associated with severe weight loss (low BMI) are predisposed to amenorrhea.

A urine pregnancy test is the initial test recommended; if positive, a serum human chorionic gonadotropin (HCG) level should be done. A baseline blood chemistry profile should be ordered to rule out hepatic or renal disease. Primary amenorrhea is often caused by chromosomal abnormalities, thus genetic testing may be helpful in determining etiology. Tests that may assist in determining the cause of secondary amenorrhea include thyroid function testing, follicle-stimulating hormone (FSH), luteinizing hormone (LH), and prolactin level testing. Further evaluation for secondary amenorrhea may include androgen studies, including total testosterone level and dehydroepiandrosterone sulfate levels, a progesterone challenge test, and measurement of prolactin and LH levels. Laboratory abnormalities and persistent amenorrhea should be evaluated by a gynecologist.

Premenstrual Syndrome (PMS)

Premenstrual syndrome describes a group of psychological and physical symptoms that occur cyclically beginning during the luteal phase of menstruation, normally 14 days after the last cycle. Most women experience mild symptoms that occur frequently with menses; however, approximately 5% of women have symptoms that are more severe and more likely to impact daily living. Although the etiology is not clearly defined, researchers do agree on the following: fluctuations in ovarian steroids impact neurotransmitter release, and the cyclic nature (not quantifiable levels) of estrogen and progesterone are responsible for symptoms associated with PMS.

Symptoms

Presentation often includes mood changes such as depression, hostility, crying episodes, anxiety, irritability, relationship conflict, increased or decreased libido, and feelings of being unable to cope. Physical symptoms may include gastrointestinal bloating, nausea/vomiting, and constipation; respiratory system rhinitis, asthma, hoarseness, and sore throat; breast tenderness, swelling, and heaviness; headaches/migraines; fatigue; backache; joint pain; lower extremity edema; weight gain; pelvic or lower abdominal pain; and food cravings. For diagnosis, symptoms should occur only during the luteal phase of the menstrual cycle.

Management

The following lifestyle changes are recommended to decrease symptoms: dietary reduction in salt, sugar, caffeine, and alcohol intake; regular aerobic exercise; and stress reduction techniques. Calcium and magnesium supplements may assist in symptom control. Treatment: The FNP may administer the SSRIs fluoxetine, sertraline, paroxetine, and/or citalopram to assist in relieving tension, dysphoria, and irritability. For patients with severe symptoms who do not respond to the lifestyle and pharmacological measures listed above, ovulation suppression therapy with danazol may be recommended.

Dysmenorrhea

Dysmenorrhea is painful menses, a disorder of menstruation that affects many women. It may be primary, in which no pelvic abnormality is identified, or secondary, which is usually accompanied by some form of pelvic pathology. Primary dysmenorrhea usually begins one to two years after menarche and is associated with ovulatory cycles. Primary dysmenorrhea pain usually starts 24 hours before menses begin and lasts for 48 to 72 hours. The goal of managing primary dysmenorrhea is to relieve pain. Secondary dysmenorrhea is usually seen in women between 40 and 50 years and may be caused by a number of pathological conditions, including endometriosis, uterine leiomyomas, pelvic inflammatory disease (PID), and endometrial polyps. Secondary dysmenorrhea pain may begin a week or more prior to menses and may last a few days after menstruation stops.

Symptoms

Patients with dysmenorrhea complain of sharp, stabbing lower abdominal pain with cramping, nausea, anorexia, low back pain, fatigue, and bowel changes.

Management

First-line therapy for dysmenorrhea includes aspirin every four hours starting before menses. This is beneficial because of the antiprostaglandin activity of the drug. Dietary changes, avoidance of caffeine, exercise, and smoking cessation are recommended. Application of heat to the lower abdomen is often helpful in pain management. The mainstay of therapy is ibuprofen 400 to 800 mg by mouth three to four times a day. Combined oral contraceptives (COCs) may be prescribed to relieve cramping by inhibition of arachidonic acid production and ovulation. The goal of managing secondary dysmenorrhea is to alleviate symptoms as well as to identify and treat the underlying cause.

Pregnancy and Lactation

Pregnancy

Pregnancy produces physiologic changes in a woman's body that begin at the time of conception. During reproductive years, a hormonal feedback loop consisting of the pituitary gland, the hypothalamus, and the ovaries provides hormonal regulation and a hospitable environment for embryo fertilization, transport, and implantation in the uterus to occur. When pregnancy occurs, this hormonal regulation changes to incorporate production and sustenance of needed elements for fetal growth and maternal health throughout gestation.

During pregnancy, changes occur in every system in the body, not only the reproductive system. Cardiovascular changes include an increase in blood volume of 30–50% with increased cardiac output. Respiratory changes include an increase in respiratory rate and, late in pregnancy, dyspnea as the growing uterus displaces the diaphragm. Skin changes include the development of striae, which are darkened lines on the abdomen, hips, and breasts as well as darkening of the face and areola of the breasts (chloasma gravidarum). Gastrointestinal changes include a slowing of peristalsis with increased flatus, constipation, and decreased bowel sounds. Dyspepsia may occur due to altered esophageal and gastric muscle tone. A predisposition to the development of gallstones occurs as the digestive system slows down, and combined with increased cholesterol saturation, this increases the risk for cholecystitis during pregnancy.

Pregnancy normally lasts 285 days, or 40 weeks, and this period is termed *gestation*. The date of delivery may be estimated by determining the first day of the last menstrual period, adding seven days, subtracting three months, and adding one year. This calculation is termed Nägele's rule and is fairly accurate for women who have regular 28-day menstrual cycles.

Pregnancy is divided into trimesters, and fetal development is characteristically considered based on trimester. The first 12 weeks are a critical period in fetal development as major organ systems are formed and exposure to toxins during this time could result in catastrophic harm. Toxins include illicit drugs, alcohol, environmental exposures, certain viruses, over-the-counter medications, and some prescription medications.

Continued hormonal changes throughout pregnancy maintain and support the pregnancy. The growing infant receives all nutrition via the placenta, which also serves as a potential portal for harmful substances in the mother's bloodstream.

Pregnancy is a time of vulnerability, not only for the baby, but also for the woman as her body undergoes the major changes brought about by pregnancy. Table 12.1 provide a summary for GTPAL acronym interpretations.

CLINICAL PEARL

Here's an example of how to interpret a woman's GTPAL:

Susan is 35 weeks pregnant. This is her second pregnancy. She delivered a healthy baby girl at 37 weeks with her first pregnancy. What is this woman's GTPAL?

Applying the scenario into the GTPAL acronym:

Right now, Susan's GTPAL is G2, T1, P0, A0, L1 (because she has not yet delivered her second baby). Once she delivers her second baby, her GTPAL will be G2, T2, P0, A0, L2.

Gravida, Term Births, Preterm Births, Abortions, and Living Children (GTPAL)

GTPAL is an acronym commonly documented in a woman's obstetrical history. FNPs need to be comfortable interpreting the acronym.

Table 12.1. GTPAL

Gravidity	The number of pregnancies conceived. For example, the gravidity of a woman with 3 pregnancies would be gravida: 3. A nulligravida would be someone who has never been pregnant (gravida: 0).
Viability	The term used when the fetus reaches i) 20 weeks gestation or ii) weight 500 g and above. The term is established for assigning pregnancy parity and does not reflect the survivability of the fetus.
Parity	The number of viable pregnancies completed PAST the 20 weeks gestation
T	The number of full-term infants
P	The number of preterm infants
A	The number of abortions
L	The number of living children delivered

Lactation and Breastfeeding

Lactation is the process of milk production and secretion from the breasts in response to an infant's need for nourishment. Changes in breast anatomy and physiology are coordinated through a complex feedback system that allows the maternal breast to produce milk in quantities and with specific qualities required by her infant. Breastfeeding is recommended as the preferred method of providing nourishment by the American Academy of Pediatrics (AAP), the American Academy of Family Physicians (AAFP), as well as the American Dietetic Association. Human milk is the ideal food for babies, and mothers are encouraged to exclusively breastfeed for the first six months. Breast milk contains nutrients needed for growth and development as well as immune substances that offer protection for the infant against infections. Breastfeeding provides many physical, psychological, and emotional benefits for both mother and baby.

Some contraindications to breastfeeding include maternal diagnosis of HIV (except in some developmentally deprived areas of the world), an infant with galactosemia, and herpetic lesions on the mother's nipple or breast. Women who are breastfeeding need additional calories with adequate calcium, fruits, and vegetables to support her health and the quality of breast milk during this time.

Mastitis

Mastitis occurs most commonly during lactation and involves inflammation and or infection in one area of the breast. Mastitis usually develops from six weeks to six months postpartum and happens when bacteria enter the breast tissue via cracked nipples or when milk ducts become plugged, leading to stasis of milk within breast tubules. The most common organisms associated with infectious mastitis include *Staphylococcus aureus*, *Escherichia coli*, *Enterobacteriaceae*, *Mycobacterium tuberculosis*, and *Candida albicans*.

Symptoms

Symptoms include localized, unilateral breast tenderness, erythema, and warmth, which may be accompanied by fever and flu-like symptoms.

Management

Management of mastitis includes continuation of breastfeeding, increased fluids, good nutrition, bed rest, application of moist heat, and anti-inflammatory medications. Antibiotics may be indicated based on causative etiology.

Menopause

The term *menopause* refers to cessation of menses. This is not a pathologic state, but rather an expected phase of a woman's reproductive history. The definition of menopause is based on the patient's report of no menstrual period for at least one year. The average age of menopause in the United States is 51 years; however, the usual age range is between 48 and 55 years.

During menopause, circulating levels of estrogen continue to decline, and the body begins to produce estrone instead of estradiol. Estrone levels remain fairly constant throughout menopause while testosterone levels decrease. Women who are obese will usually exhibit higher levels of circulating estrogens because of increased adipose tissue. However, these women, too, are subject to vasomotor symptoms associated with decreased estrogen levels.

Symptoms

Symptoms include vasomotor symptoms of hot flashes, night sweats, and insomnia. Vaginal dryness and atrophy are commonly reported as well, and this may lead to bleeding as well as pain with intercourse. Areas of sexual functioning that undergo change with menopause include a decrease in sexual responsiveness and activity, dyspareunia (pain with intercourse), and diminished sexual desire (libido). Physical examination findings include evidence of vaginal atrophy and bone demineralization and osteoporosis associated with menopause.

Management

Lifestyle modification measures include aerobic exercise, weight loss, limited alcohol intake, dressing in layers, smoking cessation, and stress reduction. A diet high in complex carbohydrates and fiber, low in fat, and high in antioxidants is recommended.

Vaginal dryness complaints should be addressed with a Pap smear (initially) and urinalysis to rule out pathology. Topical applications of estrogen are beneficial in reducing symptoms. Products include the estradiol vaginal ring, which has little systemic estrogen absorption and can be used long-term. Short-term use of estrogen vaginal cream may be helpful as well. Water-soluble vaginal lubricants are available over the counter and may be used in conjunction with estrogen-containing products to alleviate vaginal dryness.

Emotional symptoms such as irritability or depression and anxiety should be addressed with treatment based on symptomatology. Selective serotonin receptor inhibitors (SSRIs) work well in relieving hot flashes and may also prove beneficial in alleviating emotional symptoms.

CLINICAL PEARL

Current recommendations for the use of hormone therapy are limited to the treatment of moderate to severe menopausal symptoms including hot flashes and sleep disturbances. Use of hormone therapy may increase the risk for cardiovascular disease.

HEALTH CARE NEEDS OF LESBIAN, GAY, BISEXUAL, AND TRANSGENDER (LGBT) INDIVIDUALS

According to a 2021 Gallup poll, approximately 5.6% of the general population of the United States identify as lesbian, gay, bisexual, or transgender. This number is up from 4.5 % identified in 2017. This population includes individuals from various ethnic backgrounds, socioeconomic statuses, and educational levels.

There are specific and unique health care needs related to individuals who identify as LGBT and often significant barriers to accessing care. Research demonstrates that individuals who identify as LGBT experience disproportionate rates of infectious disease transmission, substance abuse, chronic disease risk, psychiatric disorders, and suicide. Domestic and intimate partner violence (IPV) incidents are often underreported or unacknowledged in this population.

Cultural awareness, competence, and compassion among clinicians provide the foundation for gaining trust and providing quality health care for LGBT patients. Because the complexities of meeting the health care needs of individuals who identify as LGBT are great, providers must work proactively to remove barriers and improve access to care for all individuals. Pervasive systemic discrimination has been cited as one explanation for the overall rates of poorer access to quality care and patient reluctance to seek care.

Health care providers often have little to no specific education on caring for individuals who identify as LGBT. Therefore, it is imperative that clinicians become familiar with the unique health care needs of this population and actively pursue opportunities to increase knowledge. In particular, health care providers should feel comfortable assessing the following:

- History of intimate partner violence
- Mental health status (evaluate for suicidal ideation)
- Social history regarding participation in high-risk behaviors such as illicit drug use, alcohol abuse, and multiple sexual partners
- Sexual behavior history including type of activity such as oral/anal, insertive/receptive and number of current partners
- Immunization history and human immunodeficiency virus (HIV) screening and status

One important component of effective communication is using gender-neutral language such as "partner" instead of husband, wife, girlfriend, or boyfriend. Other terms nurse practitioners should know include:

- Men who have sex with men: MSM
- Transgender: broad term for individuals whose gender identity is different from their natal gender. Address individuals based on gender identity (the gender they identify with), rather than natal gender. For example, a transgender woman living as a woman at the present time should be referred to as "she" or "her" or any other pronoun of their choosing. Likewise, a transgender man currently living as a man should be referred to as "he" or "him" or any other pronoun of their choosing.

Transgender identity is not a psychiatric disorder; however, these individuals require counseling and support to navigate the serious challenges they face within a society that views them as different. Many transgender individuals may opt to undergo hormone replacement therapy or surgical interventions to more closely align their bodies with their gender identity.

Although individuals who identify as LGBT experience unique health care needs, they also require health maintenance and disease prevention services to stay healthy.

CLINICAL PEARL

Younger MSM (ages 13–24 years) are the most affected subpopulation for new HIV diagnoses in the United States, as compared to other subgroups by ethnicity, age, and sex.

Gynecologic Conditions and Sexually Transmitted Infections

Endometriosis

Endometriosis is a chronic, painful disease associated with abnormally placed and implanted endometrial tissue. With endometriosis, uterine tissue lies outside the uterus and continues to respond to ovulatory hormones. Endometriosis significantly impacts fertility. Current data reveals that it can take up to nine years for a woman to be correctly diagnosed with endometriosis because symptoms resemble those of many other abdominal and reproductive disorders.

Endometriosis occurs during a woman's reproductive phase and is staged as follows: stage I (minimal disease) reflects isolated implants without evidence of adhesion, stage II (mild) is considered with superficial implants less than 5 cm in aggregate without adhesions, stage III (moderate) disease manifests as multiple superficial and invasive implants that may or may not involve the ovaries, stage IV (severe) disease demonstrates multiple superficial and invasive implants with dense adhesions as well as large ovarian endometriomas.

Symptoms

The primary symptom is recurrent abdominal or pelvic pain; this pain may range from mild to severe and debilitating. Other symptoms include pain with intercourse, urination, or defecation; fatigue; constipation or diarrhea; and nausea. The patient often has a history of autoimmune disorders. Physical examination findings include tenderness of the posterior fornix area; palpable nodules may or may not be appreciated with abdominal examination.

Management

The goals of managing endometriosis include reduction or relief of pain, slowing and shrinking endometrial growths, preventing recurrence, and preserving fertility. For mild disease, oral contraceptives are beneficial in reducing pain; NSAIDs along with oral contraceptives work well for these individuals. More severe disease requires laparoscopic exploration and possible ablation of endometrial growths. Drugs that may be used in moderate to severe disease include nafarelin nasal spray, leuprolide, and goserelin, which are gonadotropin-releasing hormone (GnRH) analogs that suppress ovulation. These medications are used for three to six months. Pharmacological treatment alone is insufficient for moderate to severe disease and does not improve fertility. Surgical interventions are the only methods by which fertility is improved and symptoms are reduced or relieved.

CLINICAL PEARL

Direct visualization of endometrial implants is the only method for definitive diagnosis; this is usually accomplished via exploratory laparotomy.

Vaginitis

Vaginitis is a broad term used to describe a group of several conditions affecting the vagina, some of which may be sexually transmitted. These conditions have overlapping symptoms of vaginal irritation, pruritus, and an unusual or malodorous vaginal discharge. The normal pH of the vagina is 4.5 or less. This acidic environment works to prevent infection by many pathogens. However, changes in the pH often lead to an environment favorable for the growth or overgrowth of pathogens. Table 12.2 provide a summary for etiologies, pathophysiology, symptoms, and management of vaginitis.

Table 12.2. Etiologies, Pathophysiology, Symptoms, and Management of Vaginitis

Etiology	Pathophysiology	Symptoms	Management
Vulvovaginal candidiasis	An overgrowth of *Candida albicans* causing irritating symptoms of pruritus and discharge. Conditions that predispose the patient to the development of candidiasis include pregnancy, diabetes mellitus, obesity, tight clothing, and excessive moisture.	Itching of the vaginal area along with a thick white discharge. There is vaginal erythema and irritation on examination. Microscopic examination of discharge with 10% potassium hydroxide reveals hyphae and spores.	Topical azole medication for 1 to 3 days. Women with more severe symptoms should be treated for 7 to 14 days with a topical agent and be given 3 doses of fluconazole, 3 days apart. Commonly used topical agents include clotrimazole, miconazole, and butoconazole.
Trichomonas vaginalis	Caused by a protozoan pathogen that can infect the vagina and lower urinary tract in women and the lower genitourinary tract in men. This is a sexually transmitted infection.	Itching and a malodorous frothy, greenish discharge. There is diffuse erythema of vaginal tissues and red macular lesions may be seen on the cervix. Under microscopic examination of discharge, motile organisms with flagella are seen.	Nitroimidazole medications are the only agents effective against *T. vaginalis*. Recommended treatment is metronidazole 2 g orally as a single dose or tinidazole 2 g orally as a single dose.
Bacterial vaginosis	Polymicrobial infection of the vagina that is not sexually transmitted. Often, an overgrowth of anaerobic bacteria is responsible for symptoms.	Grayish, frothy discharge with a pH of 5.0–5.5, which is abnormally alkaline. An amine-like odor is noted with alkalinization with 10% potassium hydroxide. On a saline wet mount under a microscope, epithelial cells that are covered with bacteria are seen. These are called "clue cells."	Metronidazole orally for 7 days, clindamycin vaginal cream for 7 days, or metronidazole vaginal gel for 5 days. Other regimens include clindamycin ovules intravaginally and tinidazole.

Human Papillomavirus (HPV) and Genital Warts

Human papillomavirus infection is the most common sexually transmitted infection (STI) in the United States. HPV infection is not a reportable disease; therefore, the exact number of cases is unknown. Almost all sexually active individuals will become infected with HPV at some point in their lives, though most are not aware of the infection. Most HPV infections clear spontaneously.

There are more than 100 known serotypes of HPV, but only around 40 are capable of infecting humans. The two types of HPV that cause 70% of all cervical cancers are HPV 16 and HPV 18. Transmission rate is high; an estimated 60% of individuals who have sex with an infected partner will develop HPV.

Symptoms

Genital warts in women are seen around the entrance to the vagina, but may also be present on the cervix, perineum, and perianal area. HPV lesions appear as soft, small, papillary swellings that appear warty. These lesions may occur singly or in clusters. Growths may also be flat and are usually flesh-colored or slightly darker with Caucasian women, black with African American women, and brown with Asian women. As the infection becomes chronic, lesions begin to resemble cauliflower and are grouped in large clusters. Lesions are typically painless unless they are large enough to cause irritation.

Management

Most HPV types that are clinically important can be prevented through vaccination. Although there are three vaccines that prevent HPV infection, only one (Gardasil 9) is available for use in the United States. This vaccine protects against HPV types 16 and 18 (which cause most cervical cancers), types 6 and 11 (predominantly responsible for genital warts), as well as five additional types of HPV now known to be associated with the development of cervical cancer (types 31, 33, 45, 52, and 58). Treatment is directed toward removing anogenital warts associated with acute HPV infection and relieving discomfort. Treatment usually involves provider-administered cryotherapy in a clinical office and topical therapy applied by the patient between visits. Topical treatment options applied by the patient include:

- Imiquimod 3.75% or 5% cream
- Podofilox 0.5% gel or solution
- Sinecatechins 15% ointment

In addition to cryotherapy, lesions may also be removed by tangential scissor excision, tangential shave excision, curettage, laser, or electrosurgery. Another topical treatment option is Trichloroacetic acid (TCA) or bichloroacetic acid (BCA) 80–90% solution. These last two solutions are caustic agents that must be applied in a provider's office.

Chlamydia Infection

Chlamydia is the most common reportable sexually transmitted infection in the United States. The causative pathogen is *Chlamydia trachomatis* bacteria. The highest prevalence of infection is seen in women ages 15 to 24 years of age. The prevalence is highest in Black women. Risk factors for chlamydia include multiple sexual partners and failure to use condoms. Annual screening for chlamydia is recommended for all patients in the age group of 12–24. Screening for chlamydia infection includes nucleic acid amplification testing (NAAT), direct immunofluorescence, nucleic acid testing, cell culture, and immunoassay.

Symptoms

Women are usually asymptomatic; however, symptoms reported include postcoital bleeding, vaginal spotting, purulent vaginal discharge, pain with intercourse, lower abdominal pain, and urinary frequency. The symptoms of chlamydia often resemble those of a urinary tract infection. Physical examination findings may include abdominal tenderness, cervical friability, mucopurulent discharge, cervical motion tenderness, and adnexal fullness.

CLINICAL PEARL

Routine vaccination is recommended for children aged 11 to 12 years but can be given as early as age 9. The vaccine is also recommended for all individuals ages 13 to 26 years who have not been previously vaccinated. The number of vaccine doses is based on age. Children and adolescents between the ages of 9 and 14 years require only two doses, while individuals between the ages of 15 and 26 years require three doses. Note: Vaccination is a primary prevention measure.

CLINICAL PEARL

Current recommendations are to treat concurrent gonorrhea infections when chlamydia is identified.

Management

First-line treatment for chlamydia is azithromycin 1 g orally as a single dose or doxycycline 100 mg orally twice a day for seven days.

Gonorrhea Infection

Gonorrhea is caused by an aerobic Gram-negative diplococcus, *Niesseria gonorrhoeae*, and is the second most commonly reported STI, after chlamydia. These two infections often occur together. Annual screening for gonorrhea is recommended for all sexually active women younger than 25 years. Gonorrhea is most commonly transmitted through sexual activity with genital-to-genital contact. Gonorrhea may also be transmitted with oral-to-genital contact and anal-to-anal contact. In females, sites of infection include the urethra, vagina, cervix, oropharynx, and Skene's and Bartholin's glands. Women are often asymptomatic.

Symptoms

When reported, symptoms may include pain with intercourse, lower abdominal pain, a change in vaginal discharge, or unilateral edema of the labia. On examination, there may be evidence of a rectal infection, a vaginal infection, or an oropharyngeal infection, which presents similarly to strep pharyngitis.

Management

First-line treatment recommendation is ceftriaxone 250 mg IM in a single dose or cefixime 400 mg orally in a single dose. Alternative treatment includes another single-dose injectable cephalosporin plus azithromycin orally.

Cancer in Women

Breast Cancer

Breast cancer is the most commonly occurring type of cancer in women after skin cancer. Statistical data demonstrate that one in every eight women will develop breast cancer. Although treatment modalities have improved and survival rates have risen, breast cancer remains one of the most feared cancers for women in the United States. Risk factors include an age over 50 years, a history of smoking, a positive family history of breast cancer, genetic mutations (BRCA1, BRCA2), early menarche, late menopause, delayed childbearing, a personal history of cancer, alcohol consumption, a high-fat diet, and lack of exercise.

Symptoms

CLINICAL PEARL

Most breast cancers (60%) occur in the upper outer quadrant of the breast, including the tail of Spence.

Early disease: single, non-tender mass with poorly-defined margins; mammographic abnormality without palpable mass. Late disease: nipple retraction, axillary lymphadenopathy, erythema, edema, and pain in affected breast; on palpation, mass is adherent to chest wall or skin.

Management

Follow recommended screening guidelines: The American Cancer Society recommends mammography screening for women at average risk beginning at age 45 and continued annually. Mammography may be offered to women starting at age 40 if they desire to be screened.

Endometrial Cancer

Endometrial cancer is cancer that arises from the endometrial lining of the uterus. The majority of these cancers are adenocarcinomas and account for a large percentage of cases of postmenopausal uterine bleeding. The average age at diagnosis is 60 years, however 25% occur before menopause.

Symptoms

Atypical cells on endometrial biopsy are a key prognostic factor in the diagnosis of endometrial cancer. The most common presentation of endometrial cancer is a postmenopausal woman with a complaint of painless abnormal uterine bleeding. Physical examination is normal; however, endometrial biopsy reveals hyperplasia with atypical cells.

Management

Primary prevention measures in women with chronic anovulation include the administration of progestin or a progesterone-containing regimen. These agents protect against endometrial hyperplasia and carcinoma development. Management includes early identification and establishment of diagnosis. Endometrial cancer has a high cure rate if treated early.

Ovarian Cancer

Although tumors of the ovaries are common, most are benign. However, ovarian cancer is the leading cause of reproductive system death. Germ-line genetic mutations have been discovered that are associated with epithelial ovarian tumors, such as BRCA1, BRCA2, and a hereditary colorectal cancer gene. Risk factors include advanced age; a positive family history of ovarian, breast, or colon cancer; early menarche; nulliparity; late menopause; a history of high-fat diet, smoking, and inactivity; or a history of prolonged use of fertility drugs. Several types of ovarian malignancies are recognized; however, tumors arising from the epithelial layer of the ovary have the poorest prognosis.

Symptoms

Patients may be asymptomatic or have vague symptoms such as back pain, constipation, and bloating. Pelvic pressure, discomfort, and urinary symptoms develop as the tumor enlarges. Other symptoms include nausea and vomiting, gas, indigestion, rectal pressure, pain with intercourse, abnormal vaginal bleeding, and weight loss. On pelvic examination, decreased cervical and adnexal mobility, a pelvic mass, adnexal fullness, and ovarian pain with a bimanual exam may be noted.

Management

There are no screening tools or recommendations for routine screening for ovarian cancer at the present time. For patients at risk for ovarian cancer, annual pelvic exam Pap smear, transvaginal ultrasound, and serum CA-125 may be beneficial in assisting in early identification.

Cervical Intraepithelial Neoplasia (CIN)

Cervical cancer is the most common cancer in women worldwide and the 14th most common cancer in women in the United States. Anatomy of the cervix predisposes patients to abnormal cell growth because the squamocolumnar junction is an area of high cell proliferation. During childhood, this area is found on the exposed vaginal portion of the cervix. At puberty, hormonal

CLINICAL PEARL

International Federation of Gynecology and Obstetrics (FIGO) staging is used to determine disease involvement: stage I is confined to the uterine corpus, stage II demonstrates involvement of the cervix, stage III is regional spread of disease to the pelvis, and stage IV refers to disease that has spread outside the pelvis. Treatment is based on the stage of the disease.

CLINICAL PEARL

Human papillomavirus (HPV) infection of the cervix carries a high association with the development of CIN, thus prevention of HPV with available vaccines is the first step in prevention. Gardasil is recommended for all girls and women aged 9 to 26 years. Current recommendations are for boys and young men to receive the vaccine as well in order to prevent penile cancers associated with HPV.

influences cause this margin of tissue to move closer to the epithelium, creating a "transformation zone" of tissue prone to metaplasia. This is where most cervical neoplasia is found. Areas of high cell turnover are high-risk areas for the development of metaplasia, or abnormal cell growth.

Symptoms

Screening with an annual Pap smear beginning at age 21 is designed to identify areas of dysplasia early, when complete cure is achievable.

Management

Current U.S. Preventive Services Task Force (USPSTF) recommendations are screening for cervical cancer in women ages 21 to 65 years with cytology assessment every three years. Women ages 30 to 65 may opt for cytology and HPV screening every five years. Colposcopy follow-up in one year is recommended for women with ASC-US and a negative HPV screen. Patients with CIN are managed by a gynecologic oncologist.

Practice Questions

1. An 18-year-old female presents with concerns that she may have "caught something" from her boyfriend. She tells the FNP that yesterday she started feeling a "stinging" sensation in the genital area. She denies any abnormal discharge, itching, pain, or lesions. On examination, the vaginal area is free of lesions, erythema, or discharge. Which of the following sexually transmitted infections may present in this way?

   (A) gonorrhea
   (B) chlamydia
   (C) bacterial vaginosis
   (D) herpes simplex virus (HSV)

2. Oral contraceptives may decrease the activity of which of the following classes of medication?

   (A) oral anticoagulants
   (B) antibiotics
   (C) anti-seizure medication
   (D) corticosteroids

3. A 25-year-old female presents with a chief complaint of allergies. During the visit, the patient tells the FNP that recently she has been having pain during intercourse. This is a new problem for her and she is worried. Many conditions may cause dyspareunia; however, which of the following does not?

   (A) multiple pregnancies
   (B) vaginal atrophy
   (C) chlamydia infection
   (D) vulvovaginitis

4. The average age of menopause for women in the United States is:

   (A) 40 years.
   (B) 48 years.
   (C) 51 years.
   (D) 60 years.

5. One barrier method of contraception is the diaphragm used with a spermicidal gel or foam. Women who use this form of birth control are at increased risk for:

   (A) vaginal candidiasis.
   (B) urinary tract infection.
   (C) postcoital bleeding.
   (D) cervical friability.

6. A 21-year-old female presents with a complaint of genital warts. She states they have been there for several months but seem to be getting bigger. She is worried about the appearance of the warts and tells the FNP she heard about a vaccination for warts. The FNP discusses Gardasil and Cervarix with her and informs her that:

   (A) since she has already been exposed to HPV, she is not eligible for the vaccine.
   (B) since she is already sexually active, she should not receive the vaccine.
   (C) she is in the recommended age group to receive the vaccine.
   (D) she needs to wait until her HPV has cleared before receiving the vaccine.

7. A patient has been diagnosed with a gonococcal infection. The FNP is aware that coinfection with which of the following is common?

   (A) candidiasis
   (B) chancre
   (C) syphilis
   (D) chlamydia

8. Breast cancer is a leading cause of morbidity and mortality in women. Which of the following is considered a risk factor for the development of breast cancer?

   (A) Asian ethnicity
   (B) smoking
   (C) having large breasts
   (D) drinking one glass of alcohol a day

9. Most breast cancers are found in which anatomical area of the breast?

   (A) upper outer quadrant
   (B) upper inner quadrant
   (C) beneath the nipple and areola
   (D) lower inner quadrant

10. Vulvovaginal candidiasis is seen more often in which group of women?

    (A) adolescents
    (B) women with frequent urinary tract infections
    (C) women with diabetes
    (D) women who are vegetarian

11. Which of the following is NOT a risk factor for the development of ovarian cancer?

    (A) early menarche
    (B) late menopause
    (C) nulliparity
    (D) multiple pregnancies

12. The definitive method of diagnosing endometriosis is:

    (A) transvaginal ultrasound.
    (B) laparoscopic surgery.
    (C) pelvic examination.
    (D) measuring serum hormone levels.

13. What is the preferred method of screening for chlamydia?

    (A) nucleic acid amplification testing (NAAT)
    (B) culture
    (C) urine testing
    (D) pelvic examination without cytology

14. A 17-year-old female presents with a chief complaint of a yellowish vaginal discharge that has a strong odor. She reports she has been sexually active with a new partner for about two months. She tells the FNP that they use condoms "most of the time." Her last menstrual period was one week ago. A wet mount of vaginal secretions shows few clue cells, moderate lactobacilli, no yeast, few white blood cells, and numerous mobile trichomonads. Based on these findings, what is the appropriate treatment for this patient?

    (A) terconazole vaginal cream one application for seven days
    (B) fluconazole 150 mg orally as a single dose
    (C) metronidazole 2 g orally as a single dose
    (D) metronidazole vaginal gel one application for five days

15. A 65-year-old postmenopausal woman presents in the office with complaints of vaginal dryness and dyspareunia. She also reports some stress incontinence and urinary frequency. Her last menstrual period was 10 years ago. What is the most common cause of her symptoms?

    (A) cystocele
    (B) bacterial vaginosis
    (C) urinary tract infection
    (D) atrophic vaginitis

Answer Explanations

1. **(D)** The first symptom of HSV infection is usually a tingling or stinging sensation in the genital area. This prodromal symptom occurs at the site of inoculation and precedes the development of the characteristic vesicular rash. Gonorrhea (choice (A)) in females is often asymptomatic; however, when symptoms are reported, they may include dyspareunia (pain with intercourse), lower abdominal discomfort, a change in vaginal discharge, or unilateral labial pain. Chlamydia (choice (B)) is also asymptomatic in many women and may go undetected. Symptoms that are reported include vaginal spotting, postcoital bleeding, purulent vaginal discharge, or urinary symptoms. Bacterial vaginosis (choice (C)) is not considered a sexually transmitted infection, but its presence is a risk factor for the development of an STI.

2. **(A)** Several classes of medication may have decreased therapeutic activity when combined with oral contraceptives. These include oral anticoagulants, benzodiazepines, acetaminophen, and oral hypoglycemic agents. Certain antibiotics (choice (B)), anti-seizure medications (choice (C)), and oral corticosteroids (choice (D)) may decrease the effectiveness of, or interact with, oral contraceptives.

3. **(A)** A history of multiple pregnancies is not associated with pain during intercourse. There may be laxity of genital tissues and problems achieving orgasm after several pregnancies. The other conditions listed—vaginal atrophy associated with aging (choice (B)), chlamydia infection (choice (C)), and vulvovaginitis (choice (D))—are all associated with a risk for dyspareunia.

4. **(C)** The average age for menopause in women living in the United States is 51 years. Perimenopause often begins 5 to 10 years before menopause.

5. **(B)** Women using a diaphragm with spermicidal gel or foam are at an increased risk for the development of a urinary tract infection. The etiology is believed to be related to pressure on the urethra by the diaphragm itself. It is also thought that spermicidal foam or gel may cause mucosal changes in the genital area that may predispose the patient to the development of a urinary tract infection. Vaginal candidiasis (choice (A)) results from an overgrowth of *Candida albicans* and is commonly seen in patients with diabetes or obesity or in those who are immunocompromised. Postcoital bleeding (choice (C)) and cervical friability (choice (D)) are seen with many vaginal and sexually transmitted infections.

6. **(C)** HPV infection is the most common sexually transmitted infection. The Centers for Disease Control (CDC) recommendations are that individuals between the ages of 13 to 26 years who have not been previously vaccinated for HPV should receive the vaccination. Ideally, females should receive the vaccine before they become sexually active. However, females who are already sexually active may obtain some benefit from the vaccine as several serotypes are covered; therefore, choice (B) is incorrect. Because this patient has genital warts, she has been infected with HPV serotypes 6 and 11. These two types are not associated with the development of cervical cancer. However, the vaccine would offer protection against HPV serotypes that cause cancer. CDC recommendations are that both girls and boys receive the immunization at age 11 or 12. This provides protection prior to exposure to the virus. The vaccine is recommended, even if the individual has known exposure to HPV, or presents with genital warts, as it protects against multiple types of the virus (choices (A) and (D)).

7. **(D)** Gonococcal infection and chlamydia are often seen in the same patient. Because of this, testing is usually done for both conditions at the same time. First-line treatment for gonococcal infection includes rocephin 250 mg IM single dose, and for chlamydia it includes azithro-

mycin 1 g orally single dose. Other STIs (choices (A), (B), and (C)) may be present with gonococcal infection; however, the most commonly seen condition is chlamydia.

8. **(B)** Risk factors for breast cancer include smoking, obesity, high-fat diet, two or more drinks of alcohol per day, a family history of a first-degree relative with breast cancer, and age over 50 years. There is no evidence that being of Asian ethnicity (choice (A)), having large breasts (choice (C)), or drinking one glass of wine daily (choice (D)) poses an increased risk for breast cancer.

9. **(A)** Most (approximately 60%) of breast cancers are located in the upper outer quadrant of the breast, including the area called the tail of Spence.

10. **(C)** Risk factors for the development of vulvovaginal candidiasis include diabetes mellitus, obesity, immunocompromised status, pregnancy, and use of oral contraceptives.

11. **(D)** The most significant risk factor for development of ovarian cancer is a positive family history of the disease. Other risk factors include nulliparity, early menarche, late menopause, use of fertility drugs, and presence of BRCA1 or BRCA2 genetic mutations. Multiple pregnancies are not considered a risk factor for ovarian cancer.

12. **(B)** Endometriosis is a leading cause of chronic pelvic pain in women and occurs when endometrial tissue abnormally implants in areas outside the uterus. The only method for making a definitive diagnosis of endometriosis is via laparoscopic exploration. Ablation of lesions may also be accomplished during exploration if indicated. Endometriosis may cause scarring and adhesions of the pelvic organs. If organ enlargement has occurred, this may be found on transvaginal ultrasound (choice (A)); however, this is not definitive proof of endometriosis. A pelvic examination (choice (C)) should be done on all women with complaints of lower abdominal pain or abnormal menses and may elicit lower abdominal tenderness. However, many conditions other than endometriosis may produce tenderness, including ectopic pregnancy and ovarian cysts. Measuring serum hormone levels (choice (D)) is of no benefit when evaluating for the presence of endometriosis. These levels may be important in determining the phase of the menstrual cycle or in ruling out pregnancy.

13. **(A)** The preferred method of screening for chlamydia infection is NAAT. This test is more specific and sensitive than other available tests (choices (B), (C), and (D)) and provides fast results. The test is done using a vaginal swab of secretions and may be collected by the patient herself or by the clinician during a pelvic examination.

14. **(C)** Metronidazole 2 g orally as a single dose is the appropriate treatment for trichomoniasis. Terconazole (choice (A)) and fluconazole (choice (B)) are used in the treatment of candidiasis. Metronidazole gel (choice (D)) does not effectively treat this sexually transmitted infection.

15. **(D)** Reduced estrogen levels associated with menopause cause a thinning of the vaginal epithelium. The pH is usually increased because of lactic acid production leading to an environment favorable for pathogen growth. Women with atrophic vaginitis report pain with intercourse, vaginal soreness, occasional spotting, and vaginal dryness. A cystocele (choice (A)) is a herniation of the bladder through the wall of the vagina. Bacterial vaginosis (choice (B)) is a common cause of vaginal discharge and is not considered a sexually transmitted infection. Risk factors for bacterial vaginosis include the presence of menstrual bleeding, a new sexual partner, douching, and lack of condom use. Symptoms of a urinary tract infection (choice (C)) include urinary frequency, dysuria, an odor to the urine, and lower abdominal cramping.

PART III
Mental Health

13

Mental Health Disorders

The term *mental health disorders* refers to conditions that affect emotional, neurologic, and behavioral development; stress and altered coping; and psychiatric illness. Mental health disorders are a frequent reason for seeking care, and as the nationwide shortage of mental health providers continues to grow, clinicians in family medicine will see even more patients with a chief complaint related to a mood disorder or other mental health problem. Mental health disorders can be challenging to manage and they often come in "multiples," making diagnosis and treatment difficult. Disorders of mood and thought impact all areas of a patient's life. Fortunately, there are many available options for management. These conditions affect people of all ages, from childhood through old age. Occasionally, these disorders are identified only incidentally to other patient presentations but may be identified as the most imperative for treatment.

Generalized Anxiety Disorder (GAD)

Anxiety is the most common psychiatric disorder in the United States, and prevalence varies widely across the globe. Research demonstrates that rates of generalized anxiety disorder are higher in higher-income countries than in developing nations. This finding corresponds to a broader pattern of higher rates of mental health disorders in wealthier countries around the world. Unlike many other mental health diagnoses, diagnosis of GAD prior to adulthood is uncommon (however, anxiety disorders themselves are common in children), and prevalence is higher in females and those who are younger than 60 years, unemployed, less educated, and less affluent when compared with national standards. Historically, anxiety is considered a condition with only minimal impact on daily living; however, recent studies indicate that the presence of GAD is a cause of significant disability and loss of work time.

Symptoms

Individuals with GAD present with motor tension, hypervigilance, autonomic hyperactivity, and anxiety or worry. This anxiety is excessive and has a significant negative impact on life. Somatic symptoms associated with anxiety include headache, shakiness, abdominal discomfort, sweating, palpitations, and shortness of breath.

Management

Management of GAD begins with patient education, including symptom recognition, triggers, and decreased use of stimulants such as caffeine. Education also focuses on teaching relaxation techniques and increasing individual self-awareness.

Pharmacological management includes short-term use of benzodiazepines for acute symptoms, with the caveat that comorbid depressive symptoms may be made worse by these medications. It is important to remember that these medications are often sedating and require managed withdrawal. Buspirone is a 5-HT 1A (subtype of 5-HT serotonin receptor) partial agonist indicated for management of anxiety. This agent does not have the muscle-relaxant, anticonvulsant, sedative-hypnotic properties that are associated with benzodiazepines. Buspirone has a delayed onset of action, and there is limited data on its long-term effectiveness; however, it is a viable option to benzodiazepine medications.

Long-term management of GAD includes the use of selective serotonin reuptake inhibitors (SSRIs), which are very helpful in patients who also have depression. Examples of frequently used SSRIs include citalopram, escitalopram, paroxetine, sertraline, and venlafaxine. Reported side effects and adverse reactions for this class include nausea, diarrhea, headache, weight gain, and sexual dysfunction. Citalopram, unlike the other agents, has been associated with prolongation of the time between the start of the Q-wave and the end of the T-wave (QT segment) on electrocardiograms (ECG). One caution when prescribing SSRIs is that these medications, in the presence of bipolar I disorder, may exacerbate symptoms and should be ruled out prior to prescribing.

Other medications used in the management of GAD include the selective norepinephrine reuptake inhibitors (SNRIs) and tricyclic antidepressants (TCAs). The SNRI medications are more likely to produce jitteriness and activation than the SSRIs, thus there is an increased risk of suicide when drug levels are increasing. Patients and caregivers are cautioned to be alert for the onset of suicidal thoughts during this period. Tricyclic medications have a propensity to cause drowsiness, anticholinergic effects, sexual dysfunction, weight gain, and cardiac arrhythmias.

The goal of GAD management is to reduce or relieve symptoms and promote effective self-care and improvement of the everyday activities of daily living. Cognitive behavioral therapy (CBT) is a very effective modality in the long-term management of GAD and works synergistically with prescribed medications. GAD7 screening questionnaire is a tool to monitor progress in managing GAD.

Major Depressive Disorder (MDD)

Major depressive disorder is a common, burdensome, costly disorder that is seen worldwide. Pharmacological and nonpharmacological modalities are effective in managing the disorder; however, due to a severe shortage of psychiatric and mental health providers, medications have become the mainstay of therapy. Major depressive disorder most often occurs along with anxiety disorder.

Risk factors associated with MDD include thyroid disorders, positive family history (genetic link), psychosocial factors such as stressful life events, unemployment, and individual temperament. Screening for depression may be accomplished using the Patient Health Questionnaire 2 (PHQ 2), which consists of two questions:

1. Over the past two weeks, how often have you been bothered by feeling little interest or pleasure in doing things?
2. Over the past two weeks, how often have you been bothered by feeling down, depressed, or hopeless?

This simple screening is effective in identifying individuals who may need further evaluation. The Patient Health Questionnaire 9 (PHQ 9) consists of a checklist of nine symptoms and is scored based on the patient's report of symptom frequency over the past two weeks. The Geriatric Depression Scale (GDS) is a validated screening tool for use with elderly individuals. Depression is seen in children also, and rates of depression increase with age. For instance, the risk of depression in early adolescence is around 5%, but this rises to 20% by late adolescence. Screening for suicidal thoughts, ideation, or plans should be performed in all patients with MDD.

Symptoms

For a diagnosis of MDD, the *Diagnostic Statistical Manual 5* (DSM-5) requires that the patient exhibit either depressed mood or anhedonia (loss of pleasure in doing things) along with other symptoms such as change in appetite, insomnia or hypersomnia, loss of energy, feelings of worthlessness or guilt, apathy for most activities, difficulty concentrating, and recurrent thoughts of death or suicide. Adults and elderly persons with MDD may demonstrate feelings of hopelessness, withdrawal and social isolation, psychomotor retardation (slowed movement), vegetative behavior, somatic complaints of pain, anxiety, agitation, irritability, hypersomnia or insomnia or obsessive feelings of guilt and worry. Very young children with MDD may demonstrate a lack of energy, speech and motor development delays, sadness, withdrawal, sleep problems, poor appetite, and weight loss. School-age children may demonstrate anger, irritability, and externalizing behavior such as difficulty handling aggression, reckless behavior, or hyperactivity. Symptoms of MDD during adolescence include fatigue, hopelessness, impulsivity, antisocial behavior, substance abuse, hypersexuality, and aggression. One symptom is seen throughout all age groups with MDD, and that is a sense of hopelessness and despair.

Management

The goal of management of MDD is remission of symptoms. Psychotherapy and/or antidepressant medications are first-line recommendations. Classes of medications include the SSRIs, SNRIs, TCAs, and antianxiety medications. Dose limitations are in place for patients with renal or liver disease or seizure disorder. Although individual response to specific agents is unique, SNRIs tend to be more activating and carry a higher risk of completed suicide within the first few weeks of therapy.

Bipolar Disorder (BD)

Bipolar disorder is a spectrum of disorders including bipolar I (BD I) and bipolar II (BD II). Bipolar disorder is a continuum of mood disorders with movement from depression to mania. BD I is associated with insomnia (decreased need for sleep), grandiosity, flight of ideas, distractibility, increased activity level, pressured speech (increased talkativeness), impulsivity, and thoughtlessness or poor judgment. To meet the diagnostic criteria for BD I, the patient must have had at least one episode of mania in their lifetime. This episode may have been preceded by depression and may be followed by depression or hypomania. BD II disorder requires at least one hypomanic episode and one major depressive episode with no history of mania. Onset of symptoms occurs in prepubescent children, adolescence, or adulthood.

Symptoms

BD presents with elevated mood which may be demonstrated as euphoria or irritability and/or dysphoria, which is a depressed mood. Approximately 25% of patients with BD have episodes of pure mania, around 40% experience mixed episodes, and around 10–25% demonstrate "rapid cycling" with abrupt shifts from depression to mania. Manic episodes, if untreated, may last from three to six months with rapid, early escalation of symptoms. Older adults may demonstrate irritability rather than elevated mood.

Management

Management goals are the remission of current symptoms, the prevention of future episodes, and the return to previous level of function. BD is managed in collaboration with psychiatry. Lithium remains the pharmacological agent of choice in management of this disorder; however, this medication is associated with many adverse effects and drug interactions and requires controlled serum levels. Other medications with indications for BD include valproic acid, carbamazepine, and lamotrigine. Management and control of comorbid disorders is critical in meeting therapeutic goals for BD.

CLINICAL PEARL

The most common comorbidity with depression is anxiety. All patients presenting with depression should be asked about previous episodes of mania or hypomania.

Schizophrenia Spectrum Disorders

Schizophrenia is a serious mental illness that is characterized by disturbances of perception (hallucinations), affect (blunted or inappropriate), thinking (delusions), and cognition (impaired working memory). The World Health Organization lists schizophrenia as a leading cause of disability in developed nations. The disorder is characterized by frequent relapses, social and vocational exclusion, and mental and physical comorbidities. Different classifications of psychotic disorders include mania with psychosis, schizoaffective disorder, schizophrenia with one of several subtypes with acute or insidious onset, and delusional disorder. Schizophrenia typically presents in men in their early 20s. For women, symptoms may appear in the late 20s or early 30s. Most individuals demonstrate subtle symptoms for years before a diagnosis is made.

Symptoms

Patients are seen with abrupt or insidious onset of positive symptoms (active abnormal symptoms), including delusions, hallucinations, and disorganized behavior and thinking. The hallmark of positive symptoms is delusions. Delusions are fixed beliefs held by the patient and cannot be changed, even when presented with conflicting evidence. Negative symptoms of schizophrenia are signaled by a diminishment or lack of normal characteristics, such as a marked decrease in emotional expression. Reduced eye contact, blunted movement of hands, and blank facial expressions are characteristic. The cognitive impairments associated with schizophrenia are frequently seen early in life and present a steady decline after other symptoms emerge. Depression and thoughts of suicide may follow a psychotic episode.

Management

Individuals with schizophrenia are managed by psychiatrists with management goals of controlling positive and negative symptoms and assisting the patient with other coexisting needs such as homelessness, unemployment, and victimization.

Substance-Related or Behavioral Addictions

Substance-abuse disorders include a core triad of behavioral, cognitive, and physiological symptoms. Terms that are important to know include *intoxication*, which occurs shortly after the agent is consumed. Intoxication is considered to be reversible, as the effects wear off over time. *Withdrawal* from a substance causes functional impairment brought about by the cessation or reduction of the amount of the substance. Sporadic or intermittent utilization of alcohol or drugs without adverse consequences is called *use*. *Dependence* may be physical and/or behavioral in nature and is manifested by physical symptoms associated with withdrawal. Patients exhibit pathological patterns of use and obtaining the substance.

Substances that are legal and subject to addictive behaviors include tobacco and alcohol. Illegal or prescription-only agents include cannabis, heroin, cocaine, opioids, hallucinogens, sedatives, stimulants, and anxiolytics. Newer evidence has determined one common thread associated with addiction, which is the presence of a pathologic, neurophysiologic propensity or risk. The highest prevalence rates for substance abuse occur in individuals between 18 and 24 years.

Symptoms

Major symptom criteria for substance-use disorders include impaired control, risky use, social impairment, tolerance, and withdrawal. Routine screening for substance use and abuse is recommended in all primary care settings.

Management

The first management goal is abstinence, and this often requires controlled withdrawal and detoxification measures. Signs and symptoms of withdrawal may begin shortly after substance cessation. Alcohol withdrawal symptoms include tremors, nausea, sweating, and cognitive changes and often begin within 6 to 12 hours after the last drink. Untreated alcohol withdrawal may be fatal. Following detoxification, individuals require a sustained period of rehabilitation, including education, support, and possibly psychotropic drugs. Management of substance-related and behavioral addictions is accomplished in specialty care settings with clinicians specifically trained in the management of these complex disorders.

Acute Suicide Risk

Around the globe, there are 800,000 completed suicides every year. Countries that are lower to mid income have higher rates of suicide than more affluent countries. Suicide occurs throughout the life span and is the second leading cause of death for individuals aged 15–29 years worldwide. In the United States, the highest rates of completed suicide occur in males aged 15–24 years and over the age of 65 years.

Attempted suicide and completed suicide are a potential complication of many mental health disorders, including bipolar disorder and depression. Other risk factors for suicide include male gender, substance abuse, chronic illness, loss of social support, advancing age, death of spouse, history of sexual abuse, previous suicide attempt, and the availability of means to commit suicide.

Symptoms

Individuals who are contemplating suicide may talk about their intent or may resist sharing their intentions with others. As primary care providers, one of the most valuable screening interventions is to directly ask the patient about suicidal thoughts and plans. Contrary to popular opinion, asking about suicide does not "plant the idea" of suicide and increase risk. In fact, many individuals who do complete suicide were seen by a health care provider within the six months prior to the event but were not asked about suicidal thoughts.

Management

Providing an environment of caring and trust allows an individual to verbalize thoughts and feelings and provides an opportunity for the provider to assist and intervene. For providers who encounter individuals contemplating suicide, the primary goal is to provide for the patient's safety. The reduction or elimination of immediate danger, the provision of physical support by not leaving the patient alone, the involvement of caregivers or family members, and an urgent referral to psychiatric care are indicated for all individuals who express suicidal intent.

Mental Health Disorders in Children and Adolescents

Emerging data reveals an increase in the incidence and prevalence of mental health disorders affecting children and adolescents. Despite the availability of effective treatments for children with mental health disorders, diagnosis is often delayed, placing these patients at risk for long-term complications associated with chronic mental health disease. Mental illnesses usually begin in childhood, and studies of children held in juvenile detention centers have demonstrated remarkably high rates of illness in this population.

Autism Spectrum Disorder (ASD)

Autism spectrum disorder is a complex neurodevelopmental disorder that is characterized by varying degrees of problems in social communication and interaction. Children with ASD may have some degree of intellectual disability and most have a degree of cognitive impairment.

Symptoms

For a diagnosis of ASD, the individual must have demonstrated characteristic symptoms early in life along with some intellectual disability classified as mild, moderate, severe, or profound. In general, children with ASD present with problems involving social interaction with others, communication problems, and decreased language skills. These children often have unusual ways of relating to people, objects, and events. Speech is usually restricted, repetitive, or echolalic. Behaviors are stereotyped. Infants with ASD may be passive and non-engaging, although ASD may not be diagnosed until later in life. Toddlers have delayed speech, lack of social relatedness, decreased eye contact, and lack of reciprocity of interaction. These children often prefer to be alone and exhibit persistent and insistent behaviors such as rocking or hand flapping.

Management

The American Academy of Pediatrics recommends screening at 18 and 24 months in all children. Early intervention services should be initiated for children with ASD, and patients may be managed in psychiatric or primary health care settings. Treatment includes extensive parental education and supportive programs based on the unique needs of each child.

Anxiety Disorders in Children

Anxiety disorders are common during childhood and may be associated with separation anxiety, phobias, panic attacks, obsessions and compulsions, and generalized anxiety. Distinguishing a normal level of anxiety (which is seen in all people) from an abnormal level requires exploring details related to the anxiety itself. The FNP should determine the object of worry, the degree of distress involved, and the degree, if any, of impairment associated with the anxiety as well as the child's coping skills. Studies have shown that children who are confident and eager to try new situations at age five are less likely to suffer with anxiety in adulthood, while those who are more passive, shy, and fearful are at greater risk. The focus of anxiety is often age-specific; toddlers are fearful of monsters, the dark, and being alone while school-age children worry about injury and natural disasters. Because young children have difficulty expressing emotions, anxiety may go unnoticed in young patients.

Symptoms

Children and adolescents with an anxiety disorder may present with somatic complaints or may present with symptoms of anxiety that are situation-specific, such as going to school. Children with high levels of anxiety are at risk for depression, substance abuse, and suicidal ideation as they age.

Management

Management of anxiety in children begins with education provided to the patient and family. Supportive counseling and cognitive behavioral therapy (CBT) are very effective in children and younger adolescents. Psychopharmacologic treatment is reserved for individuals with severe symptoms and those who do not respond to nonpharmacological measures.

Fears and Phobia

Fear is defined as a state of apprehension or anxiety in response to a perceived threat. A phobia may be described as a persistent, irrational, extreme fear that may be triggered by certain people, objects, or situations. During late infancy and toddlerhood, children begin to demonstrate signs of being fearful of certain things. This is a normal part of childhood development and serves as a protective response. Specific fears vary by age. Phobias to specific things or situations affect approximately 5% of children and may require medical or psychiatric management. Again, the important factor in assessing anxiety is the degree of disturbance caused by the symptoms.

During infancy, fear may be related to a sense of loss of physical support (falling) or unexpected or excessive stimuli such as loud noises. Toddlers often fear being separated from a parent, experiencing physical injury, and encountering strangers. During the preschool years, the child's imagination is awakening and may bring about fears of monsters, the dark, animals, or being alone. This fear of darkness and certain animals may extend into the school-age years, along with school-related fears. As a child enters adolescence, fear of bodily injury, social fears, and concerns about political upheaval predominate. It is important to remember that most fears are transient and often disappear. These fears do not predict the child will have mental health problems as an adult.

Symptoms

It is important to separate normal fears associated with daily living from abnormal fears and phobias. When fear produces a negative impact on functioning, evaluation should be performed and management initiated. Symptoms associated with phobias include a significant amount of extreme fear or dread that is experienced when the situation or thing is encountered. Phobias are problematic when they interfere with daily functioning.

Management

Management focuses on cognitive-behavioral therapy, contingency management (e.g., development of a plan for managing the phobia if other measures fail), and family interventions. Psychologists and psychiatrists who specialize in the management of these disorders should coordinate care for these children and adolescents.

Eating Disorders

Abnormal behaviors associated with eating occur secondary to dysmorphism, which is altered body image. Anorexia nervosa (AN) and bulimia nervosa (BN) are the two most commonly occurring eating disorders, although there are many others such as pica, rumination disorders, and those associated with infancy. Eating disorders are extremely complex conditions with multifaceted etiology and pathophysiological associations. An important consideration in these disorders is the lasting physiological and mental health complications and comorbidities that occur in conjunction with these conditions.

Anorexia nervosa is associated with the highest mortality rate of all mental health disorders, with a five-year mortality rate of 15–20%. Most patients die of malnutrition, electrolyte imbalance, and suicide. Because these illnesses are so complex and management is correspondingly complex, requiring team care and coordination, primary care providers play an important role in screening and identification. Both disorders affect more females than males, and symptoms usually begin during mid to late adolescence; however, cases prior to puberty do occur and may be particularly devastating. Athletes have a higher risk for eating disorders, particularly athletes who compete in sports classified by weight divisions (e.g., wrestling), long distance running, and those activities with a strong emphasis on flexibility and aesthetic lines (e.g., ice skating, gymnastics, dancing). Additional risk factors include higher socioeconomic status, chronic disease (e.g., diabetes mellitus, cystic fibrosis, depression), previous obesity, a history of abuse, and the presence of personality disorders. These children often have parents who focus on weight and fitness and place pressure on them to excel. As with most mental health disorders, evidence suggests a strong genetic component.

Symptoms

Patient presentations are variable and related to the underlying disorder. These individuals express the belief that self-worth is intrinsically tied to body image. Criteria for diagnosis of anorexia nervosa include a refusal to maintain body weight at the 85th percentile for age and height or a failure to gain weight. Individuals express an intense fear of becoming "fat" and may engage in repeated weight-loss behaviors, such as exercising and extreme portion control with eating. Binging and purging episodes may occur with AN but are more common with bulimia nervosa. Individuals with anorexia are unable to realistically assess their body size and shape and do not see themselves as severely underweight.

Patients with bulimia nervosa are often average weight or overweight. Binging and purging is a classic presentation for this disorder. Common findings with both disorders include menstrual irregularity, weight fluctuation or loss, guilt associated with eating, a fixed highly structured daily schedule, intolerance to cold, constipation, diarrhea, abdominal bloating, and sore throat and dental erosion (common with BN). Physical findings include altered growth, fluid retention, Russell's sign (e.g., abrasions, calluses on knuckles from inducing vomiting), thinning hair or alopecia, hypotension, muscle atrophy, and mental sluggishness.

Management

Management is coordinated by psychiatric specialists skilled in treating these complex disorders. Patients often require inpatient management, and relapses are common.

Practice Questions

1. The Patient Health Questionnaire 2 (PHQ 2) is a brief screening tool for depression used frequently in outpatient care. Which of the following statements completes one of the questions in the PHQ 2? Over the past two weeks, how often have you been bothered by:

   (A) feeling little interest or pleasure in doing things?
   (B) thoughts about hurting yourself?
   (C) wanting to sleep all the time?
   (D) having no appetite?

2. Your patient is a 52-year-old male who is seen infrequently in your clinic. He presents today with a chief complaint of "not feeling well." On assessment, you notice jaundice and abdominal distention. One differential diagnosis is hepatitis; however, based on his social history, you also suspect alcohol abuse. Which of the following will be helpful in assessing alcohol abuse?

   (A) administering the Patient Health Questionnaire 9 (PHQ 9)
   (B) asking the patient directly about alcohol use
   (C) ordering liver enzymes testing
   (D) ordering a CT of the abdomen

3. Peak symptoms of alcohol withdrawal are usually seen how long after the last drink of alcohol?

   (A) less than 12 hours
   (B) 12 to 24 hours
   (C) 24 to 48 hours
   (D) more than 48 hours

4. Very young children with depression may demonstrate all of the following symptoms, EXCEPT:

   (A) sleep problems.
   (B) withdrawal.
   (C) speech and motor development delays.
   (D) weight gain.

5. QT prolongation is a risk with higher doses of which of the following agents used in the treatment of major depressive disorder?

   (A) citalopram
   (B) sertraline
   (C) venlafaxine
   (D) fluoxetine

6. The pharmacological agent buspirone has:

   (A) significant antianxiety action.
   (B) low abuse potential.
   (C) a rapid onset of action.
   (D) a severe withdrawal syndrome when withdrawn suddenly.

7. Major depressive disorder in adults often presents with all the following, EXCEPT:

   (A) psychomotor retardation.
   (B) irritability.
   (C) cardiac palpitations.
   (D) increased feelings of guilt.

8. Which of the following statements is true regarding anorexia nervosa?

   (A) Onset is usually in the mid to late 20s for men and women.
   (B) The disease affects men and women equally.
   (C) Patients with anorexia nervosa are aware of their extreme thinness.
   (D) Depression is often a comorbid disorder.

9. Rates of depression among adolescents between 13 and 18 years of age:

   (A) increase with age.
   (B) decrease with age.
   (C) plateau at age 15 years.
   (D) plateau at age 10 years.

10. Evidence indicates that asking adolescents about suicidal thoughts and plans:

   (A) may precipitate thoughts of suicide.
   (B) may damage the patient-provider relationship.
   (C) may prompt the adolescent to share thoughts with the provider.
   (D) may cause the adolescent to be reluctant to share concerns.

11. Signs of major depressive disorder (MDD) may include:
    Select all that apply.

   (A) slowed movements.
   (B) complaints of muscle pain.
   (C) headaches and body aches.
   (D) feelings of sadness or hopelessness.

12. The most common comorbidity with depression is:

   (A) substance abuse.
   (B) behavioral disorders.
   (C) obsessive-compulsive disorder (OCD).
   (D) anxiety.

13. The usual first-line medication class used in the management of an initial episode of depression is:

   (A) tricyclic antidepressants (TCAs).
   (B) monoamine oxidase inhibitors (MAOIs).
   (C) selective serotonin reuptake inhibitors (SSRIs).
   (D) calcium channel blockers (CCBs).

14. Which of the following characteristics is present in bulimia nervosa?

    (A) food restriction
    (B) binge eating
    (C) excessive exercise
    (D) refusal to maintain body weight at the 85th percentile for age and height

15. Among the following choices, which constitutes the highest risk for suicide?

    (A) a positive family history
    (B) having suicidal thoughts
    (C) preparation for suicide with a detailed plan
    (D) exhibiting persistent sadness

Answer Explanations

1. **(A)** The PHQ 2 is not used to diagnose depression but is a useful screening tool that is easily administered in most clinical settings. The screen is scored from 0–6 based on the patient's selection of level or degree of concern. In most settings, a score of 3 or above indicates the need for a more in-depth evaluation. The Patient Health Questionnaire 9 (PHQ 9) is often used to follow up on a positive PHQ 2. The first question in the PHQ 2 is "Over the past two weeks, how often have you been bothered by feeling little interest or pleasure in doing things? The second question in the PHQ 2 is "Over the past two weeks, how often have you been bothered by feeling down, depressed, or hopeless?" Choices (B), (C), and (D) are not included in this brief screening.

2. **(B)** Asking the patient directly about alcohol use has proven to be an effective method of screening for alcohol abuse in primary care. An example of an appropriate question is: "How often in the past year have you exceeded the maximum daily limit for alcohol?" This limit is specific for men and women. The PHQ 9 (choice (A)) is a screening tool used in the evaluation of depressive disorders. Liver enzymes may be elevated in cases of alcohol addiction (choice (C)); however, other causes of this elevation are possible, such as hepatitis. Ordering a CT of the abdomen (choice (D)) may reveal structural abnormalities but is not helpful in evaluating for alcohol abuse and addiction.

3. **(A)** Withdrawal symptoms from alcohol cessation begin within 6–12 hours of the last drink. During this period, individuals will experience headaches, anxiety, nausea, and stomach pains. Within the next 12–48 hours (choices (B) and (C)), symptoms escalate to confusion, increased heart rate and blood pressure, and increase in body temperature. In hours 48 to 72+ (choice (D)), withdrawal symptoms may include tremors, shakes, seizures, hallucinations, delirium tremens (DTs), and possibly death.

4. **(D)** Symptoms associated with depression vary by age, and very young children may have difficulty describing how they are feeling. Very young children with depression often demonstrate sleep problems (choice (A)), withdrawal (choice (B)), speech and motor development delays (choice (C)), lack of pleasure in play, sleep problems, low energy, increased talk about death or suicide, anorexia, and loss of weight.

5. **(A)** Citalopram, sertraline (choice (B)), venlafaxine (choice (C)), and fluoxetine (choice (D)) are all selective serotonin reuptake inhibitors (SSRIs); however, only citalopram carries a higher risk for inducing ECG changes such as a prolonged QT interval. Prior to starting citalopram, consider a baseline ECG and measurement of the QT interval in patients with heart disease. Thrombocytopenia has also been reported with citalopram.

6. **(B)** Buspirone is a second-line agent indicated for the treatment of anxiety. This medication is less effective in managing anxiety than benzodiazepines (choice (A)) and has a delayed onset of action (choice (C)). Unlike the benzodiazepines, withdrawal of buspirone is unlikely to cause symptoms (choice (D)). Contrasted with benzodiazepines, buspirone has a lower abuse potential and is not a scheduled drug.

7. **(C)** Symptoms of depression in adults include feelings of hopelessness, withdrawal and social isolation, psychomotor retardation (slowed movement) (choice (A)), irritability (choice (B)), increased feelings of guilt (choice (D)), and hypersomnia or insomnia. Because of the psychomotor retardation, cardiac palpitations are unlikely to be seen in adults with depression.

8. **(D)** Depression is a frequent comorbid condition with anorexia nervosa (AN), which is a complex eating disorder associated with body dysmorphism and a refusal to maintain a minimally normal body weight. Despite what the mirror indicates, these individuals see themselves as fat and will go to almost any length to lose weight. Onset of AN is usually before young adulthood (choice (A)). Females are affected more often than males (choice (B)). They are unaware that they are extremely thin and have a disease (choice (C)). Patients with AN may fail to achieve expected weight and height gains and begin restricting food intake. AN may be associated with binge-purging cycles during which the patient eats a large amount of food very quickly and then induces vomiting. Serious physical complications associated with AN include amenorrhea, electrolyte abnormalities, and starvation. Ten percent of individuals with AN experience sudden death as a result of cardiac arrest, starvation, or suicide.

9. **(A)** Rates of depression among adolescents increase with age from an approximate 5% incidence in the early teen years to a 20% incidence in late adolescence.

10. **(C)** A provider directly asking an adolescent about suicidal thoughts or plans demonstrates to the teen that the provider cares about them and may promote open communication. Asking about suicide does not "plant the idea" of suicide in the adolescent (choice (A)), strengthens the patient-provider relationship (choice (B)), and does not cause the adolescent to be reluctant to share concerns (choice (D)).

11. **(A, B, C, D)** Symptoms associated with major depressive disorder include decreased interest in most activities, insomnia or hypersomnia, psychomotor retardation (choice (A)), vague complaints of muscle pain or body aches (choice (B)), headaches (choice (C)), change in appetite, loss of energy, behavioral agitation, feelings of sadness or hopelessness (choice (D)), and recurrent thoughts of death or suicide.

12. **(D)** While substance abuse (choice (A)), behavioral disorders (choice (B)), and OCD (choice (C)) may occur with major depressive disorder, anxiety is the most common comorbidity. Anxiety and depression often exacerbate each other, making management challenging.

13. **(C)** Guidelines in the management of major depressive disorder recommend the use of SSRIs as first-line agents for a first episode of depression. TCAs (choice (A)) may be used for individuals who did not have symptom response with SSRIs or SNRIs. MAOIs (choice (B)) are rarely used because of an extensive side effect profile and drug interactions. CCBs (choice (D)) are used as antihypertensive drugs or for cases of mild anxiety.

14. **(B)** Bulimia nervosa is a body dysmorphic disorder that occurs in individuals who are usually of average weight or are overweight. The disease is characterized by episodes of binge eating during which the individual will consume large quantities of food in a short amount of time. This is followed by extreme guilt and often purging by taking laxatives or inducing vomiting. Food restriction (choice (A)), excessive exercise (choice (C)), and refusal to maintain body weight at the 85th percentile for age and height (choice (D)) are characteristic of anorexia nervosa, not bulimia.

15. **(C)** Risk factors for acute suicide include bipolar disorder, history of a family member committing suicide (choice (A)), having persistent suicidal thoughts (choice (B)), and depression (choice (D)). However, having a detailed plan for committing suicide presents the highest risk among these choices.

PART IV
Pediatrics and Adolescents

14

Caring for Pediatric Patients

Pediatric patients span the ages from birth to 18 years. During this period of time, growth and development occur in a sequential manner; however, growth rates are entirely individual. Growth is an increase in size, whereas development indicates the increase and refinement of overall function and skill. An important role of the FNP in primary care is surveillance of growth and development throughout infancy and childhood. Early identification of developmental delay or decreased growth patterns may provide for early intervention and improved outcomes. This chapter discusses normal growth and developmental milestones, primary care surveillance, and illnesses common to pediatric patients. Also covered in this chapter are age-specific assessment techniques and a brief review of the developmental milestones associated with different age groups. Table 14.1 summarizes behavioral milestones associated with the age group from birth to two years old.

Table 14.1. Growth and Developmental Milestones (Birth to Two Years of Age)

Age	Expected Behaviors
0–1 month	Sleeps 16 hours/day; breastfed infants feed more frequently than formula-fed infants Transitions from alertness, feeding, and sleep; may lift head briefly when prone
1–3 months	Develops capacity to self-soothe; demonstrates cues when hungry; demonstrates increased visual acuity; can lift head when prone; begins to coo
4–5 months	Begins to roll over; reaches for/grasps rattle; can bring objects to mouth; plays with feet; turns in response to sound; demonstrates improved head control; smiles spontaneously; copies facial expressions; very social
6–8 months	May have 6–12 hour periods without being fed; begins solid food; begins scooting and crawling; likes to play with others; responds to other people's emotions; may be afraid of strangers; responds to name; babbles; sits without support
9–12 months	Begins to use "pincer grasp" to pick items up, such as cereal pieces; pulls to stand up; begins to "cruise" around furniture; says "mama" and "dada" not specific to correct parent; understands "no"; uses finger to point at objects; has favorite toy; comprehends object permanence Stands alone; may begin taking steps; crawls up and down stairs
15 months	Can say 1–3 words; walks well; can bend over to pick things up
18 months	Likes to hand things to others; afraid of strangers; can have temper tantrums; points to show things to others; says several single words; can walk up steps using rail
24 months	Demonstrates more independence; copies adults and older children; commonly demonstrates parallel play; follows simple instructions; points to things in a book
36 months	Learns to take turns when playing; dresses and undresses self; understands "mine," "his," and "hers"; can follow 2–3 step instructions; separates easily from parent; climbs and runs well; can ride a tricycle; speaks 3–4 word sentences
48 months	Enjoys trying new things; plays make-believe; can say first and last name; tells stories; names colors and some numbers; draws a person with 2–4 body parts; hops and stands on one foot; uses scissors

The administration of vaccines is considered a primary prevention measure. Primary prevention is the most effective form of health care as it prevents a condition from developing. Table 14.2 shows the most common recommended vaccines from birth through 18 years.

Secondary prevention includes screening tests, which aim to identify problems in the early stages when treatment may be more effective. Tertiary prevention includes measures that are directed toward improving function and preventing further deterioration associated with problems in later stages that have become chronic in nature.

Table 14.2. Recommended Vaccines from Birth through 18 Years*

Type of Vaccine	Birth	2 mos	4 mos	6 mos	9 mos	12–15 mos	18 mo	2–3 yrs	4–6 yrs	7–10 yrs	11–12 yrs	13–15 yrs	16–18 yrs
Hepatitis B vaccine	X	X		X									
Rotavirus vaccine		X	X	X									
Diphtheria, acellular pertussis vaccine		X	X	X		X (15–18)							
Haemophilus influenza type B vaccine		X	X	X		X							
Pneumococcal conjugate vaccine		X	X	X		X							
Inactivated polio vaccine		X	X	X (6–18)									
Influenza vaccine				X		Annually							
Measles, mumps, rubella, varicella vaccine						X			X				
Human papillomavirus vaccine											3-dose series		
Meningococcal vaccine											X		Booster

*Based on CDC guidelines.

Developmental Surveillance

Primary care management of pediatric patients includes developmental surveillance, which incorporates principles of growth and development as well as recognition of developmental red flags. Red flags are findings that may signal conditions that negatively impact health. Pediatric health care is intrinsically family care, as parental education is crucial in supporting parents as they care for their growing children.

Newborn to One Year (Piaget's Theory of Development: Sensorimotor Stage)

During this period, rapid growth and development of all body systems occurs. The infant progresses from the helpless state of a newborn to the relatively independent state of a toddler who is able to walk, run, climb, and explore.

Neonatal/newborn assessment at birth should include a general survey of physical characteristics along with Apgar scoring, which includes heart rate, respiratory effort, muscle tone, reflex irritability, and color. The FNP should do an assessment of body temperature and an assessment of gestational age, which includes body length, weight, and head circumference. The assessment should include an examination of the umbilical cord, which should contain two arteries and one vein.

Common findings at birth or in the newborn period include milia, which are firm, pearl-colored, opalescent white papules often scattered over the face and forehead. Within the oropharynx, these lesions are called Epstein pearls. Milia are self-limiting, and no treatment is needed. Cutis marmorata is a fine, lacy, red or blue cutaneous pattern occurring over most of the body. The condition is a response to low environmental temperatures and is benign and self-limiting.

Conditions of the Head, Face, and Eyes

- **Caput succedaneum:** a diffuse soft-tissue swelling of the scalp; underlying bruising may be present. The condition results from trauma as the head descends through the birth canal. Edema crosses cranial suture lines. Caput succedaneum is self-limiting and resolves over several days.
- **Cephalhematoma:** a collection of blood within the subperiosteal area that does not cross the suture lines of the cranium. The condition appears hours after delivery and resolves within weeks to months; no treatment is needed.
- **Cleft lip and palate:** a fetal development failure of embryonic structure closure. The cleft (or opening) may be unilateral or bilateral and may involve only the lip or may include the soft and hard palate and uvula. Bifid uvula may signal underlying submucosal cleft.
- **Congenital lacrimal duct obstruction (dacryostenosis):** the incomplete development of the lacrimal duct. The condition resolves spontaneously within six months in most infants.

Respiratory Conditions

- **Respiratory distress syndrome (RDS):** a syndrome seen with surfactant deficiency occurring in premature infants. Tachypnea, grunting, intercostal retractions, nasal flaring, and duskiness and/or cyanosis may be seen. RDS requires supportive care and mechanical ventilation.
- **Transient tachypnea of newborn (TTN):** retained amniotic fluid with diminished lung compliance. The condition is self-limiting and usually resolves within 24–48 hours.
- **Meconium aspiration:** term or post-term infants; aspiration of meconium occurs as a result of fetal distress; tachypnea, retractions, grunting, and cyanosis appear within hours of delivery. The condition may resolve spontaneously in otherwise healthy infants but may require suctioning and mechanical ventilation.

Cardiac Conditions

- **Atrial septal defect (ASD):** an acyanotic disorder characterized by an opening between the left and right atria, occurring in the septum. A heart murmur associated with an ASD is usually not heard until the child is two or three years of age. Small defects may close spontaneously; however, larger defects may require intervention.

- **Ventricular septal defect (VSD):** an acyanotic defect due to an opening in the ventricular septum. A heart murmur can be heard after birth, and the infant may develop signs of congestive heart failure. When small defects are found, they are assessed for changes every six months throughout the first year and then annually. A VSD may close spontaneously or remain open, requiring medical management.

- **Aortic dilation:** a condition in which there is an enlargement of part of the aorta. This finding is often a precursor to acute aortic dissection, which is usually fatal. Aortic dilation is a finding often associated with the genetic condition Marfan syndrome. This syndrome is also associated with the characteristics of tall stature; long, thin extremities; myopia; and retinal detachment. Connective tissue problems associated with Marfan syndrome include abnormalities of the pectus and hyperextension of joints. Along with aortic dilation, mitral valve prolapse is also a common cardiac finding.

- **Transposition of the great arteries (dextro-transposition, d-TPA):** a cyanotic defect in which the aorta communicates with the right ventricle and the pulmonary artery communicates with the left ventricle. Cyanosis develops immediately or soon after birth and requires an immediate referral to a pediatric cardiologist.

- **Tetralogy of Fallot (TOF):** a cyanotic defect that is a combination of four anatomical defects, including pulmonary valve stenosis, right ventricular hypertrophy, ventricular septal defect, and overriding aorta. TOF has a variable presentation ranging from mild to severe. The infant presents with cyanosis at birth, which increases with time, and with heart murmur. TOF requires an immediate referral to a pediatric cardiologist for management. Tetralogy of Fallot episodes, also known as "tet" episodes, occur with hypercyanosis present; the infant should be held in the knee-chest position until the episode resolves.

Gastrointestinal Conditions

- **Esophageal atresia and tracheoesophageal fistula:** a blind pouch of the esophagus with or without a fistula, or opening, into the trachea. Esophageal atresia may be associated with a history of maternal polyhydramnios, excessive oral secretions, choking, cyanosis during feedings, and vomiting. Esophageal atresia is a surgical emergency, requiring emergent referral to a pediatric surgical gastroenterologist.

- **Diaphragmatic hernia:** the herniation of abdominal contents into the thoracic area. The condition presents with varying degrees of respiratory distress. The infant should be positioned with head and chest higher than the abdomen. Diaphragmatic hernia requires an immediate referral to a pediatric specialist.

Hematologic Conditions

- **Jaundice:** a yellow-orange pigment that develops in the skin secondary to the accumulation of bilirubin. Free bilirubin is neurotoxic at high levels. Pathologic (nonphysiologic) jaundice appears within the first 24 hours of life and results from widespread autoimmune hemolysis. Jaundice may require an exchange transfusion. Physiologic jaundice appears first on the head and face during the first week of life; the condition appears clinically with a bilirubin

> **CLINICAL PEARL**
>
> Severe jaundice in the newborn period may lead to kernicterus, which is a neurological disorder secondary to increased levels of unbound bilirubin. This neurological disorder causes severe mental retardation and seizures.

of 5 mg/dL or higher and clears spontaneously in one to two weeks. Jaundice may require phototherapy. Breast milk jaundice may appear secondary to relative dehydration in breast-feeding infants. This condition occurs after seven days of age, peaks at two to three weeks, and may take a month to clear.

Musculoskeletal Conditions

- **Developmental dysplasia of the hip (DDH):** an anatomic abnormality of the hip joint in which the femoral head and acetabulum do not align properly, leading to abnormal growth of the bones involved. Screening tests include the Ortolani and Barlow tests that should be performed during the neonatal period before the second or third month of life, when muscles and ligaments surrounding the joint begin to tighten. In addition to positive findings on Ortolani and Barlow screening tests, other indicators include thigh-fold asymmetry and leg-length discrepancy (Galeazzi's sign). DDH requires referral to a pediatric orthopedic specialist. Splinting with a harness is the usual treatment.

Early Childhood (Piaget's Theory of Development: Preoperational Stage)

During the early childhood period, which includes toddlers and preschoolers (ages two to four years), rapid growth and development continue as the child increases in cognitive, psychosocial, and motor abilities. The American Academy of Pediatrics (AAP) suggests that autism screenings should be part of standard 18 and 24-month well-child checkups. Safety education for parents is key during this time as young children love to explore but have no sense of danger or risk. Injuries are common. Table 14.3 describes the characteristic features of different types of development at this stage.

Table 14.3. Growth and Developmental Milestones (Early Childhood)

Type of Development	Characteristics
Dental Development	A complete set of 20 deciduous teeth is present at 3 years of age; growth and development of permanent teeth occurs within the gums.
Neurologic Development	Fine and gross motor skills improve and sensory function increases.
Cardiovascular Development	The heart rate typically slows as the heart develops and grows in size and functional capacity. Innocent murmurs are common. Hemoglobin level stabilizes at 12–15 g/dL during this period.
Pulmonary Development	Abdominal respirations continue until the age of 5 or 6 years. The respiratory rate decreases to around 30 breaths per minute.
Gastrointestinal Development	Salivary glands reach adult size by age 2; increased stomach capacity occurs; however, small children may need a snack between meals because of small stomach size. The liver matures and is able to store vitamins, produce glycogen, and produce amino acids and ketone bodies.
Renal Development	Kidneys increase in size and move deeper into the pelvic area. Urine excretion increases to 600–750 mL/day by the age of 5 years.
Cognitive Development	Vocabulary and articulation increase. Speech gradually becomes understandable to others. Semantics (understanding the meaning of words) increases dramatically during this time.

CLINICAL PEARL

An annual wellness screening should be done for children in the preoperational stage with regard to physical and motor skills, language development, and social, emotional, and cognitive development.

School-Age Children (Piaget's Theory of Development: Operational Stage)

During the school-age years (5 to 12 years), children experience profound physical, emotional, and cognitive changes as they move from toddlerhood to adolescence. Children during this stage are stronger and demonstrate increased coordination of movement. Growth typically occurs in "spurts," which span weeks, followed by times of quiescent or slowed growth. Table 14.4 describes the characteristic features of different types of development at the operational stage.

Table 14.4. Growth and Developmental Milestones (School-Age Children)

Type of Development	Characteristics
Skin & Lymph Node Development	Tonsils and adenoids reach their largest size around 6 years old; sebaceous glands become more active as the child nears pubescence.
Head, Eyes, Ears, Mouth Development	Head size becomes more proportionate to body size; sinus cavities undergo development and increase in size; visual acuity is 20/20 by the ages of 6–7 years. The first primary teeth are lost between the ages of 5 and 6 years, and permanent teeth begin to erupt.
Pulmonary Development	The lungs continue to descend into the thoracic cavity and alveolar development is completed. Increase in phagocytic activity increases resistance to respiratory infections.
Cardiovascular Development	The heart begins to take on adult proportions in relation to separate cardiac chambers. The heart rate slows to 60 to 100 beats per minute. Atherosclerosis begins at this time.
Gastrointestinal Development	The GI system has fully matured and gained adult size.
Genitourinary Development	Regular elimination patterns are established; persistent bed-wetting becomes rare as bladder capacity expands. Changes associated with puberty begin around 10 years of age.
Musculoskeletal Development	Long bones show increased growth; the spine becomes straighter and facial bones change along with the growth and development of nasal sinuses.

Adolescents (Piaget's Theory of Development: Formal Operational Stage)

Adolescence (ages 10 years to 19 years) is typically another period of rapid changes in growth and development. As cognition increases, adolescents notice their bodies change and often wonder if they are "normal." Development of secondary sexual characteristics usually begins during middle school and often precedes emotional development.

Tanner staging is used to assess sexual maturity level and development. Breast budding, corresponding to Tanner stage 2, occurs in girls around 9 or 10 years of age. This is the first clinical sign of puberty in girls. The first sign of male puberty is testicular enlargement, which usually occurs around the age of 11 years. This change also corresponds with Tanner stage 2.

Emotional egocentrism is characteristic of adolescence and is demonstrated by a self-centered view of the world. Self-image changes along with physical and cognitive changes and concerns about "being like everyone else" take priority for many teenagers. Adolescence may be divided into three distinct stages according to age. These stages are associated with certain developmental characteristics.

Early Adolescence (10–14 Years)

Physical changes in early adolescence are extremely variable and unique to each person. During this period, you will often notice 12-year-olds who are very small physically with no obvious signs of puberty along with other 12-year-olds who have achieved sexual maturity and significant physical growth. Behavior associated with the cognitive and emotional development occurring during this stage is seen as the adolescent develops an increasing interest in peer relationships. During adolescence, many individuals begin to develop specific interests or hobbies, and fitting in with others is often a major concern.

Middle Adolescence (15–17 Years)

Physical development is nearly complete and growth slows. Individuals' concerns are less about physical changes and more about making themselves "attractive." Peer relationships are important; however, some emotional movement back toward the family is often noted. Intellectual development promotes increased creativity and problem-solving. Sexual drive emerges during this period and risk-taking and experimentation peak. Screening for sexually transmitted infections becomes an important aspect of health care surveillance along with education on transmission and prevention.

Late Adolescence (18–19 Years)

Physical, emotional, and cognitive growth are complete for most individuals during this stage, although males may continue to gain in height for a few more years. Major life decisions are often made, such as college, career choices, life partners, and lifestyle choices. Adolescents often relate to the family as adults, and the relationship itself undergoes significant changes.

Common Childhood Disorders

The following disorders are common to children from birth to 18 years of age. Some disorders may occur throughout childhood, while others are associated with specific age groups.

Croup

Croup is a self-limiting disease affecting the upper airway and is usually caused by parainfluenza type 1 virus. Occurrence of croup peaks in children between the ages of 6 and 36 months and is seen during flu season.

Symptoms

The characteristic presentation of croup is upper respiratory symptoms of inspiratory stridor with cough and hoarseness. Inflammation of the larynx and subglottis may lead to respiratory distress in young infants.

Management

Management of croup is supportive with humidified air and fluids as needed. Infants should continue to breastfeed. The illness usually resolves without sequelae.

Bronchiolitis

Bronchiolitis is a respiratory illness, usually caused by respiratory syncytial virus (RSV), and less often, adenovirus. Illness causes inflammation, edema, and necrosis of the epithelial cells of the upper airways, producing copious mucus. This communicable illness is seen most commonly from infancy to children two years of age. Severe disease is more likely in infants two to three months of age because of waning maternal antibodies. Transmission occurs through close contact with infected respiratory secretions. The virus can also live on surfaces for up to 30 minutes, thus may be transmitted by contact with surfaces in the environment such as tabletops and doors.

Symptoms

Bronchiolitis usually has an insidious onset of upper respiratory symptoms occurring over two to three days. These symptoms progress to affect the lower respiratory system over the next several days. Infants may present with wheezing and varying degrees of respiratory distress due to mucus obstruction of airways. The first 48 hours of illness are the most critical and young infants may develop apneic episodes.

Management

Management involves supportive care including hydration, antipyretics, and nebulized respiratory treatments. Younger infants may be hospitalized with continuous oxygen saturation surveillance and oxygen therapy as indicated.

Prevention of RSV is provided by administration of palivizumab, which offers some protection from severe disease. The vaccine is given in a maximum of five monthly injections to infants at risk for complications of RSV infection. Injections are provided during RSV season, usually November through March.

Infectious Diseases

Roseola Infantum (Sixth Disease)

This self-limiting illness is caused by human herpes virus (HHV) 6 and occurs in children between 7 and 24 months of age. The virus is transmitted via oral, nasal, and conjunctival routes.

Symptoms

The characteristic presentation of roseola infantum is a sudden onset of high fever of up to 103°F that lasts approximately three to five days. During this time, the infant does not seem particularly ill. When the fever breaks, a diffuse, maculopapular, rose-colored rash appears. The rash begins on the trunk and spreads outward and may last from a few hours to a few days.

Management

Management of roseola infantum is supportive with fluids and acetaminophen for fever.

Erythema Infectiosum (Fifth Disease)

Erythema infectiosum (EI) is caused by Parvovirus B19 and is seen most often in children ages 5 to 15 years. Erythema infectiosum may be transmitted vertically from mother to fetus, through respiratory secretions, and through exposure to blood or blood products. This normally self-limiting illness may be harmful to pregnant women, and fetal anomalies have been reported.

Symptoms

The illness usually begins with a prodrome of fever, headache, and malaise. Approximately 7–10 days later, an erythematous maculopapular rash appears, first on the cheeks (slapped cheek), and then progressing to the torso and limbs. The rash clears spontaneously, sometimes after a month. Rash recurrences may occur in response to heat, sunlight, exercise, stress, or trauma. Although the rash may produce mild pruritus, overall the child is not particularly ill.

Management

Care for patients with EI is supportive and includes offering fluids frequently. Patients should avoid situations that may exacerbate the rash, such as exposure to sunlight.

Varicella (Chickenpox)

Chickenpox is caused by the varicella zoster virus (VZV) and is the primary illness caused by the virus. Reactivation presents as shingles. Varicella is very contagious and is spread by direct contact, droplets, and airborne transmission; however, the overall incidence of varicella has decreased since the introduction of varicella vaccine. This illness peaks in children 10–14 years old. Varicella is usually a benign, self-limiting illness in children with a normal immune response, but can produce severe illness in those who are immunocompromised.

The varicella vaccine is given in a two-dose series. The first dose is usually given between 12 and 15 months of age with a second dose between four and six years of age. The vaccine is made from a live, though weakened, form of the virus and is very effective in preventing the disease. Individuals who have received the vaccine may still develop the illness, but the course of the illness will be much milder.

Symptoms

Children with varicella infection may have a prodromal period before the rash develops. During this stage, there may be a low-grade fever, headache, anorexia, mild abdominal pain, and listlessness. The second stage begins with the appearance of the rash, which occurs in crops of highly pruritic lesions. Lesions progress from red spots to "teardrop" vesicles, which become cloudy and umbilicate within 24 to 48 hours. Following this, scabs form over the bumps. As crops of lesions continue to erupt, lesions in different stages of healing will be seen, which is classic for this illness.

Management

Management for varicella is supportive and includes bed rest, increased fluids, acetaminophen for discomfort, and isolation until lesions have completely healed.

Mumps

Mumps is an acute viral illness caused by viruses in the *Paramyxoviridae* family. The virus is transmitted through saliva and respiratory secretions. The incubation period is from 12 to 25 days and is common during late winter and spring in children younger than 10 years.

Since the development of the mumps vaccine, there has been a significant decline in the number of cases in countries where the vaccine is regularly given. The vaccine is usually given along with the measles vaccine and rubella vaccine in a single dose. New formulations have added varicella to the mix. These vaccines are recommended at 12 to 15 months and four to six years of age.

Symptoms

A prodromal stage of fever, anorexia, headache, malaise, and muscular pain may occur approximately 24 hours before parotid swelling begins. This swelling is painful and may be unilateral or bilateral. The gland swells and fills the space below the posterior border of the mandible and the mastoid bone. This pushes the ear forward and upward and is accompanied by a severe sore throat and difficulty swallowing. Orchitis may develop in unimmunized individuals who contract the disease after puberty.

Management

Management for mumps is supportive care, such as maintaining hydration, encouraging rest, avoiding contact sports, and administering antipyretics as needed for fever. The disease is self-limiting.

Measles (Rubeola)

Measles is caused by a virus that is similar to mumps and influenza. This contagious illness affects around 20 million people every year worldwide with around 150,000 deaths. Most cases now seen in the United States occur in unvaccinated individuals who bring the virus back with them from endemic areas. Measles is a serious illness for affected children. Transmission is via respiratory droplets and fomites. Peak infection occurs in late winter and spring. The illness has an incubation period as long as 21 days, and an individual is contagious from one to two days before symptoms begin until four days after the rash appears.

Symptoms

The incubation period for measles is from 8 to 21 days, and during this time the patient has no symptoms. A prodromal stage presents with signs of an upper respiratory infection with fever along with cough, coryza, and conjunctivitis (**the three Cs of measles**). Koplik spots may be seen on the oral mucosa and are characteristic of measles. The rash appears around the fourth day and is accompanied by a rise in temperature, often to 105°F. The maculopapular rash begins on the forehead and behind the ears. The lesions enlarge and coalesce and then move downward from the face and over the entire body. Rash severity is indicative of illness severity. There is potential for the development of a hemorrhagic rash associated with disseminated intravascular coagulation (DIC), which may be fatal.

Management

Management for measles is supportive with antipyretics, rest, and a darkened room if indicated for photophobia. Bacterial superinfections may occur and are treated with antibiotics. Measles is a preventable illness, and immunization is recommended at 12 to 15 months of age and again at four to six years of age.

Rubella (German Measles/Three-Day Measles)

Rubella is an RNA virus from the *Rubivirus* family. Transmission occurs transplacentally from mother to fetus as well as through nasopharyngeal secretions. This virus is not transmitted easily and requires repeated, prolonged exposure. An incubation period of 14 to 21 days precedes the rash. This illness is more commonly seen in adolescents and young adults and occurs during winter and spring months. Lifelong immunity results from naturally occurring infection; however, asymptomatic reinfection is possible. Maternal infection during the first trimester of pregnancy is associated with a high risk for fetal congenital defects.

Symptoms

A prodromal syndrome of fever, sore throat, malaise, and headache may appear before the rash erupts. Lymphadenopathy is also seen and may present up to a week before the rash appears. The rash is an enanthem, which is an eruption involving mucus membranes (Forcheimer spots) and is characteristic for rubella infection. Appearance of discrete maculopapular lesions begins on the face and spreads to the chest and downward over the next day or two. The rash has usually cleared by day 3 of the illness. Unlike measles, there is no photophobia associated with rubella.

Management

Management for rubella is supportive. Incidence of rubella has decreased significantly since the implementation of vaccine recommendations. The rubella vaccine is given, along with mumps, measles, and varicella vaccines, at 12 to 15 months of age and repeated at four to six years of age. A pregnant woman who has not received the rubella vaccine and is nonimmune should be vaccinated immediately after delivery.

Influenza

Influenza is an orthomyxovirus with three antigenic types: A, B, and C. Types A and B are typically responsible for influenza epidemics. Influenza is highly contagious and may be transmitted through contact with droplets, nasopharyngeal secretions, direct contact, and fomites contaminated by nasopharyngeal secretions. The illness typically occurs in epidemic fashion during the winter months. Children may shed the virus longer than adults, and thus are effective vectors for disease spread.

Symptoms

Characteristic presentation of influenza is the abrupt development of high fever, chills, headache, vertigo, sore throat, dry cough, and generalized pain in the back and extremities. In young children, there are often gastrointestinal symptoms such as nausea, vomiting, diarrhea, and croup. This severe illness can develop into sepsis in infants and may require aggressive supportive measures. Rapid influenza testing is available in the outpatient setting and assists in diagnosis.

Management

Management for influenza includes supportive care and administration of antiviral medication in certain individuals at higher risk for complications. Medications with indications for management of acute illness and for prophylaxis include oseltamivir, zanamivir, and peramivir. Individuals for whom antiviral agents should be considered include:

- Children with immunosuppression
- Children under two years of age
- Children with chronic disease
- Adolescents under age 19 who receive long-term aspirin therapy
- Women who are pregnant or postpartum
- Alaska natives and American Indians
- Morbidly obese children and those living in residential facilities

Influenza can be prevented or attenuated through annual vaccination with the influenza vaccine. Administration may begin at age six months and should continue annually in children.

Infectious Mononucleosis (IM)

Infectious mononucleosis is a viral syndrome that produces sore throat, fever, and lymphadenopathy along with prolonged malaise and fatigue. Viruses most often implicated with this illness are the Epstein-Barr virus (EBV), which is part of the herpes virus family, and, less often, cytomegalovirus (CMV). Laboratory findings associated with this immune-mediated disorder include a predominance of monocytes with reactive lymphocytosis. IM is seen most often between the ages of 15 and 24 years. The virus is shed in the saliva, and transmission occurs by sharing eating or drinking utensils and by intimate kissing (and thus is called the "kissing disease").

CLINICAL PEARL

Antiviral medications are most effective when started within 48 hours of symptom onset and should be continued until symptoms have resolved. Oseltamivir is indicated for treatment of influenza in individuals two weeks old and above and for prophylaxis in those one year and older.

CLINICAL PEARL

Patients with IM should avoid contact sports during the illness and for at least six weeks after resolution of symptoms due to the possibility of splenic rupture associated with splenomegaly.

Symptoms

Patients with IM present with fever, headache, sore throat, nausea, anorexia, myalgias, and photophobia. High fevers are common in children and adolescents. Lymphadenopathy is common along with splenomegaly, which is seen in the majority of cases. The "classic triad" of symptoms associated with IM are fever, pharyngitis, and lymphadenopathy, which occur in more than 50% of cases.

Management

Management of IM includes symptom control, rest, hydration, and NSAIDs or acetaminophen for fever and discomfort. Short-term oral corticosteroids may be indicated, such as prednisone 40 mg/day for five days. Avoid the administration of aspirin during IM, as this medication causes a rash in approximately 90% of patients.

Practice Questions

1. Your patient is a six-month-old male with physical exam findings of thigh-fold asymmetry and decreased abduction of the right leg. Which test or sign is used to assess for developmental dysplasia of the hip (DDH) in this age group?

   (A) Ortolani test
   (B) Galeazzi's sign
   (C) Barlow maneuver
   (D) Adam's forward bend test

2. An 11-year-old African American male is brought to the clinic by his mother, who reports she is worried because he has been wetting the bed lately, which is unusual. The patient was potty-trained at age two and has been dry at night since that time. On physical examination, you note his BMI is 30 and his blood pressure is slightly elevated. Based on these findings, which screening test(s) would be appropriate to order first?

   (A) renal function tests
   (B) thyroid function tests
   (C) blood glucose and hemoglobin A1c
   (D) electrocardiogram

3. Your patient is a 15-year-old male who presents for a sports physical for basketball. You note that he is tall and thin with abnormally long arms and legs. He also has pectus carinatum, flat feet, and mild scoliosis. Based on these findings, you screen him for:

   (A) aortic stenosis.
   (B) aortic dilation.
   (C) mitral valve stenosis.
   (D) rheumatic fever.

4. Primary prevention is the most cost-effective form of health care. All of the following choices are examples of primary prevention, EXCEPT:

   (A) administration of pneumococcal vaccine.
   (B) education on seat belt use.
   (C) referral for early intervention services.
   (D) administration of tetanus toxoid vaccine.

5. Jean Piaget developed a theory of growth and development based on his observations of infants, children, and adolescents. Based on his theory, the stage during which individuals learn about their environment and the world around them through their senses and motor movements is called the:

   (A) sensorimotor stage.
   (B) preoperational stage.
   (C) concrete operational stage.
   (D) formal operational stage.

6. Development of the "pincer grasp" by infants is usually noted around:

   (A) 3–6 months.
   (B) 6–9 months.
   (C) 9–12 months.
   (D) 12–15 months.

7. Infants can usually sit alone without support by what age?

   (A) 3 months
   (B) 6 months
   (C) 9 months
   (D) 12 months

8. A six-month-old infant is brought to the clinic by his mother for his six-month immunizations. Which of the following conditions would cause his immunizations to be deferred today?

   (A) The child is on antibiotics.
   (B) The child's mother is pregnant.
   (C) The child has otitis media with a fever of 103°F.
   (D) The child has an older sibling with leukemia.

9. A child can usually first stand on one foot at what age?

   (A) two years
   (B) three years
   (C) four years
   (D) five years

10. A child who is 15 months old is referred to as:

   (A) a neonate.
   (B) an infant.
   (C) a toddler.
   (D) a preschooler.

11. Your patient is Sara, who was born with a cleft palate. When should Sara begin treatment for cleft palate?

   (A) immediately after birth
   (B) at one month of age
   (C) at three months of age
   (D) at six months of age

12. Max is a 17-year-old male who presents with a sore throat and is not feeling well. Rapid testing in the office along with your physical exam supports a diagnosis of infectious mononucleosis (IM). Which of the following statements is true about this condition?

    (A) Patients with IM should avoid contact sports and heavy lifting.
    (B) Patients with IM are not contagious and may return to regular activities.
    (C) Patients with IM will require prolonged antibiotic therapy.
    (D) Patients with IM are at increased risk for scarlet fever.

13. The viral exanthem called Koplik spots are pathognomonic for which illness?

    (A) erythema infectiosum
    (B) mumps
    (C) varicella
    (D) rubeola

14. Jennifer is a six-year-old patient who is brought to the clinic today by her mother, who is worried about a new rash. The mother tells you the rash is mainly on her cheeks. On examination, you note an erythematous maculopapular rash on both cheeks, along with the beginning of a rash on her upper arms and trunk. Jennifer is active and alert and in no acute distress. This presentation is consistent with:

    (A) erythema infectiosum (fifth disease).
    (B) mumps.
    (C) varicella.
    (D) rubella.

15. You are providing parental education to a mother with a six-month-old boy. When she asks you about the best games to play with him at this age, you recommend:

    (A) rolling a ball back and forth.
    (B) push-pull toys.
    (C) pat-a-cake and peek-a-boo.
    (D) playing with a stuffed animal.

Answer Explanations

1. **(B)** Because the infant is now six months old, the Galeazzi's sign, which is assessed by observing for leg-length discrepancy, is the appropriate measure to evaluate for DDH. The Ortolani test (choice (A)), which involves rotating the baby's hips through the normal range of motion and listening for a click during abduction, as well as the Barlow maneuver (choice (C)) are used to assess DDH in infants younger than three months of age. The Barlow maneuver is performed by pressing gently on the child's knees (with the child in the supine position) to place pressure on the femoral head during hip flexion. If positive, posterior sub-luxation of the hip is found. The Adam's forward bend test (choice (D)) is used to evaluate for scoliosis in children between the ages of 10 and 15 years. This test requires the child to bend over from the waist so the FNP can observe for curvature or other abnormal appearance of the spine, which may indicate scoliosis.

2. **(C)** This patient presentation suggests type 2 diabetes mellitus; therefore, you would initially order a blood glucose level and hemoglobin A1c. Normal fasting serum glucose is less than 100 mg/dL, and a normal two-hour post-prandial is less than 140 mg/dL. A patient with a fasting glucose between 100 and 125 mg/dL is considered prediabetic. Diabetes is diagnosed with a fasting glucose of 126 mg/dL or higher. Normal hemoglobin A1c level is 5% or less. An A1c of 6.5% or above is suggestive of diabetes. Higher rates of type 2 diabetes mellitus are seen in individuals of African American, Native American, Hispanic, and Asian ethnicities. Other associated factors are obesity, insulin resistance, and hypertension. Children with type 2 diabetes often present with increased thirst, polyuria, and enuresis (bed-wetting). Renal and thyroid testing (choices (A) and (B)) may be appropriate as well but would be based on initial testing and patient presentation that is indicative of renal and/or thyroid dysfunction. An electrocardiogram (choice (D)) would not be indicated by this presentation alone as this test is used to detect electrical brain abnormalities.

3. **(B)** This patient exhibits physical characteristics consistent with Marfan syndrome, which is associated with aortic dilation. Patients with Marfan syndrome are at risk for potentially fatal aortic dissection and should be screened for aortic abnormalities immediately. Marfan syndrome is a genetic disorder characterized by tall stature, long limbs, myopia, retinal detachment, spontaneous pneumothorax, connective tissue abnormalities including pectus deformities, and joint hyperextensibility. Aortic root dilatation and mitral valve prolapse/regurgitation are commonly seen in patients with this condition. Children with severe con-nective tissue involvement should be restricted from strenuous physical activities and should avoid football and other sports involving frequent physical contact, such as basketball. Aortic stenosis (choice (A)) is a narrowing of the aorta that may occur on the valve itself, above the valve, or below the valve. In this disorder, the stenotic aortic valve is usually bicuspid instead of tricuspid. Mitral valve stenosis (choice (C)) is seen with a history of ischemic heart disease, endocarditis, rheumatic heart disease, and other valve abnormalities. Stenosis is a narrowing of the valve orifice that causes impedance to blood flow, producing a murmur. Rheumatic fever (RF) (choice (D)) is an autoimmune disorder occurring after a streptococcal infection, usually of the oropharynx or tonsils. The inflammatory process of RF involves the heart, joints, central nervous system, and subcutaneous tissues. Long-term effects on most tissues are usually minimal, but cardiac involvement is often severe with valvular fibrosis and scarring.

4. **(C)** Referral to early intervention resources is a form of tertiary prevention. Tertiary prevention includes activities that help limit progression of an already established disease and improve the patient's quality of life. Primary prevention measures include interventions such as vaccines (choices (A) and (D)), which help prevent the occurrence of disease or illness. Secondary prevention measures include screening programs with the goal of early disease identification. Providing education regarding the use of seat belts (choice (B)) constitutes a form of primary prevention as this measure is aimed at preventing injuries related to motor vehicle use.

5. **(A)** Infants typically learn about their environment through motor activity and by using their senses. According to Piaget, this is the sensorimotor stage and usually lasts from birth to age two years. The preoperational stage (two to seven years) (choice (B)) is characterized by egocentrism and reasoning that is based on concrete objects within the environment. During the concrete operational stage (7–12 years) (choice (C)), children are able to begin more complex thought processes and understand that symbols can represent concrete objects. Children and adolescents in the formal operational stage (13–18 years) (choice (D)) begin to be able to think abstractly and develop a range of possible solutions for problems.

6. **(C)** The pincer grasp is a method whereby babies learn to pick things up using two digits, and this develops around 9–12 months. Prior to this (choices (A) and (B)), infants use a scraping motion to move objects nearer but lack the dexterity to pick them up. Appearance of the pincer grasp and other developmental milestones are used for evaluating cognitive, motor, and neurological systems. By age 12 months or older (choice (D)), a child should have already developed the pincer grasp.

7. **(B)** By 6 months of age, babies have developed the motor and neural control to sit alone without support (if even for a few seconds). An infant who is 3 months old (choice (A)) has improved head control but lacks overall body support to sit alone. Infants at 9 and 12 months old (choices (C) and (D)) should be sitting alone without support, but this should have first been seen around 6 months of age.

8. **(C)** There are relatively few reasons to defer immunizations in children. A child with acute otitis media and a fever of 103°F should have vaccines deferred until illness has resolved. A child who is taking antibiotics (choice (A)), a child whose mother is pregnant (choice (B)), and a child with a sibling with leukemia (choice (D)) may receive immunizations.

9. **(B)** A young child usually has the gross motor development to be able to stand on one foot at three years of age. Gross motor and neural development have not progressed by age two years (choice (A)) to enable a child to perform this activity. A four- or five-year-old child (choices (C) and (D)) should have demonstrated the ability to stand on one foot at an earlier age.

10. **(C)** A 15-month-old is referred to as a toddler. The neonatal period (choice (A)) is considered the first time period from birth through the first 28 days of life. Infancy (choice (B)) is typically from birth to 12 months. Preschool children are ages three to five years (choice (D)).

11. **(A)** Cleft palate will impact nutritional intake; thus, management of the condition should begin immediately after birth. Surgery is indicated; however, the timing is individualized based on the type and degree of the cleft. Early management begins with implementation of specialized nipples and feeding techniques. Nutritional management must begin before one month of age, therefore the other choices, (B), (C), and (D)), are incorrect.

12. **(A)** IM is caused by Epstein-Barr virus (EBV) in the majority of cases. The illness is widespread and older children and adolescents in the United States would test positive for EBV. The virus is transmitted through personal contact, usually from deep kissing, sexual activity, or exchange of saliva through sharing eating and drinking utensils. IM is a disease of lymphoid tissue and causes pronounced lymphadenopathy. Enlargement of the spleen leads to splenomegaly and an increased risk for splenic rupture. During active disease and for six weeks afterward, individuals should avoid contact sports and heavy lifting. The illness is very contagious, making choice (B) incorrect, and occurs in episodic fashion during the year. Antibiotics (choice (C)) are not indicated in the management of IM because the etiology is viral. Scarlet fever (choice (D)) is an illness associated with group A streptococcus infection and is caused by erythrogenic toxin. Symptoms include sore throat, high fever, headache, chills, malaise, and edematous tonsils. A rash appears one to five days after symptoms begin and is characterized by red, fine papules that blanch with pressure and feel like sandpaper.

13. **(D)** Koplik spots are white macular lesions found along the gums and cheek mucosa of infants with measles (rubeola). Erythema infectiosum (EI) (choice (A)) is also known as fifth disease and presents with a rash that occurs in three stages beginning around 7–10 days after the prodromal period. An intense red eruption begins on the cheeks ("slapped cheek") and is characteristic of EI. The second stage develops as a lace-like maculopapular rash beginning on the trunk before moving to the arms and legs (third stage). Mumps (choice (B)) is a generalized illness caused by a virus that is characterized by enlargement of the salivary glands. A rash is not a usual characteristic of mumps. Varicella (choice (C)), known as chickenpox, is highly contagious and presents with a rash beginning on the face, scalp, or trunk. Lesions develop in crops that are highly pruritic and begin as spots on the skin. These spots progress to vesicles (fluid-filled blisters) that scab over and umbilicate. Characteristic findings associated with varicella include the presence of all three types of lesions simultaneously.

14. **(A)** Erythema infectiosum is a viral illness that presents with an intensely red rash beginning on the cheeks ("slapped cheek" appearance). The rash then spreads downward to the body and limbs in a sequential manner. This is a self-limiting childhood disorder. Mumps (choice (B)) is a generalized viral illness that presents with painful enlargement of the salivary glands. Varicella (chickenpox) (choice (C)) presents with an intensely pruritic maculopapular rash, which begins on the scalp face or trunk. Lesions become vesicular and teardrop-shaped before becoming cloudy and then scab over. Rubella (choice (D)) is an acute viral illness seen in childhood that produces lymphadenopathy followed by a rash, which presents as discrete maculopapular lesions. This illness is a self-limiting viral infection seen in childhood.

15. **(C)** Pat-a-cake and peek-a-boo games are appropriate for a parent to play with a six-month-old infant. Rolling a ball (choice (A)) requires eye-hand coordination that is not yet present in a six-month-old. These infants are not yet walking, therefore push-pull toys (choice (B)) would not be much fun. Playing with a stuffed animal (choice (D)) usually requires some degree of "pretend" and is therefore not a good option for an infant of this age.

PART V
Geriatrics

15

End-of-Life Issues and Team-Based Management

Advances in medical technology in the diagnosis and treatment of chronic disease have dramatically increased life expectancy globally as the death toll continues to fall for many of the most common illnesses and diseases. In the United States, an anticipated continuing surge in the demand for health care services is expected due to these advancements in care. The baby boomer generation is now entering retirement and, along with increased life expectancy, it portends a growing population of elderly adults with concomitant health needs as they age. This chapter will discuss demographics surrounding aging as well as care issues specific to older individuals.

Demographics

There are four classifications of older adults based on age. Young-old adults are those 65–75 years old. Middle-old are from 76–84 years, and the oldest-old are from 85–99 years. The oldest group are the centenarians, who are 100 years and above. The group of oldest-old is the fastest growing population segment in the United States, with numbers expected to exceed nine million by 2030.

Four out of five older adults have one or more chronic diseases. Forty percent of the women are widowed, and approximately 60% of older adults live within a community setting. The major sources of retirement income for older adults are derived from Social Security (the most important source of income), private/government pension accounts, part-time job earnings, and personal assets. It has been reported that approximately 45% of adults ages 65 and older have incomes listed as twice below the poverty thresholds under the supplemental poverty measures released in 2015. About 36 million falls are reported among older adults each year. The American Geriatrics Society/British Geriatrics Society guideline recommends screening all adults aged 65 years and older for fall risk annually.

Medicaid

Medicaid was first implemented in 1965 with the intention of providing basic health coverage for low-income individuals and families receiving government welfare benefits. Medicaid also provides assistance to low-income Medicare beneficiaries through dual eligible benefits. Such benefits allow Medicaid to provide assistance with Medicare monthly premiums and cost sharing services, as well as coverage for any long-term services and support (LTSS), which are excluded in the Medicare benefits. Note that the cost of Medicaid is subsidized by the federal government and the participating state government. Therefore, Medicaid programs can vary from state to state, and *not* all states provide the Medicaid program for all low-income adults below a certain income level.

Medicare

Medicare was first implemented in 1965 with the intention of providing basic health coverage for older adults aged 65 years and above regardless of their income level and medical health history. Since then, the program has shifted the reimbursement mechanism from fee for service to the value-based payment reimbursement. There are four parts of Medicare that cover specific services, as outlined in Table 15.1.

Table 15.1. Medicare Services

Medicare Part Name	Covered Services
Medicare Part A	Also known as "Hospital Insurance Program." It covers inpatient hospital utilization, skilled nursing facilities, home health, and hospice care services.
Medicare Part B	Also known as "Supplemental Medical Insurance Program." This is a voluntary program with monthly premiums. It covers medically necessary outpatient medical services, including home health and a preventative wellness program and/or annual wellness exam, conducted by health care providers.
Medicare Part C	Also known as "Medicare Advantage Program." Beneficiaries may enroll in private health plans and have the same access to Medicare Part A and Part B health benefits, in addition to Part D prescription drug coverage. Examples of these plans include health maintenance organizations (HMOs), preferred provider organizations (PPOs), provider-sponsored organizations (PSOs), and private fee-for-service (PFFS) plans.
Medicare Part D	Also known as "Medicare Prescription Drug Benefit." The benefits are delivered through private health plans contracted with Medicare (Medicare Part C). Note: Medicare Part D benefits only cover prescriptions that are listed on the formulary list of preferred drugs. The formulary list is updated annually and can be downloaded from the Centers for Medicare and Medicaid Services (CMS) website.

Physical Changes Associated with Aging

As we age, our body systems change. Table 15.2 shows the physical changes associated with aging related to each body system.

Table 15.2. Physical Changes Associated with Aging

Key: ↓ = decrease, ↑ = increase

Body/System	Changes
EENT	Ears: ↓ hearing acuity (high frequency) Eyes: ↓ visual acuity (screen for cataracts) ↓ lens flexibility ↓ tear production ↑ intraocular pressure (this test should be conducted as part of the annual wellness screening for glaucoma) Nose: ↓ sense of smell Mouth: ↓ oral secretion/salivation ↓ taste
Cardiac	↑ systolic blood pressure ↓ ejection fraction ↑ atrial fibrillation ↑ syncopal events

Continued

Table 15.2. Physical Changes Associated with Aging *(Continued)*

Key: ↓ = decrease, ↑ = increase

Body/System	Changes
Pulmonary	No changes in total lung capacity ↑ residual volume ↓ vital capacity ↓ FEV1 (resulting in shortness of breath)
Liver	↓ liver size/mass ↓ perfusion (↓ metabolic clearance of drugs due to reduced efficacy of cytochrome P450 enzyme) ↑ cholesterol level and LDL
Renal	↓ renal size/mass
Gastrointestinal	↓ gastric emptying (↑ gastritis, ↑ GERD) ↓ production of prostaglandins ↓ GI absorption (↓ folic acid, B12, calcium) ↑ episodes of constipation
Musculoskeletal	↓ muscle mass, muscle strength (osteoporosis/osteopenia) ↑ cartilage degeneration (osteoarthritis, degenerative joint disease) ↑ compression of spine (kyphosis)
Integumentary	↓ skin sensitivity ↓ collagen and subcutaneous fat tissues ↓ skin elasticity, fragile skin with remarkably slow healing process, prone to superficial skin infection ↑ skin atrophy
Endocrine	↑ insulin levels with mild peripheral insulin resistance ↑ fluctuation of circadian rhythm (sleep disturbance, fatigue) Male: ↓ production of testosterone and dehydroepiandrosterone (DHEA) Female: ↓ estrogen and progesterone due to menopause
Immune	↓ T-cells (prone to developing infections) Note: less likely to have presentation of fever during infections
Neurologic	↓ cognition (↑ processing time) ↓ refluxes ↓ dopamine receptors (Parkinson's disease)

PHARMACOKINETIC CHANGES

Due to the aging of body systems, older adults may not be able to metabolize the conventional medications and dosages for antipsychotics, tricyclic antidepressants (TCAs), and benzodiazepines. For a complete list, readers are encouraged to visit the American Geriatrics Society (AGS) website for a detailed explanation of the Beers criteria.

Health Maintenance

The U.S. Preventive Services Task Force (USPSTF) (2014) recommends a variety of clinical preventive services specifically for adults 65 years and older. These recommendations are based on evidence-based clinical research. Each recommendation has an assigned letter grade (A, B, C, or D). Practitioners are strongly encouraged to offer and provide recommended services with Grade A and B. Grade C recommendations should only apply to selected patients depending on their circumstances. The USPSTF discourages providers from implementing services with Grade D recommendations. Table 15.3 provide some examples of recommended screening for adults 65 and older.

Table 15.3. Examples of Recommended Screenings for Adults 65 and Older*

Screening Type	Additional Information
Annual wellness visit (AWV)	Conducted annually for all patients
Abdominal aortic aneurysm (AAA)	One-time screening by ultrasound for men 65–75 years who have smoked at least 100 cigarettes or 5 packs in their lifetime as well as anyone with a family history of AAA
Alcohol misuse screening and counseling	For patients who currently drink more than 2 drinks per day
Bone density test	Every 2 years for women who are estrogen deficient with a risk for osteoporosis
Cardiovascular disease (behavioral therapy)	For obese patients
Cardiovascular screenings (cholesterol, lipids, triglycerides)	Lipid panel once every 5 years for patients without any signs or symptoms of cardiovascular disease
Colorectal cancer screening	Colonoscopy every 10 years for all patients
Diabetes screening	Glucose or GTT twice per year for patients with risk factors for diabetes; once per year for patients who were previously screened and not diagnosed with prediabetes
Diabetes self-management training	For diabetic patients
Glaucoma test	Conducted annually for all patients
Hepatitis C screening	Once in a lifetime for patients born between 1945 and 1965
Annual lung cancer screening	Low dose CT for patients from 55 to 77 years of age with a tobacco smoking history of at least 30 packs per year, and for current smokers or former smokers who have quit smoking within the last 15 years
Smoking and tobacco use cessation	For patients currently smoking and using tobacco products
Influenza vaccine	Conducted annually for all patients
Hepatitis B shot	For patients in high-risk groups
Pneumococcal vaccine	Prevnar 13, or Pneumovax 23 as needed; consult CDC recommendations
Shingles vaccine	Zoster recombinant for all patients

*For complete recommended immunization schedules, please visit the CDC website.

Clinical Assessment

Common geriatric assessment components carried out in a primary care setting include current living environment, caregiver support, screening for cognition and mood (depression), safety (risk of falls), polypharmacy, review of over-the-counter medications list, and end-of-life care arrangements.

Physiological Changes

Many physiological changes occur with aging, and these changes impact disease, quality of life, response to treatment, and caregiving needs for older individuals. The APRN caring for elderly patients should be cognizant of common findings associated with aging, as well as findings that may be pathological and require management. Older individuals with illness or disease often present with atypical symptoms as compared with younger adults. For example, bacterial infections may present with hypothermia instead of fever. Confusion and other cognitive changes are frequently seen with illness in older adults.

Medication-Related Changes

Medications commonly used in this population may precipitate chronic problems. For example, long-term use of over-the-counter Prilosec (one of the proton-pump inhibitor (PPI) class of medications) is associated with the depletion of micronutrients, including iron and vitamin B12; an increased risk of fractures (wrist, hip, spine, forearm); an increased risk of contracting pneumonia; and increased episodes of *C. difficile* colitis and/or diarrhea. Many older adults use non-steroidal anti-inflammatory drugs (NSAIDs) such as ibuprofen to treat chronic pain and discomfort associated with osteoarthritis. Long-term use of these agents may lead to chronic, slow gastrointestinal bleeding, predisposing the individual to anemia.

End-of-Life Care

Hospice is a model of transition from palliative care. It is designed for terminally ill patients who are in the final stages of disease progression. A majority of hospices are home-based services, while some hospices provide specialized inpatient beds located within the hospital facility. The focus of hospice is on comfort care, and not curative care. There is also respite care service. This very limited service enables the primary caregiver to recharge and rest while another caregiver provides services for one day.

Hospice Care Criteria

Life-sustaining equipment during an emergency is not part of hospice service. The patient must consent to begin and receive hospice care services and have a life expectancy of six months or less, and the service must be documented with an official written hospice care order created by a physician.

Hospice Team

Hospice team members consist of registered nurses, home health aides, hospice physician(s) and/or nurse practitioner(s), social workers, and clergy.

Advance Care Planning

There are two types of advanced directives, a living will and a durable power of attorney. A living will is a legal document drafted and based on the types of medical treatment the patient requests in the event he or she is not able to provide a consent form due to medical issues. A durable power of attorney is also known as a health care proxy. This is a document that dedicates a person or persons who will make the medical health decisions on behalf of the incapacitated patient.

Practice Questions

1. Among the retiree age group population, the fastest growing age group is those:

   (A) 51 to 60 years.
   (B) 61 to 70 years.
   (C) 71 to 80 years.
   (D) 85 to 99 years.

2. Which of the following immunizations is/are recommended for adults 65 years and above? Select all that apply.

   (A) influenza vaccine
   (B) shingles vaccine
   (C) pneumococcal vaccine
   (D) human papillomavirus vaccine

3. Age-related changes in the pulmonary system in an elderly adult include all of the following, EXCEPT:

   (A) an increase in systolic blood pressure.
   (B) a decrease in atrial fibrillation events.
   (C) an increase in syncopal episodes.
   (D) a decrease in ejection fraction.

4. Age-related changes in the gastrointestinal system of an elderly adult include all of the following, EXCEPT:

   (A) an increase in gastrointestinal absorption.
   (B) a decrease in gastric emptying.
   (C) an increase in episodes of constipation.
   (D) a decrease in production of prostaglandins.

5. Side effects of long-term use of proton-pump inhibitors (PPIs) include all the following, EXCEPT:

   (A) a reduced risk of developing C. *difficile* colitis.
   (B) an increased risk of fractures.
   (C) a reduced absorption of iron.
   (D) an increased risk of contracting pneumonia.

6. Which of the following resources is reported as the most important income resource for older adults?

   (A) government pension
   (B) personal savings
   (C) Social Security
   (D) private pension investment account

7. All the following statements accurately describe the Medicaid program, EXCEPT:

   (A) Medicaid provides health coverage that covers all low-income adults below a certain income level.
   (B) Medicaid provides health coverage for some low-income people, families, and children in all states.
   (C) Medicaid provides health coverage for some pregnant women and the elderly.
   (D) Medicaid provides health coverage for some people with disabilities.

8. A 67-year-old female presents at the clinic for her wellness visit. Which Medicare plan would cover the wellness visit?

   (A) Medicare Part A
   (B) Medicare Part B
   (C) Medicare Part C
   (D) Medicare Part D

9. A 65-year-old male presents at the clinic for a sinus problem. Upon your assessment, you conclude that the patient will begin a course of antibiotic treatment. Which Medicare plan will cover the cost of the prescription?

   (A) Medicare Part A
   (B) Medicare Part B
   (C) Medicare Part C
   (D) Medicare Part D

10. The United States Preventive Services Task Force (USPSTF) recommends that practitioners offer recommended services with which of the following letter grade(s)?

    (A) A only
    (B) A and B
    (C) A, B, and C
    (D) A, B, C, and D

11. Common geriatric assessment measures performed in the primary care setting include all the following, EXCEPT:

    (A) screening for depression.
    (B) screening for cognition changes.
    (C) ordering lab for complete blood count with differentials.
    (D) medication reconciliation.

12. The primary goal of hospice is:

    (A) providing comfort care.
    (B) hastening of death.
    (C) improving the activities of daily living.
    (D) enabling the primary caregiver to rest.

13. Which of the following statements is true related to hospice care?

   (A) Life-sustaining equipment during an emergency is part of the hospice service.
   (B) Patients must have a life expectancy of six months or less, with an official written hospice care order by a physician.
   (C) Patients in the first stage of prostate cancer are eligible for hospice care service.
   (D) Patients do not need to consent to hospice care service.

14. Hospice team members consist of:
   Select all that apply.
   (A) a registered nurse.
   (B) home health aides.
   (C) a hospice physician and/or nurse practitioner.
   (D) social workers.
   (E) legal counsel.

15. Elements of advance directives can include all the following, EXCEPT:

   (A) a living will.
   (B) a durable power of attorney.
   (C) a health care proxy.
   (D) a primary beneficiary on the patient's life insurance policy.

Answer Explanations

1. **(D)** There are four classifications for older adults based on their age group: young-old, 65–75 years; middle-old, 76–84 years, oldest-old, 85–99 years; and centenarians, 100 years and above. Oldest-old is the fastest growing segment in the United States, with the population projected to exceed nine million by 2030.

2. **(A, B, C)** Please refer to Table 15.3 Examples of Recommended Screenings for Adults 65 and Older. Human papillomavirus (HPV) vaccine (choice (D)) is more appropriate for the age groups between 9 and 45 years old.

3. **(B)** Age-related changes in the pulmonary system in an elderly adult include an increase in systolic blood pressure, making choice (A) true; an increase in syncopal events, making choice (C) true; and a decrease in ejection fraction, making choice (D) true as well. Age-related changes in the pulmonary system in an elderly adult include an increase, not a decrease, in atrial fibrillation events, making choice (B) false and thus the correct answer.

4. **(A)** Age-related changes in the gastrointestinal system of an elderly adult include a decrease in gastric emptying (with an increase in gastritis and GERD) (choice (B)), an increase in episodes of constipation (choice (C)), and a decrease in the production of prostaglandins (choice (D)). These changes also include a decrease, not an increase, in gastrointestinal absorption (specifically folic acid, B12, and calcium), making choice (A) false and thus the correct answer.

5. **(A)** Long-term use of the PPI class of medications is associated with an increased risk of fractures (wrist, hip, spine, forearm), so choice (B) is true. It is also associated with the depletion of micronutrients, including vitamin B12 and iron, making choice (C) true, and with an increased risk of contracting pneumonia, making choice (D) true as well. The PPI class of medications is associated with *increased* episodes of *C. difficile* colitis and/or diarrhea, not with a reduced risk of those conditions, making choice (A) false and thus the correct answer.

6. **(C)** The most important source of retirement income reported for older adults is derived from Social Security. Other sources include government pension accounts (choice A)), personal assets (choice (B)), private pension accounts (choice (D)), and part-time job earnings.

7. **(A)** Medicaid provides health coverage for some low-income individuals, families, and children, some pregnant women and the elderly, and some people with disabilities, making choices (B), (C), and (D) true. The cost of Medicaid is subsidized by the federal government and the participating state government. Therefore, Medicaid programs can vary from state to state. Not all states provide the Medicaid program for all low-income adults below a certain income level, making choice (A) false and thus the correct answer.

8. **(B)** The patient's wellness visit would be covered by Medicare Part B, also known as the supplemental medical insurance program. This is a voluntary program with monthly premiums. Coverage includes "medically necessary" outpatient medical services, including home health, and a preventative wellness program and/or annual wellness exam, conducted by health care providers.

9. **(D)** Medicare Part D, also known as the Medicare prescription drug benefit, will cover the cost of the patient's prescription. The benefits are delivered through private health plans contracted with Medicare (Medicare Part C, choice (C)). Note: The benefit only covers prescription(s) that are listed on the formulary lists of preferred drugs. The formulary list is updated annually and can be downloaded from the Centers for Medicare and Medicaid Services (CMS) website. Medicare Part A (choice (A)) is also known as the Hospital Insurance Program. It covers inpatient hospital utilization, skilled nursing facilities, home health, and hospice care services. Medicare Part B (choice (B)) is also known as the Supplemental Medical Insurance Program. This is a voluntary program with monthly premiums. It covers "medically necessary" outpatient medical services, including home health and a preventative wellness program and/or annual wellness exam, conducted by health care providers.

10. **(D)** Each USPSTF recommendation has an assigned letter grade (A, B, C, or D). Practitioners are strongly encouraged to offer or provide recommended service(s) with Grade A (choice (A)) and B (choice (B)). Grade C (choice (C)) recommendations should only apply to selected patients depending on their medical circumstances. Providers are discouraged from implementing service(s) with Grade D recommendations (choice (D)).

11. **(C)** Common geriatric assessment in a primary care setting includes an assessment of current living environment, caregiver support, safety (risk of falls), a screening for mood (e.g., depression) and cognition, making choices (A) and (B) true, and polypharmacy, or medication reconciliation, making choice (D) true as well. Unless there are concerns for possible infections, a complete blood count with differentials is not an appropriate lab test for all clinical visits, making choice (C) false and thus the correct answer.

12. **(A)** Hospice care is designed for terminally ill patients entering the final stages of the disease process. Hospice focuses on comfort care, not hastening of death (choice B)) or improving the activities of daily living (choice (C)). It includes respite care service, a very limited service that enables the primary caregiver to rest while another caregiver cares for the patient for one day (choice (D)).

13. **(B)** To enter hospice care, the patient must have a life expectancy of six months or less, with an official written hospice care order by a physician. Life-sustaining equipment during an emergency (choice (A)) is not part of hospice service. Patients with stage 1 prostate cancer (choice (C)) are not eligible for hospice care. The patient must consent to receive hospice care services (choice (D)).

14. **(A, B, C, D)** Hospice team members consist of a registered nurse, home health aides, a hospice physician and/or nurse practitioner, social workers, and clergy. Legal counsel (choice (E)) is not a member of the hospice team.

15. **(D)** There are two types of advanced directives. One type is a living will, making choice (A) true. A living will is a legal document drafted and based on the types of medical treatment the patient requests in the event he or she is not able to provide a consent form due to medical issues. The other type of advance directive is a durable power of attorney, making choice (B) true. A durable power of attorney is a legal document in which an agent is assigned to legally make health care decisions on behalf of the patient in the event that the patient is deemed incapable of making and executing health care decisions. A durable power of attorney is also known as a health care proxy, making choice (C) true as well. A primary beneficiary is the person or entity named to receive a benefit and is determined by the account holder. It is not part of an advance directive, making choice (D) false and thus the correct answer.

PART VI
Professional Issues

16

Advanced Practice Role: Issues, Legal, and Decision-Making

Role of the Advanced Practice Registered Nurse

The role of the advanced practice registered nurse (APRN) in the United States health care system continues to evolve and expand to meet rising needs. As highly trained, educated health professionals, APRNs are at the forefront of changes on a national level that place an emphasis on improving access to care and providing safe and effective high-quality care that is truly patient-centered, with improved patient outcomes. Much of the movement within the health care system toward health promotion and disease prevention is already in place within the profession of nursing. Nurses have always sought to provide high-quality care that is holistic in nature and encompasses all aspects of a patient's life. However, there are state differences in the variation of scope of practice for advanced nurse practitioners. Nevertheless, APRNs now have the challenge of assisting other clinical professions in adopting new ways of providing health care.

The role of the APRN as primary care provider is well established. Data indicate that patient outcomes and satisfaction with care provided by APRNs are the same as, or better than, care provided by physicians. The APRN role fits well into new models of care that are now being implemented. The Affordable Care Act, enacted in 2010, has made it possible for millions of previously uninsured individuals to obtain insurance; however, it has also highlighted the need for continued reform. Many people who were initially able to become insured when the law was enacted have now lost their insurance due to rising rates and high deductibles. The number of individuals without health care insurance continues to grow. Providing care for this diverse group will continue to present complex challenges to our already overtaxed health care system.

Nursing has historically been the profession willing to go into difficult places to provide care for those who need it. Moreover, nursing continues in the role of meeting needs for underserved populations. Specific areas in which APRNs are bridging care gaps include:

- Practicing family care as an integral component of primary care
- Caring for vulnerable populations who would otherwise be unable to receive care
- Providing needed mental health services in areas with a shortage of mental health providers
- Applying concepts of cultural sensitivity within diverse care situations
- Developing collaborative and interprofessional care teams
- Acting as leaders in the development of community, state, and national health initiatives
- Developing and implementing disease prevention and health maintenance programs within the communities that are most in need
- Practicing evidence-based care that is cost-effective and resource conscious
- Changing academic settings in order to remain current with student, population, and stakeholder needs
- Implementing and improving new ways to handle patient data and health records
- Becoming proactive in legislative efforts to improve patient care and removing practice barriers that limit access to care for millions of individuals

Information is power, and APRNs are the leaders among health care professionals in acquiring the information needed to change the caring landscape for populations of all sizes and types. In developing trusting, collaborative relationships with patients and their families, APRNs are able to collect valuable information to help direct care at the individual, family, and population level.

Genogram Documentation

One invaluable tool when assessing individual and population health is the genogram, which provides a pictorial representation of family relationships as well as disease prevalence within families for three generations. The genogram enables providers and patients to step back and look at health and illness within a family from previous generations. Figure 16.1 provides a list of symbols used in the development of a genogram along with their interpretations. Figure 16.1 shows the basic pedigree symbols. Table 16.1 shows the application of genogram documentation in family relationship.

Figure 16.1. Basic Pedigree Symbols

Table 16.1. Family Relationships

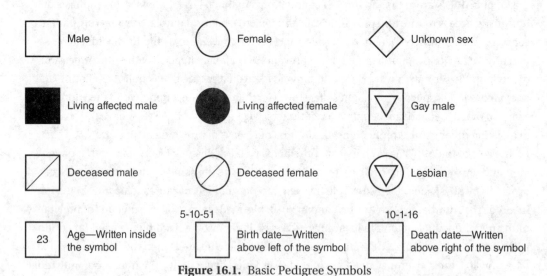

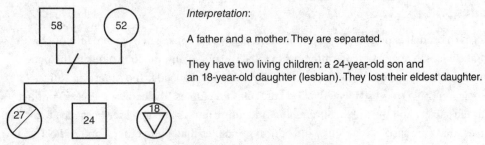

Interpretation:

A father and a mother. They are separated.

They have two living children: a 24-year-old son and an 18-year-old daughter (lesbian). They lost their eldest daughter.

Figure 16.2. Genogram Example

APRN Scope of Practice

Educational programs that offer APRN degrees continue to evolve with changing patient and population needs. Global increases in disease and a lack of enough health care providers provide the backdrop for continued growth in educational program curricula. Because of this, the APRN role has grown since the first program was developed, which focused on care for pediatric patients. Current APRN areas of practice include:

- Adult primary care
- Family primary care
- Geriatric primary care
- Neonatal care
- Obstetrics and gynecology
- Pediatric acute care
- Primary care of children from infancy through adolescence

State laws define the scope of practice for health care professionals and provide them with title protection; however, there is much variability between states. Many states have implemented legislation limiting the APRN scope of practice and providing strict oversight of APRN practice. Professional licensure is a states' granting of rights to practice nursing. Controversy exists because many rules and regulations surrounding professional licensure have led to decreased access to health care for many individuals.

APRNs who are certified in family practice often practice in the following health care settings:

- Emergency health care
- Mental health
- Oncology and palliative care
- Rehabilitation and tertiary care
- Occupational health
- Public health

Mandated collaborative agreements between APRNs and physicians are in place in many states. These agreements may be broad in scope or extremely prescriptive, with much variation. State qualifications for APRN practice include holding an unencumbered registered nurse license, successfully completing an accredited academic program appropriate to the degree of masters or doctoral and receiving certification through a national certifying body.

Ethical and Legal Issues

Nursing care emphasizes a focus on the holistic approach, as we challenge ourselves to remain current with the changes in the lifestyles of our patients. Therefore, nursing is an ongoing, evolving profession. In 2019, the Gallup organization announced that nursing was listed as the most ethical profession in the United States. In fact, nursing has been listed as the top profession for the past 18 years.

CLINICAL PEARL

APRNs must sometimes face difficult, complex, and unclear choices and decisions. When this happens, the local Institutional Ethics Committee (IEC) can be consulted for guidance.

Ethics

Ethics is a branch of philosophy that represents one's own conscience when confronted with moral choices. Nursing practice attempts to fulfill the nurse's moral obligations to the patient by incorporating personal choices based on a personal moral code. The American Nurses Association (ANA) has established a Code of Ethics for Nurses. The code serves as a contract between society and the nursing profession (including nurses and advanced practice registered nurses) that emphasizes the values and ethical principles that guide nurses' and APRNs' clinical judgments and clinical decisions. It provides guidance for carrying out their professional role when choosing between personal and professional values.

Ethical Principles of APRN Practice

The following ethical principles are part of the ANA Code of Ethics for Nurses and are common to all APRN practice.

Autonomy

This principle underscores the importance of individual free will to make informed decisions and choices without outside interference. Two examples of behaviors that may restrict the autonomy of a patient are paternalism and maternalism. These behaviors treat individuals as if they are children. Although the feelings behind these behaviors may be benevolent, they negate the rights of the individual to make decisions for themselves.

Clinical Scenario: The patient is a 78-year-old male with a recent laboratory finding of an elevated prostate specific antigen (PSA) level. The APRN discusses the meaning of the test results with the patient and then provides information regarding different treatment options to address this abnormal finding.

Discussion: The role of the APRN in this situation is to gather input from the patient and discuss all treatment options, including the option for surgery. The patient has the right to make the final decision regarding his care, and this decision should be based on the most current, evidence-based information available. The APRN is providing a setting in which the patient may make an autonomous decision about his care.

Beneficence

This principle was stated in the Nightingale Pledge (a modified version of the Hippocratic Oath) with an emphasis on "do no harm." Nurses should practice and act in the patient's best interest at all times, including while providing compassionate care.

Clinical Scenario: The APRN stops prescribing hydrochlorothiazide (HCTZ) medication to a patient with hypertension who also has chronic gouty arthritis and replaces the medicine with Losartan, a different type of antihypertensive agent.

Discussion: One risk factor associated with the medication HCTZ is elevation of serum uric acid levels. High levels of uric acid predispose an individual to the development of gouty arthritis. The antihypertensive Losartan is a weak uricosuric and can lower the serum urate level slightly. This action by the APRN is based on knowledge of pharmacokinetic properties and the ethical principle of beneficence. Note: This is not a general protocol, and the decision must be individualized.

Nonmaleficence

Nonmaleficence is the principle based on the APRN's responsibility to prevent harm to the patient. This principle involves the APRN's professional insight into individual scenarios that may occur in providing health care.

Clinical Scenario: A newly graduated APRN is told to remove a Nexplanon (etonogestrel birth control implant) from a patient. The APRN tells the collaborating physician that she has been trained neither in the subdermal implant process nor in the removal of the device and therefore is not qualified to perform this task.

Discussion: APRNs should be knowledgeable about scope of practice within their state and demonstrate professional insight into particular tasks that may or may not be within the scope of practice. *All* medical providers need to complete a training course provided by the Nexplanon pharmaceutical company before they can insert or remove the product. The APRN graduate is demonstrating the principle of nonmaleficence by not performing a procedure that she has not been trained for and one that may cause the patient harm if performed by someone unskilled in the procedure.

Veracity

The principle of veracity refers to telling the truth. The business of health care requires providers to provide information to patients regarding options for care. Veracity implies telling the entire truth, instead of providing only part of the information to be conveyed. As autonomous individuals, patients have the right to expect veracity from all health care providers.

Clinical Scenario: An APRN refers a bedbound patient to hospice care services due to the patient having advanced Stage IV small cell lung cancer (SCLC). The patient's daughter thinks that he has a very good chance of recovering and does not understand why the patient needs hospice services. The APRN explains to the daughter the patient's poor diagnosis and the role of hospice in palliative care.

Discussion: Advanced SCLC tends to spread quickly. Stage IV SCLC has a relative five-year survival rate of about 2%. The APRN is demonstrating the principle of veracity by being honest and truthful about the patient's prognosis and the role of hospice care, which requires a life-expectancy of six months or less. Note: Discussion about prognosis should include not only the family, but the patient as well.

Confidentiality

The principle of confidentiality is the obligation to respect the patient's privileged information through the protection of the patient's identity, personal information, medical history, and medical records.

Clinical Scenario: A husband comes to a clinic asking for the reason for his wife's clinical visit the past Monday. He provides her name, date of birth, and Social Security number. The front desk staff members tell the gentleman that they cannot confirm or verify any information and turn him away.

Discussion: The front desk is doing the right thing. They practiced the principle of confidentiality by not confirming or providing any information about the patient. Note: Patient rights are also protected under the Health Insurance Portability and Accountability Act (HIPAA). This act was promulgated by the federal government with the goal of protecting patient privacy and confidentiality. HIPAA applies across all health care settings and must be adhered to by all individuals who provide services to patients. It is important to know that there are instances in which sharing of a patient's medical information is not protected under HIPAA law. These instances include the following situations:

- When a medical record is subpoenaed as part of a litigation case
- When medical information is shared with a patient's insurance carrier
- When certain information is covered under a mandatory reporting statute by the state department of health (such as mandatory reporting of certain diseases)

Fidelity

The principle of fidelity encompasses the obligation of health care providers to act in ways that are fair to everyone concerned. Patients are vulnerable individuals who deserve loyalty and fairness in all interactions with health care providers.

Clinical Scenario: A 32-year-old patient presents for her annual wellness visit by herself. During the sexual history intake, the patient tells the APRN that she is also sexually active with other women, but she doesn't want her husband to know. The APRN tells the patient that the APRN will not discuss the matter with anyone and informs her that her information is protected under HIPAA law.

Discussion: The APRN is exercising the concept of fidelity by reassuring the patient that all health information is private and by not disclosing the information to the patient's husband.

Justice

Justice is the concept of fair and equal treatment to everyone, including equal distribution of goods and services and the principle of the provision of nonjudgmental care to individuals in the setting of health care.

Clinical Scenario: A 51-year-old patient presents together with a police officer to evaluate a possible dislocated finger. During the initial intake, the APRN learns that the mechanism of the injury is due to a domestic violence incident during which the patient hit his wife. The APRN orders an X-ray, and the X-ray confirms a dislocated metacarpophalangeal joint in the right index finger. The APRN refers the patient to an orthopedic surgeon.

Discussion: The circumstances surrounding the patient's injury are not relevant in the treatment of this patient. The APRN is exercising the principle of justice in managing the patients' care by providing fair, equal, and nonjudgmental treatment.

Minors

Due to the complexity of legal age laws in different states, the APRN should be familiar with the local state law in the area in which he or she chooses to practice. In most states, a child under the age of 18 years is considered a minor, and information and decisions about health care are made by the child's parent or legal guardian. Therefore, the minor's parent(s) or guardian(s) may request the minor's medical records without the minor's consent (except for emancipated minors). It is important to note that there are actually two instances in which medical consent may be given by a person other than the patient. The first is when the patient is a minor, and the second is when the patient has been declared legally incompetent.

Emancipation

Emancipation is a legal process that enables a teenager to be legally independent from his or her parent or guardian. The age at which someone may become an emancipated minor varies by state. For example, the age in Connecticut is 16 years, while in Alabama the age is 18 years. Emancipated teenagers can seek medical care, enroll in school or college, and sign legal contracts under their own name without their parent's or guardian's approval. Of course, they will be responsible for paying any acquired bills and honoring any contractual agreements they have signed. Emancipated minors are also able to file a lawsuit as well as have a suit filed against them.

Malpractice

Malpractice is the failure of a professional to exercise the skills and knowledge commonly applied by the average prudent, reputable member of the same profession. The elements required to prove malpractice include the following:

1. The APRN owes the plaintiff a duty, also known as a "duty of care" (this may be established in many ways, including moving into a patient care situation, offering medical advice over the phone to friends or neighbors, texting medical advice to an acquaintance, or implying your involvement through actions in a care scenario).
2. The APRN's treatment action fell below the APRN standard of care (breach of standard of care).
3. The APRN's action caused the plaintiff's injury (proximate cause).
4. The plaintiff was injured (actual injury must have occurred).

Sources of legal risk for the APRN include activities such as entering documentation in the electronic medical record, ordering and prescribing medications, performing invasive procedures, and offering timely referrals for patients when indicated. Training activities and continuing education sessions are examples of activities that do not incur risk for the APRN.

Malpractice Insurance

There are two types of advanced practice nursing malpractice insurance available: claims-based policies and occurrence-based policies, as outlined in Table 16.2.

Table 16.2. Malpractice Insurance

Policy Type	Advantage	Disadvantage
Claims-based Policy	Lower premium $$	Only covers the APRN when the insurance policy is "active"
Occurrence-based Policy	Covers any incident that occurred while the APRN was insured	Higher premium $$$$

Clinical Scenario: An APRN who has been retired from an urgent care clinic for three years has a claim filed against him for an incident that occurred while he was employed. During his active employment time, he signed up with a claims-based policy.

Discussion: Unfortunately, his claims-based policy will not cover this claim. If he had had an occurrence-based policy, the claim would have been covered.

Statute of Limitations

Statutes of limitations are laws passed by legislative bodies in the common law system to set the maximum time limit after an event within which legal proceedings may be initiated. In general, the law requires that any medical malpractice lawsuit be initiated within two years from the date when the injury is first sustained. However, states have different time limitations for medical malpractice law, and APRNs need to be aware of the statute of limitations for the state in which they practice.

Practice Questions

1. All of the situations described below represent establishment of "duty of care," EXCEPT:

   (A) The APRN administers first aid to a child on her son's soccer team.
   (B) The APRN stops at the site of an accident and offers to help injured passengers.
   (C) The APRN calls 911 to report an unconscious individual at a restaurant where he is having lunch.
   (D) The APRN gives advice to her friend about over-the-counter medications to relieve her allergy symptoms.

2. The acronym HIPAA stands for:

   (A) Health Insurance for Patient Access and Availability.
   (B) Health Insurance Portability and Accountability Act.
   (C) Health Insurance Protection of Access and Availability.
   (D) Health Insurance Protection, Access, and Accountability.

3. There are two instances when a medical consent form may be signed by someone other than the patient. The first instance is when the patient is a minor, and the second instance is when:

   (A) the person signing the document is the spouse of the patient.
   (B) the person signing the document is the insurance holder.
   (C) the patient has been declared legally incompetent.
   (D) the patient tells the physician that the other person may sign the document.

4. Which ethical term listed below is associated with the principle of "do no harm?"

   (A) autonomy
   (B) nonmaleficence
   (C) veracity
   (D) justice

5. Sources of legal risk for the APRN include all of the following situations, EXCEPT:

   (A) prescribing medications.
   (B) performing invasive procedures.
   (C) adding documentation within the electronic medical record.
   (D) practicing skills during an in-service training session.

6. The four elements required to successfully prove malpractice include 1) duty of care, 2) breach of standard of care, 3) injury or harm to the patient, and 4):

   (A) patient is mentally competent to file a malpractice case.
   (B) injury resulted from breach of duty.
   (C) harm was intended.
   (D) the defendant is insured for malpractice.

7. All of the following statements are true regarding licensure for APRNs, EXCEPT:

   (A) Licensure ensures a minimum level of professional competency.
   (B) Licensure requires verification of the educational program and degree achieved.
   (C) Licensure grants permission for an individual to practice in a profession.
   (D) Licensure bodies review information through a nongovernmental agency.

8. The APRN's legal right to practice is derived from:

   (A) the Institute of Medicine.
   (B) the state nursing board.
   (C) national certification organizations.
   (D) the U.S. Department of Health and Human Services.

9. The ethical term used for a nurse's obligation to act in the patient's best interest is:

   (A) nonmaleficence.
   (B) beneficence.
   (C) fidelity.
   (D) veracity.

10. Maintaining patient confidentiality is the responsibility of all health care professionals. Which of the following choices indicates a breach of patient confidentiality?

   (A) An attorney subpoenas medical records for a court deposition.
   (B) An APRN gives medical information to a patient's spouse.
   (C) A doctor sends medical information to the state public health department.
   (D) A dentist's office sends medical records to insurance companies.

11. All of the following family information is normally included in a genogram, EXCEPT:

   (A) divorce.
   (B) number of children.
   (C) cause of death.
   (D) criminal history.

12. APRN scope of practice is determined by:

   (A) federal legislation.
   (B) state law.
   (C) the American Nurses Association.
   (D) national certifying bodies.

13. The principle of autonomy protects an individual's right to make their own decisions regarding their life as well as medical care. Which of the following behaviors overrides an individual's right for autonomy?

   (A) capacity
   (B) paternalism
   (C) competence
   (D) substituted judgment

14. An APRN working in an emergency department is caring for two patients. The first patient is a homeless male with advanced cirrhosis of the liver. The second patient is the mayor of the city. When the APRN provides preferential care to the mayor while neglecting care for the first patient, he or she is violating which ethical principle?

(A) veracity
(B) nonmaleficence
(C) justice
(D) beneficence

15. The Affordable Care Act was enacted in:

(A) 2000.
(B) 2005.
(C) 2010.
(D) 2015.

Answer Explanations

1. **(C)** Whenever a nurse practitioner agrees to care for another person, a "duty of care" is established. An APRN who provides first aid care to a child on her son's soccer team has, by her actions, indicated responsibility for care. This establishes "duty of care," so choice (A) is true. The APRN who stops to render aid at the site of an accident has established a responsibility to act in a manner consistent with safe, ethical care, so choice (B) is also true. Duty of care may also develop in a casual situation such as helping a friend select an allergy medication, making choice (D) true. When you move into a scene and indicate you will be caring for someone, that unspoken duty of care is present. From the choices given, the nurse practitioner calling 911 to report an unconscious individual (choice (C)) is the correct answer, as the nurse practitioner has not moved into the scene as a provider, and a duty of care has not been established.

2. **(B)** The Health Insurance Portability and Accountability Act was enacted in 1996 and provides guidelines for the management of confidential medical information. This act ensures that only individuals with a legitimate reason to do so will have access to patient information. Some legitimate reasons for accessing patient information include subpoenaing records for legal reasons and providing information to insurance carriers for the purpose of reimbursement for care. Information on diagnoses is covered by a state's mandatory reporting statute.

3. **(C)** Medical consent for treatment may only be signed by someone other than the patient if the patient is a minor or the patient has been declared legally incompetent. A spouse of a patient, even if he or she is the insurance holder (choices (A) and (B)), does not have the legal authority to sign consent for treatment. A patient telling a health care provider that it is okay for another person to provide medical consent does not constitute a legal right for them to do so (choice (D)).

4. **(B)** Nonmaleficence is the term used to describe the obligation of health care providers to "do no harm." This might be encountered when a nurse practitioner attempts a procedure for which he or she has not been trained and a patient is injured. Autonomy (choice (A)) refers to a health care provider's respect for the patient and the patient's right to make their own decisions about health care. Veracity (choice (C)) is telling the truth. Justice (choice (D)) indicates fairness in all interactions with others.

5. **(D)** There are many inherent sources of legal risk for a practicing APRN. These include prescribing medications (choice (A)), performing invasive procedures (choice (B)), and entering documentation within a medical record (choice (C)), among others. Of the choices provided, practicing skills during an in-service training session is the only scenario that does not expose the APRN to legal risk.

6. **(B)** In order to successfully bring a malpractice suit to court, the plaintiff needs to prove four things: 1) the APRN had a duty to care for the patient; 2) in caring for the patient, the APRN acted in a way that did not follow nurse practitioner standard of care; 3) injury or harm must have occurred to the patient; and 4) the injury actually resulted from the APRN's breach of duty. An injury to the patient that occurs as a result of the APRN acting in a manner not consistent with current standards of care is an element required for successful proof of malpractice, making choice (B) correct. A patient's mental capacity (choice (A)) is not a prerequisite for proving malpractice. The plaintiff does not need to prove that the APRN intended to harm the patient in order to successfully prove malpractice (choice (C)). An APRN who is insured

for malpractice is acting in a responsible manner in order to mitigate risks in malpractice situations. However, the fact of being insured (choice (D)) is not a requirement for proof of malpractice.

7. **(D)** There are many aspects to professional licensure, and nurse practitioners are required to meet many requirements to be allowed to practice. Licensure ensures the public that an APRN has a minimum level of competency, making choice (A) true; that the APRN has graduated from or successfully completed an accredited APRN educational program, making choice (B) true; and that the APRN has permission to practice in that state, making choice (C) true. Choice (D) is incorrect as licensure requirements are not reviewed through a nongovernmental agency.

8. **(B)** The nurse practitioner's legal right to practice in a state is derived from the state board of nursing. The Institute of Medicine (choice (A)) is a national organization that has long advocated for removal of practice barriers for nurse practitioners. While certification (choice (C)) is a requirement in most states, becoming certified does not meet all the requirements for practice. The U.S. Department of Health and Human Services (choice (D)) is a governmental agency overseeing health organizations throughout the nation.

9. **(B)** The ethical term used to describe a nurse's obligation to act in the patient's best interest is beneficence. Acting in the patient's best interest may involve changing the plan of care based on new information gathered. Nonmaleficence (choice (A)) is the principle of preventing harm to the patient. Fidelity (choice (C)) is about being loyal and fair. Veracity (choice (D)) refers to telling the truth.

10. **(B)** Confidentiality of patient information and health records is an obligation for all health professionals. Knowing with whom information may be shared is critical. Medical information may not be shared with a patient's spouse unless the patient has allowed the spouse to be in the room while care is being discussed, making choice (B) a breach of confidentiality and thus the correct answer. Medical records may be subpoenaed for use in litigation (choice (A)). Many diseases are subject to mandatory reporting to state health departments (choice (C)). Examples include sexually transmitted infections such as gonorrhea and syphilis. Entities and individuals with a legal right to the information include health care providers, health care agencies, and insurance companies (choice (D)).

11. **(D)** Information found in a family genogram does not include the criminal history of family members. Divorce (choice (A)), number of children (choice (B)), and cause of death (choice (C)) are components that are often included in the genogram.

12. **(B)** State law determines the APRN scope of practice. Because state laws vary, scope of practice varies throughout the United States. Federal legislation (choice (A)) determines overall health care standards for all Americans. Choice (C), the American Nurses Association (ANA), is the largest nursing organization in the United States. This organization provides guidance and education about current practice matters, but does not determine APRN scope of practice. The ANA works to advocate for nurses in the United States and is very active in federal and state governments. National certifying bodies (choice (D)) include two organizations for family nurse practitioners: the American Nurses Credentialing Center (ANCC) and the American Academy of Nurse Practitioners (AANP). These organizations produce and administer certifying examinations to qualified APRN candidates, but do not determine APRN scope of practice.

13. **(B)** The principle of autonomy promotes an individuals' right to make their own decisions regarding health care. An example of a behavior that negates an individual's right to autonomy is paternalism. This behavior is frequently seen when grown children begin to treat their elderly parents as if they are children. While often well meaning, this behavior does not allow autonomy in decision-making. Capacity (choice (A)) is a clinical judgment made about whether a patient is capable of understanding information given to them. For instance, a patient signing a consent form for surgery must have the cognitive capacity to understand the risks and benefits of the offered treatment. Competence (choice (C)) refers to a legal status. All adults are considered to be competent unless they are determined by a judge to be unable to understand or make decisions on their own. Competence is often based on psychological or medical conditions that may impair cognition. Substituted judgment (choice (D)) is used by family members or caregivers of an elderly individual to make decisions based on what they believe the patient would have chosen, if they were declared competent, alert, oriented, and able to make decisions.

14. **(C)** Justice is the ethical principle involved with treating others fairly. In a health care situation, the APRN is to provide effective, evidenced-based care to all patients. An APRN who gives preferential treatment to a patient with political clout or influence is violating the principle of justice. Veracity (choice (A)) is the principle of telling the truth. The ARPN in this scenario has not violated this principle. Nonmaleficence (choice (B)) is the commitment to providing care that "does no harm" and is not in violation in this scenario. Beneficence (choice (D)) is the principle involved with providing the best care possible to patients in the health care setting. While the APRN may be violating this principle by providing less-than-optimal care to the homeless individual, the overt violation is of the principle of justice.

15. **(C)** In March of 2010, the Affordable Care Act (ACA) was signed into law in a groundbreaking effort to produce health care reform in the United States. This act was intended to allow access to health insurance for all Americans by decreasing premium costs and eliminating preexisting condition clauses. The ACA was also enacted to improve not only access to care, but also the quality and efficiency of health care in the United States. Since the enactment of the ACA, outcomes monitoring has risen to the forefront of evaluating health care quality. It has been more than 10 years since the ACA was signed and subsequent governmental actions have been taken in an attempt to dismantle some or all of the fundamental components of the act.

17

Reimbursement

The 1997 Balanced Budget Act (BBA) enhanced the value of family nurse practitioners as Medicare began to reimburse for services provided by FNPs. Currently, the FNP is reimbursed at 85% of the physician rate for medical services provided to patients. From a business and professional sense, the mechanism of reimbursement continues to play a significant and vital role in how a business entity may sustain and continue to offer medical services. Therefore, the FNP needs to have a foundation of knowledge related to the areas of coding and billing.

Eligibility

Scope of Practice

The scope of advanced practice nurses such as family nurse practitioners varies from state to state. Some states allow independent practice, whereas other states require a collaboration practice with a physician or physicians. FNPs should be familiar with the practice environment in the state in which they plan to practice.

Claim Submission Eligibility

Several elements are required before a family nurse practitioner can submit claims to the Centers for Medicare & Medicaid Services (CMS). Figure 17.1 shows the required components in claim submission for reimbursement.

National Provider Identifier (NPI)

CMS requires all medical providers to have a National Provider Identifier when filing for medical claims. The NPI is a unique identifier for the FNP, stays with the FNP regardless of where the practice is located, and does not expire. Applying for an NPI is free through the CMS website.

Employer Provider Number

The Employer Provider Number is a unique number assigned to a medical facility, and it represents where services occur. Some insurance companies (payees) use an employer identification number (EIN) and others assign their own employer provider number to the medical facility. The FNP will need to know which employer provider number to use when submitting the claim forms.

Third-Party Credentialing

FNPs need to apply to and be credentialed by the third-party payer. This is commonly known as third-party credentialing and takes place in order to bill the insurance company for the medical services provided. Each private insurance company has their own list of requirements and forms that need to be completed to file.

Claim submission eligibility = (national provider identifier) + (employer provider number) + (credentialing by insurance company)

Figure 17.1. Claim Submission Eligibility

Coding and Billing

There are different components in coding and billing. The components include the International Classification of Diseases (ICD), the Current Procedural Terminology (CPT), the Healthcare Common Procedure Coding System (HCPCS), and the Evaluation and Management (E/M) codes. Each component is crucial, not only because they serve as the foundation blocks to complete the bill, but also as support for the maximum reimbursement.

International Classification of Diseases (ICD)

The World Health Organization (WHO) developed and maintains the International Classification of Diseases codes. The current version is known as ICD-10. The ICD codes are used to promote a systematic documentation for diagnosis, symptoms, and reasons for seeking care. When assigning the ICD codes, it is best practice to use the most specific diagnosis codes and not the symptoms codes. For example, if a patient presented with a sore throat and fever and was diagnosed with streptococcal pharyngitis, use the streptococcal pharyngitis as the main diagnosis and not the fever and sore throat.

Current Procedural Terminology (CPT)

The Current Procedural Terminology is published by the American Medical Association and is used to document the procedures and services conducted. Documentation of the CPT needs to be accurate, since it will determine the amount of reimbursement the provider will receive from the insurance company.

Healthcare Common Procedure Coding System (HCPCS)

The Healthcare Common Procedure Coding System is a set of standardized codes used by Medicare (CMS) and other health care insurance providers, including the Blue Cross Blue Shield Association and the American Dental Association. There are two types of HCPCS coding systems: HCPCS Level I and HCPCS Level II. HCPCS Level I includes the CPT codes, while HCPCS Level II includes codes for durable medical equipment, prosthetics, orthotics, and supplies (DMEPOS), ambulance services, chemotherapy drugs, Medicaid, and other services.

Evaluation and Management (E/M) Codes

The Evaluation and Management (E/M) codes are also used by Medicare (CMS) and other health care insurance providers, including the Blue Cross Blue Shield Association and the American Dental Association. These codes are used to determine the medical level of the patient encounter. In primary care, FNPs must be familiar with the level of service or services rendered. For new patients, the common level service codes for the approximate amount of time spent with a patient include 99202 (10 minutes), 99203 (15 minutes), 99204 (25 minutes), and 99205 (40 minutes or more). For established patients, the common service codes are 99212 (10 minutes), 99213 (15 minutes), 99214 (25 minutes), and 99215 (40 minutes or more). Table 17.1 shows the evaluation and management documentation components for new or established patient codes.

CLINICAL PEARL

It is the responsibility of the medical biller to use the most updated coding available. ICD and CPT are updated and published annually. HCPCS Level II is updated quarterly.

Table 17.1. Evaluation and Management (E/M) Documentation Components for New/Established Patient Codes

	99202/99212	99203/99213	99204/99214	99205/99215
Visit Type	Problem Focused	Expanded Problem Focused	Detailed	Comprehensive
History (Documented)[1,2,3]	HPI: 1–3 ROS: none PFSH: none	HPI: 1–3 ROS: 1 PFSH: none	HPI: > 4 ROS: 2–9 PFSH: > 1	HPI: > 4 ROS: > 10 PFSH: > 3
Physical Exam (Documented)	Organ system: 1 1–5 findings	Organ system: 1 6–12 findings	Organ system: 1–6 1–2 findings (each system) or 12–18 findings in 1 system	Organ system: > 9 > 18 findings
Decision-Making	Straightforward	Low complexity	Moderate complexity	High complexity
Time	10 minutes	15 minutes	25 minutes	40 minutes

[1]HPI: history of present illness

[2]ROS: review of systems

[3]PFSH: past family social history

*Note: HPI, ROS, and PFSH are part of the major components of E/M documentation.

CLINICAL PEARL

Note that E/M code level 99201/99211 (minimal) is omitted from Table 17.1, as the level of this visit is usually a nurse (medical assistant) visit.

CLINICAL PEARL

According to the 2021 CPT manual, a new patient is one who has not received any face-to-face professional services, from the physician/qualified health care professional or from another physician/qualified health care professional who belongs to the same group practice, within the past three years.

Practice Questions

1. Which of the following statements is true about the National Provider Identifier (NPI) number?

    (A) An FNP's NPI numbers differ from one state to another.
    (B) An FNP can apply for a NPI through the state board of nursing.
    (C) The NPI is a unique identifier for the FNP regardless of where the practice is located.
    (D) The NPI is renewed annually.

2. Which of the following statements is true about the Employer Provider Number (EPN)?

    (A) The EPN is a unique number assigned to a facility, and it represents where services occur.
    (B) The EPN is a universal number assigned to a facility, and it represents where services occur.
    (C) The EPN is a unique identifier for the FNP where the practice is located.
    (D) The EPN stays with the FNP regardless of the states in which the FNP practices.

3. CPT stands for:

    (A) Common Procedural Terminology.
    (B) Common Professional Terminology.
    (C) Current Procedural Terminology.
    (D) Current Professional Terminology.

4. The 1997 Balanced Budget Act (BBA) allows FNPs to be reimbursed at what percentage?

    (A) 80%
    (B) 85%
    (C) 90%
    (D) 100%

5. The International Classification of Diseases (ICD) was developed by which of the following organizations?

    (A) Healthy People 2021
    (B) World Health Organization (WHO)
    (C) Centers for Disease Control and Prevention (CDC)
    (D) The North Atlantic Treaty Organization (NATO)

6. All of the following are key components of E/M documentation, EXCEPT:

    (A) history of present illness (HPI).
    (B) review of systems (ROS).
    (C) past family social history (PFSH).
    (D) health insurance status.

7. Which of the following encounters is considered a new patient visit?

   (A) a patient who follows up with a FNP for suture removal, which had been previously sutured by a MD from the same facility

   (B) a patient who presents for a pre-op assessment

   (C) a patient who is returning for a monthly B12 shot

   (D) a patient who dropped out of care for four years without a primary care provider

8. What is the optimal E/M code for a 15-year-old new female patient who is sexually active with the onset of nausea and vomiting for the past two weeks, with a standing order to run two in-house urinalysis and pregnancy tests?

   (A) 99202

   (B) 99204

   (C) 99212

   (D) 99214

9. What is the optimal E/M code for an 89-year-old established bed-bound male patient with onset of low-grade fever and change in mental status who is recently discharged from the hospital? The FNP plans to conduct a mini-mental state examination and send his urine culture to a lab.

   (A) 99202

   (B) 99204

   (C) 99212

   (D) 99214

10. The FNP diagnosed a six-year-old patient with a right ear infection two weeks ago. The patient presents today at the office for a follow-up visit, having completed all of his medication without any adverse effects. The FNP evaluates the patient's right ear and concludes that there is no sign of new infection, and no further workup is required. What is the E/M code for this visit?

    (A) 99202

    (B) 99204

    (C) 99212

    (D) 99214

11. A patient presented at the clinic with fever, nausea and vomiting, diarrhea, and flu-like symptoms. The FNP conducted an in-house influenza A and B test. The test shows a positive result for influenza A. What is the primary diagnosis for this visit?

    (A) J10.1 influenza A

    (B) R50.9 fever

    (C) R19.7 diarrhea

    (D) R11.2 nausea and vomiting

12. The FNP diagnosed a 17-year-old patient with bilateral otitis media with effusion two weeks ago with symptomatic treatment only. The patient presents today at the office for a follow-up visit. He is complaining of bilateral frontal and maxillary sinus pressure with greenish nasal discharge. The FNP evaluates the patient's ears and concludes that there is no sign of new infection, no further workup is required. During the same visit, the FNP conducts a detailed exam and orders an occipitomental view (Waters view) of the skull and further diagnoses him for frontal sinusitis. A course of antibiotic treatment was also ordered. Summary of the documented history reveals: HPI: three components, ROS: six components, and PFSH: two components. What is the optimal E/M code for this visit?

    (A) 99213
    (B) 99204
    (C) 99212
    (D) 99214

13. Which of the following is/are components in coding and billing?
    Select all that apply.

    (A) the International Classification of Diseases (ICD)
    (B) the Current Procedural Terminology (CPT)
    (C) the Healthcare Common Procedure Coding System (HCPCS)
    (D) Evaluation and Management (E/M) codes

14. During an in-house quarterly audit, a clinic manager was reviewing a FNP patient's chart. The clinic manager noted that the FNP diagnosed her new patient with streptococcal arthritis and ordered four different lab tests during the same visit. The FNP spends approximately 40 minutes in the patient's room providing face-to-face consultation. Under the history section, there are only two components listed under the HPI section and nothing (0) listed for the ROS and PFSH sections. Physical exam showed one recorded finding under the musculoskel-etal system. What is the optimal E/M code that can be billed for this visit?

    (A) 99201
    (B) 99202
    (C) 99203
    (D) 99204

15. All of the following orders require the use of the Healthcare Common Procedure Coding System (HCPCS) when filing for Medicare patients, EXCEPT:

    (A) glucose meter.
    (B) crutches.
    (C) cam walker boot.
    (D) amoxicillin antibiotic prescription.

Answer Explanations

1. **(C)** The National Provider Identifier (NPI) is a unique identifier for the FNP and it stays with the FNP regardless of where the practice is located. The FNP applies for the NPI through the CMS website, not through the state board of nursing (choice (B)). NPIs do not expire, so there is no need to renew annually (choice (D)), and there is no cost to apply. The NPI number remains the same and does not differ from one state to another (choice (A)).

2. **(A)** The Employer Provider Number (EPN) is a unique identifier for the business entity where services are rendered. Different insurance companies (payees) have their own unique EPN (choice (B)). A facility may have one EPN and multiple National Provider Identifier (NPI) numbers based on the number of nurse practitioners practicing at the facility. The NPI, not the EPN, is a unique identifier that stays with the FNP regardless of where the practice is located, making choices (C) and (D) incorrect.

3. **(C)** CPT stands for Current Procedural Terminology. The CPT is published by the American Medical Association, and CPT codes are used to document the procedures and services conducted. For example, when removing a marble from the nose of a three-year-old child, the CPT code is 30300 (removal of foreign body).

4. **(B)** The 1997 Balanced Budget Act, signed by President Bill Clinton, allows the FNP to be reimbursed at 85% of the physician rate for medical services provided to patients.

5. **(B)** The International Classification of Diseases was developed by the World Health Organization. The ICD is used to identify a patient's diagnosis and reasons for seeking care. Healthy People 2021 is not a worldwide program (choice (A)). It is only available in the United States, and it identifies our nation's health improvement priorities through utilizing evidence-based national health objectives. The Centers for Disease Control and Prevention (choice (C)) is the leading public health institute of the United States. It plays a significant role in monitoring public health; fostering and promoting health safety and health research; and providing leadership, education, and training to enhance public health. The North Atlantic Treaty Organization (choice (D)) is an international alliance that consists of 29 member states from North America and Europe.

6. **(D)** Insurance status may assist in determining the charges for the patient (cash pay versus commercial insurance); however, it is not part of the E/M coding components. History of present illness (choice (A)), review of systems (choice (B)), and past family social history (choice (C)) are major components of E/M documentation.

7. **(D)** This patient dropped out of care for four years. To qualify for a new patient encounter, the patient must not have been seen at the same practice location for three years or more. The patient already established care with the MD prior to returning to see FNP (choice (A)). The patient must return to his/her primary care provider for pre-op assessment, thus this is an established patient (choice (B)). The patient who is returning for a monthly treatment service is an established patient visit (choice (C)).

8. **(B)** For new patients, the common level service codes with the approximate amount of time spent with a patient include 99202 (10 minutes), 99203 (15 minutes), 99204 (25 minutes), and 99205 (40 minutes). With new patient care, the FNP will need additional face time to evaluate the HPI, PMFH, ROS components and evaluate the results from the in-house lab test. The presented scenario will also require additional workup, and because the patient is a teenage female, this could be GYN, GI, or GU etiology related. Thus, 99204 is the appropriate choice.

(Exam tip: Since this is a new patient, the presented options should trigger you to ignore 99212 (choice (C)) and 99214 (choice D)), which are codes for established patients. 99202 (choice (A)) is not appropriate, as the FNP will need the HPI, PHFH, ROS components to justify the lab testing. Thus, by using 99202, the FNP is under code for the visit and the facility will not be receiving the optimal reimbursement.

9. **(D)** For established patients, the common service codes are 99212 (10 minutes), 99213 (15 minutes), 99214 (25 minutes), and 99215 (40 minutes). In this scenario, the FNP will need additional time for the additional workup, and because the patient is elderly, bedbound, and recently discharged from the hospital, this could be MRSA, GI, or GU etiology. The FNP also plans to order a MMSE and urine culture for the patient. Thus, 99214 is the appropriate choice. (Exam tips: Since this is an established patient, the presented options should trigger you to ignore 99202 (choice (A)) and 99204 (choice (B)), which are codes for new patients.) 99212 (choice (C)) is not appropriate, as the FNP will need the HPI, PHFH, ROS components to justify the MMSE exam and lab testing. Thus, by using 99202, the FNP is under code for the visit and the facility will not be receiving the optimal reimbursement.

10. **(C)** For established patients, the common service codes are 99212 (10 minutes), 99213 (15 minutes), 99214 (25 minutes), and 99215 (40 minutes). In this scenario, the FNP does not need additional workup. Evaluation of the right ear shows no sign of infection, and the patient has no new symptoms. Thus, 99212 is the appropriate choice. (Exam tips: Since this is an established patient, the presented options should trigger you to ignore 99202 (choice (A)) and 99204 (choice (B)), which are codes for new patients.) 99214 (choice (D)) is not appropriate, as the FNP only rechecks the patient's ear. There is no other chief complaint or new illness presented in this visit. If the FNP uses 99214, the FNP is up-coding the visit and the facility may trigger an audit from the insurance agency for possible fraud.

11. **(A)** Since the in-house test shows a positive result for influenza type A, this should be the primary diagnosis for this visit. Other options (choices (B), (C), and (D)) are related to the symptoms and should not be coded as the primary diagnosis for this visit.

12. **(D)** The minimum documented history components required for the E/M of 99214 are HPI: four components, ROS: two components, and PFSH one component. 99204 (choice (B)) is for new patient encounters. 99212 (choice (C)) only requires documentation of one component under the HPI category, and 99213 (choice (A)) requires only one documented HPI component and one documented ROS component.

13. **(A, B, C, D)** All four choices are foundation components in submitting a claim for maximum reimbursement.

14. **(B)** Due to the lack of documented information under HPI, ROS, and PFSH, the best optimal E/M for this new patient visit is 99202. 99201 (choice (A)) is commonly reserved for a medical assistant visit. 99203 (choice (C)) requires only one documented HPI component and one documented ROS component. The minimum documented history components required for the E/M of 99204 (choice (D)) are HPI: four components, ROS: two components, and PFSH: one component.

15. **(D)** Medication prescription is not part of the health care common procedure, and it does not require HCPCS code. However, choices (A), (B), and (C) are part of the health care common procedure and require specific HCPCS codes.

PART VII
Research and Theory
(For ANCC Test-Takers Only)

18

Research, Theory, and Evidence-Based Practice

Research is one of the vital foundation blocks in the field of nursing practice. While not all nurses are conducting research, the evidence-based practice (EBP) used daily by many nurses is the result of work gathered and compiled by researchers. There are different types of research, and each one focuses on and uses a variety of different discipline methods to validate or solve problems related to the nursing field. Nurses with a DNP or PhD degree are prepared to conduct research. Prior to conducting any research or projects, it is important for the researcher to seek approval from institutional review boards.

Research

Research Populations

This is generally a collection of individuals or samples that provide some form of data to assist a researcher in designing and determining the content of their research questions. Because research normally involves human participants, an informed consent form is necessary before the gathering of research information can be implemented.

Informed Consent

Participants should complete an informed consent form before any research project begins. The consent form should describe the purpose of the study, the risks, discomfort, and benefits to the subject for participating in the study, any reward or compensation the subject will receive for participating, how the participant's privacy and personal information will be protected, whom to contact if the participants have concerns about the study, and the ability for participants to withdraw from the study at any time without punitive consequences.

Vulnerable Populations

Recruiting participants is a major step for moving forward with and conducting research. Subjects/participants who fall under the category of "vulnerable populations" require paperwork in addition to the completion of an informed consent form. Vulnerable populations include infants and children under the age of 18 (minors), pregnant women, persons with impaired cognition or impaired decision-making capacity, undocumented immigrants, homeless populations, and prisoners.

Institutional Review Boards (IRB)

The role of institutional review boards is to protect the rights and safety of research participants. This includes both human and animal subjects. There are different requirements based on the types of subjects recruited for the research. The IRB office is usually well established within large academic institutions. For facilities that do not currently have an IRB office, the researcher may contact other local IRB offices to initiate an approval prior to beginning a research project.

CLINICAL PEARL

At any time, participants have the right to withdraw from the study even if they have given consent to participate in the research.

269

Research Data

There are two types of research data: primary data and secondary data. **Primary data** is collected directly from the actual source. One example would be reviewing a patient's past medical history through verifying the records with your patient during their clinical visit. **Secondary data** is a set of data usually compiled and interpreted by someone else. For example, a nurse practitioner may want to review the number of new flu cases reported by the Centers for Disease Control and Prevention (CDC) in neighboring states in order to anticipate the total amount of flu test kits and vaccines the clinic will need to order in advance. Therefore, the nurse practitioner would utilize the secondary data compiled by the CDC to assist in the decision-making process.

Types of Research

Prospective

Prospective research is conducted in present time with an anticipated cut-off time. For example: An FNP researches the use of antibiotics in conjunction with the treatment for flu from November of the current year to February of the following year.

Retrospective

Retrospective research usually makes use of preexisting data. For example: An FNP working on a quality improvement project reviews the patient's past five years of medical diagnosis and treatment history.

Longitudinal

Longitudinal studies follow a group of the same subjects/participants for specific measurements or data collected over many years.

Quantitative

A quantitative study evaluates quantifiable data as part of the data analysis. For example: An FNP evaluates a patient's vital signs and food intake calories. Quantitative studies use deductive reasoning to determine an answer or solution upon evaluating the generalization data, from a general to specific topic.

Qualitative

A qualitative study evaluates the data gathered as words (nonnumerical data). For example: An FNP reviews interview transcripts. Qualitative study uses inductive reasoning, with the aim to identify concepts and phenomena, from a specific to general topic.

Research Design

There are multiple types of research designs. **Experimental research** is the gold standard in the field of research design. There are three components: randomized sampling of participants (recruiting participants in a randomized control environment with a predetermined plan), a control group (baseline), and an intervention group (outcome). For example, a pharmaceutical company is evaluating the efficacy of Drug X, a drug that reduces blood pressure in an acute setting. A total of 100 participants were randomly selected from a group of 1,000 participants. Of the selected

100 participants, 50 participants are assigned to Group A and Group B, respectively. Group A is a control group, and the participants would be given a placebo drug. Group B is an intervention group in which the participants receive Drug X. At the end of the study, the blood pressure readings from Group A and Group B would be used to evaluate the efficacy of Drug X.

Quasi-experimental research design is similar to experimental research design. One difference is that it uses a convenient sampling technique where there is no randomization among the research participants.

IMPORTANT TERMINOLOGY

SENSITIVITY: The proportion of people with disease who have a positive result.

EXAMPLE: If a test is highly sensitive and the test result(s) shows "negative," you can be certain that the tested subject does not have a disease.

SPECIFICITY: The proportion of people without a disease who have a negative test result.

EXAMPLE: If a test is highly specific and the test result is "positive," you can be confident that the tested subject has the disease.

HYPOTHESIS: The prediction of the research phenomenon.

EXAMPLE: In evaluating the efficacy of weekly face-to-face meetings in a weight-loss support group, the researcher hypothesized that the participants in the face-to-face meeting each week would lose more weight when compared to the other participant group that met only once a month. In this scenario, the researcher hypothesized that participating in a weekly face-to-face meeting would result in greater weight loss.

NULL HYPOTHESIS: A statement that indicates there is no significant relation between the variables of the study.

Using the example from the previous scenario, the null hypothesis could be stated as: There is no significant difference in weight loss reduction between participants who met in the weekly face-to-face meeting versus the participants who met face-to-face monthly.

N: A variable representing the total number of participants involved in the study; represents the number of subjects in a group.

EXAMPLE: A total of 100 participants were recruited and assigned equally into Group A and Group B. Research literature may present the information as ($N = 100$, $n = 50$, $n = 50$).

VARIABLE: Research variables represent a specific characteristic that can be measured. There are two types of variables: independent and dependent variables.

INDEPENDENT VARIABLE: A variable that can be manipulated and is not affected by the outcome.

DEPENDENT VARIABLE: A variable that results from the manipulation of independent variable(s).

EXAMPLE: An FNP studies the influence of the total number of hours participants spent on the treadmill and its effect on body weight. The independent variable is "hours spent on the treadmill," and the dependent variable is "body weight."

Theory

Nursing theory is derived from an organized framework that assists nurses in practicing efficiently in the field. Nursing theory influences how nurses communicate, provide patient care, and make daily clinical decisions. In the research field, nursing theory can also play a major role in providing a strong foundation framework for any research topic.

A theory evolves over a long period of time. The process of the scientific method in the development of a theory includes observation, logical hypothesis, testing, dissemination, and replication.

Nursing Philosophies

Nursing philosophies present nursing phenomena through analysis, reasoning, and logical approach. While nursing philosophies may be difficult to understand due to their abstract nature, the challenge presented to nurses should inspire them to discover and appreciate the concepts and theories. The following are some of the most common nursing philosophies the FNP should understand:

- **The philosophy of Florence Nightingale:** Nightingale's philosophy of health and healing principles remain the foundation of nursing practice today with focus on the following three major relationships: environment to patient, nursing to environment, and nursing to patient.
- **Theory of Human Caring (Jean Watson):** Watson's transpersonal caring relationship serves as the foundation of her theory. The core concepts of the theory include a relational caring for self and others.
- **Theory of Bureaucratic Caring (Marilyn Anne Ray):** The core concept of Ray's theory is the influence of organizational structure in caring.
- **The Primacy of Caring (Patricia Benner and Judith Wrubel):** The Banner and Wrubel theory proposes that caring for someone is the primary action in care as it establishes the possibility of giving and receiving help.

Nursing Conceptual Models

Nursing conceptual models comprise nursing works by theorists considered to be pioneers in nursing. Each of the following comprehensive nursing models addresses the metaparadigm concepts of person, environment, health, and nursing.

- **Four Conservation Principles (Myra Estrin Levine):** The goal of Levine's model is to adapt and maintain wholeness using the principles of conservation (energy, structure, personal integrity, and social integrity).
- **The Science of Unitary and Irreducible Human Beings (Martha Rogers):** Rogers's model emphasizes that nurses should view the patient as a whole, with dignity.
- **Self-Care Deficit Theory of Nursing (Dorothea Orem):** Orem's model is made up of three other related theories: the theory of self-care (focus on oneself, "I"), the theory of self-care deficit (focus on "you" and "me"), and the theory of nursing system (focus on "we," as a part of the community). The core concept of the theory focuses on persons and relationships rather than on individuals.
- **Theory of Goal Attainment (Imogene M. King):** King's model focuses on nurses and patients working together in a setting and taking actions to achieve their goals together. The focus is on the personal system, and not on organization as a whole. For example, soliciting the patient's opinion as part of the plan of care in managing the patient's health outcomes.

- **System Model (Betty Neuman):** Neuman's model is usually presented in a model diagram where the human being is viewed as an open system that interacts with internal and external environmental stressors.
- **Adaptation Model of Nursing (Sister Callista Roy):** Roy's model indicates that the individual will strive to adapt to a stressor they face from their surroundings as a form of survival. The adaptation will influence the individual's daily activities of living, health outcome, and quality of life.

Evidence-Based Practice (EBP)

Nurses are expected to implement evidence-based practice as part of their daily clinical role. The evidence-based information derived from various academic resources includes results from multiple clinical experiments, multisite studies, and expert recommendations. Through EBP, nurses can evaluate the improvement of medical knowledge, patient care, and quality outcomes.

Evidence-Based Programs and Policies

There are multiple resources that provide information related to EBP programs and policies. It is the responsibility of the FNP to stay informed with the clinical changes while providing the optimal medical care for their patients.

Advisory Committee on Immunization Practices (ACIP)

The Advisory Committee on Immunization Practices is composed of medical and public health experts who evaluate the current scientific evidence based on diseases related to immunization through vaccinations. Their experts develop recommendations on immunizations that help control diseases in the United States. For more information, visit the CDC website.

CDC Guidelines and Recommendations

Accessible through the CDC website, the CDC Guidelines and Recommendations provide a resource page for medical providers, patients, and consumers. The guidelines and recommendations are developed through collaboration with different health care organizations, agencies, and CDC federal advisory committees. For more information, visit the CDC website.

Prevention of HIV/AIDS, Viral Hepatitis, STDS, and TB through Health Care

An information website providing valuable knowledge on current practice and policies with the aim to prevent the spread of HIV/AIDS, viral hepatitis, STDs, and TB infections. For more information, visit the CDC website.

Compendium of Proven Community-Based Prevention Programs

This program was released by the Trust for America's Health (TFAH) and the New York Academy of Medicine (NYAM). The organization highlights 79 evidence-based disease and injury prevention programs that have saved lives and improved health.

Prevention Status Reports

This website highlights the top 10 public health problems and concerns for all 50 states and the District of Columbia. For more information, visit the CDC website.

United States Preventive Services Task Force (USPSTF)

This is an independent nonfederal panel of experts that evaluates current scientific evidence focusing on clinical preventative health care services. The USPSTF develops recommendations for primary care providers in clinical and health care settings and systems. The information is available for everyone to review including patients and caregivers. More information is available at *https://www.uspreventiveservicestaskforce.org/Page/Name/home.*

Treatment Guidelines

There are many different types of treatment and prevention guidelines provided by different organizations. These guidelines serve as a practice recommendation. It is the responsibility of the FNP to stay current and make informed decisions in adopting recommendations into his or her practices. As an example, the 2014 JNC-8 was based on the SPRINT trial results. However, many experts still urge a conservative go-slow treatment approach. Ultimately, some medical providers may opt to use the JNC-7 recommendation as opposed to the JNC-8. Utilization of treatment guidelines is always with consideration of individual patient characteristics and presentation, which serve as the foundation for patient-centered treatment approaches.

Grading Definition

The USPSTF assigns letter grades (A, B, C, D, I) per their clinical practice recommendations, as outlined in Table 18.1.

Table 18.1. USPSTF Grades and Interpretations*

Grade	Interpretation (Suggestions for Practice)
A	The net benefit is substantial and the USPSTF suggests health professionals offer/provide the service.
B	The net benefit is moderate to substantial and the USPSTF suggests health professionals offer/provide the service.
C	The net benefit is small and the USPSTF suggests health professionals offer/provide the service based on individual circumstances.
D	There is no net benefit and the USPSTF suggests health professionals discourage the use of the service.
I	The USPSTF is unable to determine the balance of benefits and harms. If the health professional provides the service, patients should understand that benefit and safety standards are undetermined.

*For more information, visit: *https://www.uspreventiveservicestaskforce.org/Page/Name/grade-definitions.*

> **CLINICAL PEARL**
>
> In a primary care setting, nurse practitioners should offer clinical services aligned with recommendations of grades A and B by the USPSTF. Grade C services should only be offered to patients with individual circumstances, as the net benefit is small.

Practice Questions

1. Which of the following is an example of the collection of primary data?

    (A) An FNP reviews de-identified data from a research data warehouse.
    (B) A grandfather tells an FNP that he thinks his grandson's immunization shots are up to date.
    (C) An FNP asks a patient to describe the mechanism leading to the patient's fall.
    (D) A patient rephrases to an FNP the possible side effects of the patient's current prescription after reading customer reviews on a website.

2. Which of the following is the role of an institutional review board (IRB)?

    (A) The IRB's role is to protect the research participants' rights and safety.
    (B) The IRB is responsible to contact the researcher prior to conducting any research.
    (C) The IRB's role is to protect the researcher's findings.
    (D) The IRB is responsible for enforcing the validity of research.

3. Which of the following statements is accurate about informed consent?

    (A) A participant must complete the research activity upon signing the informed consent form.
    (B) An informed consent form must be signed by the participants before participating in a research project.
    (C) The researcher can counter sue the participants if they decide to withdraw from the research.
    (D) Disclosing any benefits or possible adverse emotional distress from participating in the informed consent is optional.

4. When ordering a culture and sensitivity on a urine sample, the FNP understands that the antibiotic sensitivity report will provide information on:

    (A) the specific types of antibiotics that will work against the strain.
    (B) the types of possible strains presented in the urine.
    (C) the specific list of nutrient deficiency from the body.
    (D) the specific amount of protein and leukocytes in the urine.

5. All of the following are considered vulnerable populations, EXCEPT:

    (A) middle school soccer players.
    (B) undocumented immigrants.
    (C) school bus drivers.
    (D) pregnant women.

Questions 6 and 7 are based on the following clinical scenario.

An FNP initiates a study to determine the influence of the total number of minutes patients spent on the treadmill and its effect on heart rates at her clinic.

6. Which is the independent variable in this scenario?

    (A) the nurse practitioner
    (B) the clinic
    (C) the total number of minutes patients spent on the treadmill
    (D) the heart rates

7. Which is the dependent variable in this scenario?

    (A) the nurse practitioner
    (B) the clinic
    (C) the total number of minutes patients spent on the treadmill
    (D) heart rates

8. All the following components meet the criteria for a gold standard in an experimental research design, EXCEPT:

    (A) incorporating randomizing sampling.
    (B) incorporating convenience sampling.
    (C) establishing a control group.
    (D) establishing an intervention group.

9. Which of the following theorists is related to self-care deficit theory?

    (A) Dorothea Orem
    (B) Betty Neuman
    (C) Imogene M. King
    (D) Martha Rogers

10. All the following concepts are related to the personal system in Imogene King's theory, EXCEPT:

    (A) body image.
    (B) activities of daily living.
    (C) organization.
    (D) perception.

11. Resources for patients and guardians about lung cancer screening can be found at which of the following organization's websites?

    (A) United States Preventive Services Task Force (USPSTF)
    (B) Advisory Committee on Immunization Practices (ACIP)
    (C) Compendium of Proven Community-Based Prevention Programs
    (D) Prevention Status Reports

12. Resources for nurse practitioners in the use of vaccines can be found at which of the following organization's websites?

    (A) United States Preventive Services Task Force (USPSTF)
    (B) Advisory Committee on Immunization Practices (ACIP)
    (C) Compendium of Proven Community-Based Prevention Programs
    (D) Prevention Status Reports

13. The USPSTF recommends that clinicians offer clinical services aligned with the following grades:

    (A) grade A only.
    (B) grades A and B.
    (C) grades A, B, and C.
    (D) grades A, B, C, and D.

14. Match the following USPSTF recommended grades with the correct definitions:

Grade	Interpretation
A	( ) There is no net benefit; discourage the use of the service.
B	( ) Net benefit is small; offer/provide the service based on individual circumstances.
C	( ) Net benefit is moderate to substantial; offer/provide the service.
D	( ) Net benefit is substantial; offer/provide the service.
I	( ) Unable to determine the balance of benefits and harms; if the service is provided, patients should understand benefits/safety standards are undetermined.

15. All the following resources could serve as the primary resource for the FNP when researching a specific health topic related to the current clinical practice, EXCEPT:

    (A) United States Preventive Services Task Force (USPSTF).
    (B) Advisory Committee on Immunization Practices (ACIP).
    (C) Consumer Report in *Health* magazine.
    (D) Centers for Disease Control and Prevention (CDC).

Answer Explanations

1. **(C)** Primary data is collected directly from the actual resource. It is usually verifiable. In choice (C), the FNP is interviewing the patient directly and seeking information on the mechanism that leads to the patient's fall. The other choices are secondary data. De-identified data (choice (A)) is secondary data because there is no mechanism to verify the accuracy of the presented data. A patient's memory recall on immunization (choice (B)) is not primary, unless there is a written vaccination record. Anyone can post their review on the Internet (choice (D)), and there is no authentication for the provided information. This type of information is usually misleading to patients.

2. **(A)** The role of an institutional review board is to protect the research participants' rights and safety. It is the researcher's responsibility to contact the IRB and initiate any IRB application prior to conducting research, not the other way around (choice (B)). The IRB is not responsible for protecting the researcher's findings (choice (C)) or for enforcing the validity of research (choice (D)).

3. **(B)** All participants should complete an informed consent form before any research project begins. The following components should be listed on the consent form: the purpose of the study, the risk/discomfort and benefits to the subject for participating, any reward or compensation to the subject for participating in the study, how the participant's privacy and personal information will be protected, whom to contact if the participants have concerns about the study, and the ability for participants to withdraw from the study at any time without punitive consequences.

4. **(A)** When ordering a culture and sensitivity (C&S), the report will provide a list of organisms (strains) cultured from the specimen. Frequently, the report will also provide a list of antibiotics that are susceptible to the strains. The C&S utilizes quantifiable testing techniques and are most commonly order in the primary and urgent care clinics setting. Urine culture will only provide the types of strains presented in the urine (choice (C)). Urine analysis can be used to detect the presence of protein or leukocytes in the urine (choice (D)). There are many testing available when comes to evaluating the nutrient deficiency from the body. For example: CBC, nutritional test, vitamin panel testing and mineral panel testing (choice B)).

5. **(C)** In conducting a research project, vulnerable populations have additional paperwork and consent requirements. Vulnerable populations include infants and children under the age of 18 (minors) (choice (A)), undocumented immigrants (choice (B)), pregnant women (choice (D)), persons with impaired cognition or impaired capacity decision making, homeless populations, and prisoners.

6. **(C)** An independent variable is a variable that can be manipulated and has a role in determining the findings of the outcome. Based on the given scenario, the total number of minutes patients spent on the treadmill is the independent variable.

7. **(D)** The dependent variable is a variable that results from the manipulation of an independent variable(s). In this scenario, the total number of minutes spent on the treadmill (the independent variable, choice (C)) will influence the heart rates (the dependent variable, choice (D)).

8. **(B)** One of the major differences between a quasi-experimental research study and an experimental research study is the recruiting mechanism. Quasi-experimental research uses convenience sampling. Experimental design study uses randomized sampling (choice (A)), in addition to having control and intervention groups (choices (C) and (D)).

9. **(A)** Dorothea Orem developed the self-care deficit theory of nursing. The core concept focuses on persons and relationships rather than individuals. Betty Neuman (choice (B)) is known for her system model. Neuman's model is usually presented in model diagrams with the human being viewed as an open system that interacts with internal and external environmental stressors. Imogene M. King (choice (C)) is known for the theory of goal attainment. King's theory focuses on having nurses and patients work together to take actions to achieve their goals. Martha Rogers (choice (D)) focused on the science of unitary and irreducible human beings. The model emphasizes that nurses should view the patient as a whole, with dignity.

10. **(C)** Imogene M. King's model was the theory of goal attainment. This process is focused on the personal system, and not on organization as a whole. For example, nurses and patients work together one-on-one in a setting and take actions to set health outcome goals together.

11. **(A)** Lung cancer screening is part of the preventative health care services. Therefore, the correct answer should be the USPSTF. The ACIP (choice (B)) is composed of medical and public health experts that evaluate the current scientific evidence based on diseases related to immunization through vaccinations. The Compendium of Proven Community-Based Prevention Programs (choice (C)) is released by the Trust for America's Health (TFAH) and the New York Academy of Medicine (NYAM). The program highlights 79 evidence-based disease and injury prevention programs that have saved lives and improved health. Prevention Status Reports (choice (D)) is a website highlighting the top 10 public health problems and concerns for all 50 states and the District of Columbia.

12. **(B)** The ACIP is an organization that provides resources on immunization through vaccinations.

13. **(B)** In a primary care setting, nurse practitioners should offer clinical services aligned with the recommendation of grades A and B by the USPSTF. Grade C services (choices (C) and (D)) should only be offered to patients with individual circumstances, as the net benefit is small.

14. The correct matching of USPSTF letter grades with interpretations is as follows:

Interpretation
(D) There is no net benefit; discourage the use of the service.
(C) Net benefit is small; offer/provide the service based on individual circumstances.
(B) Net benefit is moderate to substantial; offer/provide the service.
(A) Net benefit is substantial; offer/provide the service.
(I) Unable to determine the balance of benefits and harms; if the service is provided, patients should understand benefits/safety standards are undetermined.

15. **(C)** The information retrieved from the Consumer Report in *Health* magazine should not be utilized as a primary resource in clinical practice. Choices (A), (B), and (D) are all reputable peer-reviewed reports and should be the primary resources for researching a specific health topic.

PART VIII
Practice Tests

ANSWER SHEET
Practice Test 1

1. Ⓐ Ⓑ Ⓒ Ⓓ	31. Ⓐ Ⓑ Ⓒ Ⓓ	61. Ⓐ Ⓑ Ⓒ Ⓓ	91. Ⓐ Ⓑ Ⓒ Ⓓ
2. Ⓐ Ⓑ Ⓒ Ⓓ	32. Ⓐ Ⓑ Ⓒ Ⓓ	62. Ⓐ Ⓑ Ⓒ Ⓓ	92. Ⓐ Ⓑ Ⓒ Ⓓ
3. Ⓐ Ⓑ Ⓒ Ⓓ	33. Ⓐ Ⓑ Ⓒ Ⓓ	63. Ⓐ Ⓑ Ⓒ Ⓓ	93. Ⓐ Ⓑ Ⓒ Ⓓ
4. Ⓐ Ⓑ Ⓒ Ⓓ	34. Ⓐ Ⓑ Ⓒ Ⓓ	64. Ⓐ Ⓑ Ⓒ Ⓓ	94. Ⓐ Ⓑ Ⓒ Ⓓ
5. Ⓐ Ⓑ Ⓒ Ⓓ	35. Ⓐ Ⓑ Ⓒ Ⓓ	65. Ⓐ Ⓑ Ⓒ Ⓓ	95. Ⓐ Ⓑ Ⓒ Ⓓ
6. Ⓐ Ⓑ Ⓒ Ⓓ	36. Ⓐ Ⓑ Ⓒ Ⓓ	66. Ⓐ Ⓑ Ⓒ Ⓓ	96. Ⓐ Ⓑ Ⓒ Ⓓ
7. Ⓐ Ⓑ Ⓒ Ⓓ	37. Ⓐ Ⓑ Ⓒ Ⓓ	67. Ⓐ Ⓑ Ⓒ Ⓓ	97. Ⓐ Ⓑ Ⓒ Ⓓ
8. Ⓐ Ⓑ Ⓒ Ⓓ	38. Ⓐ Ⓑ Ⓒ Ⓓ	68. Ⓐ Ⓑ Ⓒ Ⓓ	98. Ⓐ Ⓑ Ⓒ Ⓓ
9. Ⓐ Ⓑ Ⓒ Ⓓ	39. Ⓐ Ⓑ Ⓒ Ⓓ	69. Ⓐ Ⓑ Ⓒ Ⓓ	99. Ⓐ Ⓑ Ⓒ Ⓓ
10. Ⓐ Ⓑ Ⓒ Ⓓ	40. Ⓐ Ⓑ Ⓒ Ⓓ	70. Ⓐ Ⓑ Ⓒ Ⓓ	100. Ⓐ Ⓑ Ⓒ Ⓓ
11. Ⓐ Ⓑ Ⓒ Ⓓ	41. Ⓐ Ⓑ Ⓒ Ⓓ	71. Ⓐ Ⓑ Ⓒ Ⓓ	101. Ⓐ Ⓑ Ⓒ Ⓓ
12. Ⓐ Ⓑ Ⓒ Ⓓ	42. Ⓐ Ⓑ Ⓒ Ⓓ	72. Ⓐ Ⓑ Ⓒ Ⓓ	102. Ⓐ Ⓑ Ⓒ Ⓓ
13. Ⓐ Ⓑ Ⓒ Ⓓ	43. Ⓐ Ⓑ Ⓒ Ⓓ	73. Ⓐ Ⓑ Ⓒ Ⓓ	103. Ⓐ Ⓑ Ⓒ Ⓓ
14. Ⓐ Ⓑ Ⓒ Ⓓ	44. Ⓐ Ⓑ Ⓒ Ⓓ	74. Ⓐ Ⓑ Ⓒ Ⓓ	104. Ⓐ Ⓑ Ⓒ Ⓓ
15. Ⓐ Ⓑ Ⓒ Ⓓ	45. Ⓐ Ⓑ Ⓒ Ⓓ	75. Ⓐ Ⓑ Ⓒ Ⓓ	105. Ⓐ Ⓑ Ⓒ Ⓓ
16. Ⓐ Ⓑ Ⓒ Ⓓ	46. Ⓐ Ⓑ Ⓒ Ⓓ	76. Ⓐ Ⓑ Ⓒ Ⓓ	106. Ⓐ Ⓑ Ⓒ Ⓓ
17. Ⓐ Ⓑ Ⓒ Ⓓ	47. Ⓐ Ⓑ Ⓒ Ⓓ	77. Ⓐ Ⓑ Ⓒ Ⓓ	107. Ⓐ Ⓑ Ⓒ Ⓓ
18. Ⓐ Ⓑ Ⓒ Ⓓ	48. Ⓐ Ⓑ Ⓒ Ⓓ	78. Ⓐ Ⓑ Ⓒ Ⓓ	108. Ⓐ Ⓑ Ⓒ Ⓓ
19. Ⓐ Ⓑ Ⓒ Ⓓ	49. Ⓐ Ⓑ Ⓒ Ⓓ	79. Ⓐ Ⓑ Ⓒ Ⓓ	109. Ⓐ Ⓑ Ⓒ Ⓓ
20. Ⓐ Ⓑ Ⓒ Ⓓ	50. Ⓐ Ⓑ Ⓒ Ⓓ	80. Ⓐ Ⓑ Ⓒ Ⓓ	110. Ⓐ Ⓑ Ⓒ Ⓓ
21. Ⓐ Ⓑ Ⓒ Ⓓ	51. Ⓐ Ⓑ Ⓒ Ⓓ	81. Ⓐ Ⓑ Ⓒ Ⓓ	111. Ⓐ Ⓑ Ⓒ Ⓓ
22. Ⓐ Ⓑ Ⓒ Ⓓ	52. Ⓐ Ⓑ Ⓒ Ⓓ	82. Ⓐ Ⓑ Ⓒ Ⓓ	112. Ⓐ Ⓑ Ⓒ Ⓓ
23. Ⓐ Ⓑ Ⓒ Ⓓ	53. Ⓐ Ⓑ Ⓒ Ⓓ	83. Ⓐ Ⓑ Ⓒ Ⓓ	113. Ⓐ Ⓑ Ⓒ Ⓓ
24. Ⓐ Ⓑ Ⓒ Ⓓ	54. Ⓐ Ⓑ Ⓒ Ⓓ	84. Ⓐ Ⓑ Ⓒ Ⓓ	114. Ⓐ Ⓑ Ⓒ Ⓓ
25. Ⓐ Ⓑ Ⓒ Ⓓ	55. Ⓐ Ⓑ Ⓒ Ⓓ	85. Ⓐ Ⓑ Ⓒ Ⓓ	115. Ⓐ Ⓑ Ⓒ Ⓓ
26. Ⓐ Ⓑ Ⓒ Ⓓ	56. Ⓐ Ⓑ Ⓒ Ⓓ	86. Ⓐ Ⓑ Ⓒ Ⓓ	116. Ⓐ Ⓑ Ⓒ Ⓓ
27. Ⓐ Ⓑ Ⓒ Ⓓ	57. Ⓐ Ⓑ Ⓒ Ⓓ	87. Ⓐ Ⓑ Ⓒ Ⓓ	117. Ⓐ Ⓑ Ⓒ Ⓓ
28. Ⓐ Ⓑ Ⓒ Ⓓ	58. Ⓐ Ⓑ Ⓒ Ⓓ	88. Ⓐ Ⓑ Ⓒ Ⓓ	118. Ⓐ Ⓑ Ⓒ Ⓓ
29. Ⓐ Ⓑ Ⓒ Ⓓ	59. Ⓐ Ⓑ Ⓒ Ⓓ	89. Ⓐ Ⓑ Ⓒ Ⓓ	119. Ⓐ Ⓑ Ⓒ Ⓓ
30. Ⓐ Ⓑ Ⓒ Ⓓ	60. Ⓐ Ⓑ Ⓒ Ⓓ	90. Ⓐ Ⓑ Ⓒ Ⓓ	120. Ⓐ Ⓑ Ⓒ Ⓓ

ANSWER SHEET
Practice Test 1

121. Ⓐ Ⓑ Ⓒ Ⓓ	135. Ⓐ Ⓑ Ⓒ Ⓓ	149. Ⓐ Ⓑ Ⓒ Ⓓ	163. Ⓐ Ⓑ Ⓒ Ⓓ
122. Ⓐ Ⓑ Ⓒ Ⓓ	136. Ⓐ Ⓑ Ⓒ Ⓓ	150. Ⓐ Ⓑ Ⓒ Ⓓ	164. Ⓐ Ⓑ Ⓒ Ⓓ
123. Ⓐ Ⓑ Ⓒ Ⓓ	137. Ⓐ Ⓑ Ⓒ Ⓓ	151. Ⓐ Ⓑ Ⓒ Ⓓ	165. Ⓐ Ⓑ Ⓒ Ⓓ
124. Ⓐ Ⓑ Ⓒ Ⓓ	138. Ⓐ Ⓑ Ⓒ Ⓓ	152. Ⓐ Ⓑ Ⓒ Ⓓ	166. Ⓐ Ⓑ Ⓒ Ⓓ
125. Ⓐ Ⓑ Ⓒ Ⓓ	139. Ⓐ Ⓑ Ⓒ Ⓓ	153. Ⓐ Ⓑ Ⓒ Ⓓ	167. Ⓐ Ⓑ Ⓒ Ⓓ
126. Ⓐ Ⓑ Ⓒ Ⓓ	140. Ⓐ Ⓑ Ⓒ Ⓓ	154. Ⓐ Ⓑ Ⓒ Ⓓ	168. Ⓐ Ⓑ Ⓒ Ⓓ
127. Ⓐ Ⓑ Ⓒ Ⓓ	141. Ⓐ Ⓑ Ⓒ Ⓓ	155. Ⓐ Ⓑ Ⓒ Ⓓ	169. Ⓐ Ⓑ Ⓒ Ⓓ
128. Ⓐ Ⓑ Ⓒ Ⓓ	142. Ⓐ Ⓑ Ⓒ Ⓓ	156. Ⓐ Ⓑ Ⓒ Ⓓ	170. Ⓐ Ⓑ Ⓒ Ⓓ
129. Ⓐ Ⓑ Ⓒ Ⓓ	143. Ⓐ Ⓑ Ⓒ Ⓓ	157. Ⓐ Ⓑ Ⓒ Ⓓ	171. Ⓐ Ⓑ Ⓒ Ⓓ
130. Ⓐ Ⓑ Ⓒ Ⓓ	144. Ⓐ Ⓑ Ⓒ Ⓓ	158. Ⓐ Ⓑ Ⓒ Ⓓ	172. Ⓐ Ⓑ Ⓒ Ⓓ
131. Ⓐ Ⓑ Ⓒ Ⓓ	145. Ⓐ Ⓑ Ⓒ Ⓓ	159. Ⓐ Ⓑ Ⓒ Ⓓ	173. Ⓐ Ⓑ Ⓒ Ⓓ
132. Ⓐ Ⓑ Ⓒ Ⓓ	146. Ⓐ Ⓑ Ⓒ Ⓓ	160. Ⓐ Ⓑ Ⓒ Ⓓ	174. Ⓐ Ⓑ Ⓒ Ⓓ
133. Ⓐ Ⓑ Ⓒ Ⓓ	147. Ⓐ Ⓑ Ⓒ Ⓓ	161. Ⓐ Ⓑ Ⓒ Ⓓ	175. Ⓐ Ⓑ Ⓒ Ⓓ
134. Ⓐ Ⓑ Ⓒ Ⓓ	148. Ⓐ Ⓑ Ⓒ Ⓓ	162. Ⓐ Ⓑ Ⓒ Ⓓ	

Practice Test 1

ANCC-Style

DIRECTIONS: You have 3.5 hours to answer the following 175 questions.

1. A five-year-old child presents with his father for follow-up care. He was diagnosed with acute otitis media on the previous visit and has completed the 10-day course of amoxicillin. However, the child's father reports that he is still having deep ear pain and mild fever at night. During the assessment, you note that the child's tympanic membrane is fiery red and bulging, with absence of cone light reflex. What should the FNP do next?

   (A) initiate amoxicillin/clavulanate and OTC acetaminophen treatment
   (B) initiate amoxicillin treatment and OTC acetaminophen treatment
   (C) initiate amoxicillin/clavulanate treatment
   (D) initiate amoxicillin treatment

2. Infectious mononucleosis is most commonly caused by:

   (A) cytomegalovirus.
   (B) Epstein-Barr virus.
   (C) influenza virus.
   (D) varicella-zoster virus.

3. Which of the following types of sports are best for people with exercise-induced bronchoconstriction (EIB)?

   (A) ice hockey
   (B) snowboarding
   (C) marathon running
   (D) baseball

4. For patients with COPD, research has demonstrated that supplemental oxygen may improve quality of life and decrease short-term mortality. How many hours per day must the oxygen be used in order for this benefit to be realized?

   (A) 3–5 hours
   (B) 6–10 hours
   (C) 11–14 hours
   (D) 15–18 hours

5. A 24-year-old African American male presents to the clinic for management of hypertension. There is no history of diabetes; however, the patient has stage 1 renal disease. As part of the preferred hypertension treatment, the FNP should include:
Select all that apply.

(A) thiazide diuretic.
(B) an angiotensin-converting enzyme (ACE) inhibitor.
(C) an angiotensin receptor blocker (ARB).
(D) a calcium channel blocker (CCB).

6. A 34-year-old patient presents with a positive Chvostek's sign accompanied by respiratory stridor. The blood pressure is 80/60. What is the next appropriate action for the FNP?

(A) order T3, T4, and TSH tests
(B) order a 25-hydroxycholecalciferol assay
(C) order an electrocardiography
(D) refer the patient to the emergency department

7. Match the following hormones to the correct statements.

growth hormone ( )	(A) stimulates ductal growth in the breasts
estrogen ( )	(B) stimulates alveolar lobular growth of the breasts
prolactin ( )	
corticosteroids ( )	
progesterone ( )	

8. All the following are major differential diagnoses for weight gain, EXCEPT:

(A) Cushing's syndrome.
(B) premenstrual syndrome.
(C) Graves' disease.
(D) depression.

9. Your patient is a 40-year-old female with a new diagnosis of type 2 diabetes mellitus (T2DM). You are discussing options with her, and together you decide to begin therapy with metformin. In providing education about this medication, it is important to discuss with her the risk of:

(A) nausea and vomiting.
(B) lactic acidosis.
(C) hypoglycemia.
(D) hyperglycemia.

10. The clinical term for an enlarged thyroid gland is:

(A) exophthalmos.
(B) goiter.
(C) acromegaly.
(D) organomegaly.

11. A patient who has been prescribed pioglitazone should have which of the following tests specific to this medication?

   (A) screening for microalbuminuria in one month
   (B) hemoglobin A1c in six months
   (C) liver function studies in two to three months
   (D) lipid panel in six weeks

12. All the following statements are correct about asymptomatic bacteriuria (AB), EXCEPT:

   (A) The diagnosis of AB in women is based on two consecutive clean catch voided urine specimens with isolation of the same organism in quantitative counts of $\geq$ 10,000 cfu/mL with the absence of symptoms.
   (B) The diagnosis of AB in men is based on a single clean catch voided urine specimen with isolation of a single organism in quantitative counts of $\geq$ 10,000 cfu/mL with the absence of symptoms.
   (C) There are no recommendations involving the screening and management of AB among all populations.
   (D) There is a recommendation involving the screening and management of AB among pregnant women.

13. A 24-year-old pregnant woman is diagnosed with a urinary tract infection. All of the following medications are appropriate treatments, EXCEPT:

   (A) ampicillin (Omnipen).
   (B) nitrofurantoin (Macrobid).
   (C) cephalexin (Keflex).
   (D) tetracycline (Sumycin).

14. A 65-year-old patient with a history of chronic kidney disease has a glomerular filtration rate of 16 mL/min. What is the stage of his kidney disease?

   (A) stage 1
   (B) stage 2
   (C) stage 3
   (D) stage 4

15. A common physical exam finding in a patient with a diagnosis of pyelonephritis is:

   (A) costovertebral angle (CVA) tenderness.
   (B) dysuria.
   (C) a positive Murphy's sign.
   (D) intermittent abdominal pain.

16. An FNP received a hepatitis B lab result report with the following information: HBsAg: positive, anti-HBs: negative, anti-HBeAg: positive, anti-HBe: negative, anti-HBc: IgM. The tentative diagnosis is:

   (A) hepatitis B.
   (B) body developed immunity or recovery from hepatitis B infection.
   (C) chronic hepatitis B infection with high viral replication (high risk for transmission).
   (D) chronic hepatitis B infection with low viral replication activity (low risk for transmission).

17. A father presents to the clinic with his 10-month-old baby. The father reports that the baby has been crying inconsolably and that symptoms started midmorning. The father first noted the baby crying, screaming, and drawing up his legs with periods of sleeping between episodes. The patient recently recovered from a cold. The father reports "jelly-colored stool" this morning in the patient's diaper. During assessment, the patient appears glassy-eyed and falls asleep on the examination table. The FNP notes and feels a small pea-sized mass on the right upper quadrant of the patient's abdomen. The patient's Dance sign is positive. What should the FNP suspect?

(A) intussusception

(B) constipation

(C) peritonitis

(D) colic

18. A 78-year-old patient presents to the office in a wheelchair, accompanied by his son. The son reports concern about his dad's memory problems and confusion. According to the son, the confusion fluctuates throughout the day, becoming more prominent during midmorning and early afternoon hours. The patient was recently discharged from the hospital and is recovering from a fracture of his right knee. During the assessment, the patient appears confused, unable to determine the time, date, and location. However, his vital signs are stable. Following discharge, the patient remains on his previous medications. What is the possible diagnosis?

(A) dementia

(B) depression

(C) delirium

(D) stroke

19. To assess for dementia in an elderly patient in the office setting, the FNP should use the most widely utilized tool, which is the:

(A) Delirium Rating Scale (DRS).

(B) Confusion Assessment Method (CAM).

(C) Mini-Mental State Exam (MMSE).

(D) PHQ 9.

20. A primary abortive treatment used for cluster headaches is:

(A) IV morphine.

(B) nasal sumatriptan.

(C) high liter oxygen administration.

(D) NSAID use.

21. All the following are symptoms for osteoarthritis (OA), EXCEPT:

(A) pain tends to worsen with activities.

(B) it usually affects asymmetrical joints.

(C) affected joints include hands, knees, hips, and spine.

(D) morning stiffness lasts 50 minutes or more.

22. Which of the following areas is NOT included in the 18 tender points associated with fibromyalgia?

    (A) upper frontal sinus
    (B) distal to the lateral epicondyle
    (C) mid upper trapezius muscle
    (D) upper outer quadrant of the buttock

23. A 35-year-old woman presents to the clinic with complaints of morning stiffness on the right side of the elbow with persistent aching and no history of injury. The patient has been working in her garden for the past three days. The symptoms started with soreness of the forearm muscles but gradually worsened to the point where she cannot hold a flower pruner or turn a doorknob. The FNP applied light pressure and was able to replicate the tenderness in the right elbow and wrist. What should the FNP suspect?

    (A) epicondylitis
    (B) osteochondritis dissecans
    (C) radial head subluxation
    (D) carpal tunnel syndrome

24. Which of the following tests is considered to be the most specific in the diagnosis of rheumatoid arthritis (RA)?

    (A) rheumatoid factor (RF)
    (B) anti-CCP antibodies
    (C) tumor necrosis factor-alpha (TNF-alpha)
    (D) quantitative antinuclear antibodies (ANA)

25. Your patient is a 33-year-old male who has not been feeling well. The patient reports nonspecific complaints of fatigue and malaise. On CBC with diff, the MCV is 76 (normal 80–100 fL). You order a total iron binding content (TIBC), ferritin, and serum iron levels. What are your differential diagnoses?

    (A) iron deficiency anemia and sickle cell anemia
    (B) iron deficiency anemia and thalassemia trait
    (C) iron deficiency anemia and pernicious anemia
    (D) iron deficiency anemia and anemia of chronic disease

26. A patient with HIV who reports recurring, massive diarrhea likely has:

    (A) toxoplasmosis infection.
    (B) cryptosporidiosis infection.
    (C) progressive multifocal leukoencephalopathy (PML).
    (D) cryptococcus infection.

27. Skin conditions including pruritus, hyperpigmentation, and uremic frost are commonly seen in patients with:

    (A) diabetes mellitus.
    (B) hyperthyroidism.
    (C) hepatic cancer.
    (D) chronic renal failure.

28. The chief complaint associated with pediculosis capitis is:

    (A) alopecia.
    (B) pain.
    (C) itching.
    (D) burning.

29. While teaching a 16-year-old boy how to perform a testicular self-exam, the FNP noted and felt soft and movable blood vessels that felt like a "bag of worms" under the scrotal skin. Upon further examination, there is no sign of abnormality. The FNP diagnoses the patient with varicocele. What is the treatment?

    (A) levofloxacin
    (B) ceftriaxone IM followed by oral doxycycline
    (C) amoxicillin
    (D) no treatment, continue monitoring

30. Which of the following is a recommended suppressive treatment for herpes simplex virus (HSV) infection?

    (A) abacavir
    (B) acyclovir
    (C) raltegravir
    (D) darunavir

31. During a prostate exam, you note an area of hardness on the posterior side of the gland. This finding is most consistent with which of the following?

    (A) a normal prostate gland
    (B) acute bacterial prostatitis
    (C) benign prostatic hyperplasia
    (D) prostate cancer

32. A 78-year-old male patient has a chief complaint of urethral irritation after urination. If sexually transmitted diseases and a UTI are ruled out, what might be the diagnosis?

    (A) epididymitis
    (B) chronic prostatitis
    (C) bladder cancer
    (D) asymptomatic bacteriuria

33. What is the current recommended folic acid supplement dosage during pregnancy for a healthy 27-year-old patient?

    (A) 1,000 mcg
    (B) 2,000 mcg
    (C) 800 mcg
    (D) 400 mcg

34. Primary amenorrhea is defined as:
    Select all that apply.

    (A) no menses by age 13 in girls who have not developed any secondary sexual characteristics.
    (B) no menses by age 14 in girls who have not developed any secondary sexual characteristics.
    (C) no menses by age 16 in girls who may or may not have developed secondary sexual characteristics.
    (D) no menses by age 15 in girls who may or may not have developed secondary sexual characteristics.

35. Susan is 35 weeks pregnant. This is her second pregnancy. She delivered a healthy baby girl at 37 weeks with her first pregnancy. How should the FNP document her GTPAL?

    (A) G: 2, T: 2, P: 0, A: 1, L: 2
    (B) G: 2, T: 1, P: 1, A: 0, L: 1
    (C) G: 2, T:2, P: 0, A: 0, L: 2
    (D) G: 2, T: 1, P: 0, A: 0, L: 1

36. A 60-year-old transgender patient (MTF) presents to the office for her annual physical exam. The patient tells the FNP that she has not had any gender confirmation surgery and is currently on long-term hormone replacement therapy. Which of the following items should the FNP include in this visit?
    Select all that apply.

    (A) breast examination
    (B) prostate specific antigen
    (C) digital rectal exam
    (D) Papanicolaou test

37. Selective serotonin reuptake inhibitors (SSRIs) and selective norepinephrine reuptake inhibitors (SNRIs) are very effective in the pharmacologic management of bulimia nervosa (BN). Which of the following medications is contraindicated with BN?

    (A) citalopram
    (B) bupropion
    (C) fluoxetine
    (D) sertraline

38. An FNP examines a child and suspects child abuse. What is the FNP's legal responsibility?
    Select all that apply.

    (A) The FNP should accurately document his or her findings.
    (B) The FNP should report the case to local authorities.
    (C) The FNP should assist the family in identifying community resources.
    (D) The FNP should refer the family to an appropriate support group.

39. A teenage patient has a blood pressure of 90/65 and seems drowsy, euphoric, and unable to focus. Pupils are constricted and speech is slurred. These symptoms are consistent with:

    (A) opioid intoxication.
    (B) benzodiazepine overdose.
    (C) marijuana use.
    (D) amphetamine overdose.

40. Since beginning pneumococcal vaccination in infants, which of the following is correct?

    (A) Acute otitis media (AOM) due to *S. pneumoniae* has been eradicated.
    (B) The prognosis and cure rates for AOM have improved.
    (C) There have been decreased numbers of AOM caused by *H. influenzae*.
    (D) There has been a shift in pathogenesis to fewer cases of *S. pneumoniae*.

41. A 67-year-old patient presented for his wellness exam. The FNP is reviewing his vaccination record and notices that he needs a shingles vaccine. Which Medicare plan will cover a shingles vaccination?

    (A) Medicare Part A
    (B) Medicare Part B
    (C) Medicare Part C
    (D) none of the above

42. Which of the following statements accurately describes the role of a state board of nursing?

    (A) The board of nursing determines the testing domains for the family nurse practitioner certification exam.
    (B) The board of nursing is responsible for ensuring public safety by requiring all advanced practice nurses to meet the minimum requirement qualifications.
    (C) The board of nursing sets universal practice protocols for all states.
    (D) Every year, the board of nursing initiates a job satisfaction survey to all advanced practice nurses.

43. There are five different nursing leadership types. A leader who has an ability to communicate well with others, is unusually charismatic, and has great working relationships is using:

    (A) situational leadership.
    (B) transformational leadership.
    (C) authoritarian leadership.
    (D) democratic leadership.

44. An FNP diagnosed a six-year-old patient with acute sinusitis 10 days ago. She presented today at the office for a follow-up visit. She completed all medications without any adverse effects. The FNP completed the assessment and concluded that there was no sign of new infection. What is the E/M code for this visit?

    (A) 99211
    (B) 99213
    (C) 99212
    (D) 99214

45. Which of the following represents the collection of secondary data?

    (A) An FNP asks a patient to describe the mechanism leading to his fall.

    (B) A mother presents a copy of the immunization record of her daughter.

    (C) A researcher reviews de-identified data from a research data warehouse.

    (D) A patient reads the possible side effects of his current prescription from the container label.

46. What is the first-line therapy for treating acute bacterial sinusitis in a patient who has a penicillin allergy?

    (A) trimethoprim/sulfamethoxazole

    (B) amoxicillin/clavulanate

    (C) amoxicillin

    (D) clarithromycin

47. An ill-appearing 68-year-old male presents with sudden onset of an elevated blood pressure of 170/100 and vision changes with no history of injury. The patient's symptoms were first noted yesterday evening. During the assessment, the FNP notices that the patient's right eye cornea is red and the midsized pupil is nonreactive to light. Which of the following diagnoses should the FNP consider?

    (A) retinal detachment

    (B) cataract

    (C) acute angle-closure glaucoma

    (D) conjunctivitis

48. When performing the Weber test during an assessment of hearing loss, the sound is louder in the unaffected ear in which type of loss?

    (A) conductive

    (B) sensorineural

    (C) traumatic

    (D) mixed

49. An FNP works in a clinic that sees patients from Monday to Thursday. Which of the following day(s) is NOT appropriate to offer tuberculin skin testing (TST)?
Select all that apply.

    (A) Monday

    (B) Tuesday

    (C) Wednesday

    (D) Thursday

50. Which of the following treatments is appropriate for treating a patient with mild persistent asthma?

    (A) intermittent reliever medication taken as needed

    (B) one daily controller medication

    (C) multiple daily medium-dose inhaled corticosteroid and controller medications

    (D) multiple daily high-dose inhaled corticosteroid and controller medications

51. You examine a 66-year-old male with dilated cardiomyopathy and heart failure. On examination, you expect to find all of the following, EXCEPT:

    (A) jugular venous distention.
    (B) right upper quadrant abdominal tenderness.
    (C) point of maximal impulse (PMI) at left fifth intercostal space midclavicular line.
    (D) peripheral edema.

52. What level of high-density lipoprotein (HDL) is considered cardio protective?

    (A) > 30 mg/dL
    (B) > 40 mg/dL
    (C) > 50 mg/dL
    (D) > 60 mg/dL

53. An 82-year-old male has early renal insufficiency. What lab study would be the best test to evaluate his renal function?

    (A) urinalysis
    (B) serum creatinine level
    (C) 24-hour urine measurement
    (D) glomerular filtration rate (GFR)

54. The initial presenting symptom of a bladder tumor is usually:

    (A) weight loss.
    (B) uremia.
    (C) painless hematuria.
    (D) low-grade fever.

55. While reviewing a hepatitis B report, which of the components in the report will provide information if the patent has developed immunity via vaccination?

    (A) positive HBsAg
    (B) positive anti-HBc
    (C) positive anti-HBs
    (D) positive anti-HBe

56. Esophageal adenocarcinoma usually occurs:

    (A) in the upper esophageal area.
    (B) near the upper esophageal sphincter.
    (C) at the junction of the esophagus and the stomach.
    (D) in the lower esophageal area.

57. A patient presents with a complaint of feeling dizzy. The FNP decides to do a focused assessment. Which of the following systems should the FNP evaluate?
    Select all that apply.

    (A) ear, eyes, throat
    (B) cardiovascular
    (C) integumentary
    (D) neurological

58. Which of the following medications may assist in managing tremors in a multiple sclerosis (MS) patient?

(A) carbamazepine (Tegretol)
(B) tizanidine (Zanaflex)
(C) dantrolene (Dantrium)
(D) diazepam (Valium)

59. According to the World Health Organization (WHO), a bone mineral density (BMD) greater than 2.5 standard deviation (SD) below young adult reference mean (22.5) is classified as:

(A) normal.
(B) osteopenia.
(C) osteoporosis.
(D) osteoporosis (severe).

60. A patient presents with an MCV of 108. What should the FNP order?

(A) serum iron level and TIBC
(B) serum ferritin level and TIBC
(C) vitamin B12 and folate levels
(D) folate level and serum iron level

61. The American Cancer Society uses the ABCDE mnemonic to help patients and clinicians develop awareness of skin lesions that may be cancerous. What does the "B" represent?

(A) bleeding
(B) black
(C) border
(D) benign

62. What is the preferred treatment for uncomplicated gonococcal infection in a 44-year-old female with no drug-allergy history?

(A) amoxicillin
(B) trimethoprim-sulfamethoxazole (TMP-SMX)
(C) metronidazole
(D) ceftriaxone IM plus azithromycin

63. A five-year-old boy presents with his father at the clinic with complaints of scrotal pain. The family has recently returned from a camping trip. Vital signs are stable. The patient is able to void without any concerns. Physical examination shows a mild swollen lump noted on his left scrotum, mild tenderness on palpation, and no sign of injury or infection. An in-house urinalysis is normal. The FNP diagnoses the patient with epididymitis. What is the treatment?

(A) rest and ibuprofen
(B) amoxicillin
(C) trimethoprim-sulfamethoxazole (TMP-SMX)
(D) metronidazole

64. Based on the report of the percentage of women experiencing an unintended pregnancy in the first year of birth control use, arrange the following methods from *least* effective to *most* effective.

Select all that apply.

(A) vaginal contraceptive sponge

(B) calendar calculation

(C) combination oral contraceptives

(D) postcoital control

65. A 34-year-old transgender (FTM) patient has a follow-up appointment after a gender confirmation/reassignment surgery. This is the first time the patient has visited the clinic. The patient brings his transgender partner with him into the examination room. What should the FNP do first?

(A) politely request the patient's partner leave the examination room for the patient's privacy

(B) introduce herself as an FNP and ask the patient which pronouns they use

(C) review the procedure history chart, perform the examination, and tell the patient and his partner the examination findings

(D) review the procedure history chart, perform the examination, and tell the patient directly the examination findings

66. Individuals with major depressive disorder (MDD) who are treated with SSRIs will likely report which of the following within the first six months of treatment?

(A) increased libido

(B) weight gain

(C) sleep disorders

(D) high blood sugar levels

67. A patient presents with erosion of the nasal septum with continuous oozing of blood. The tissue is macerated as well. Which of the following is a likely cause?

(A) chronic sinusitis

(B) severe allergic rhinitis

(C) cocaine abuse

(D) improper use of intranasal spray

68. A three-month-old infant is diagnosed with dermatitis of the diaper area. The rash is bright red with satellite lesions. Based on this finding, the rash should be treated with:

(A) zinc oxide.

(B) topical antifungal cream.

(C) topical antibacterial cream.

(D) low-potency hydrocortisone cream.

69. A 14-year-old male comes to the office with a complaint of leg pain. He has no history of injury. His mother tells you he has been going through a growth spurt and she thought he was just having "growing pains." When the mother noticed a "bump," she wanted to have it checked out. The patient tells you that the pain is worse when he squats or climbs stairs and gets better with rest. On exam, you note a tender bony mass on the anterior tubercle. This presentation is consistent with:

    (A) Klinefelter syndrome.
    (B) Osgood-Schlatter disease.
    (C) meniscal tear.
    (D) ligamentous injury.

70. An 89-year-old patient presents for his wellness exam. His medical history includes hypertension and gout. He has smoked a half pack of cigarettes per day for the past 30 years. Which of the following should an FNP recommend?

    (A) aspirin for the prevention of cardiovascular disease
    (B) no recommended screening
    (C) colorectal cancer screening
    (D) lung cancer screening

71. When administering the Mini-Mental State Exam (MMSE), what activity are you performing?

    (A) assessing for cognitive impairment
    (B) screening for delirium
    (C) screening for depression
    (D) assessing for Parkinson's disease

72. Which of the following organizations grants the APRN the legal right to practice?

    (A) the Institute of Medicine
    (B) state board of nursing
    (C) national certification organizations
    (D) the U.S. Department of Health and Human Services

73. A husband comes to a clinic asking for the reason his wife visited the clinic last Monday. He provides her name, date of birth, and Social Security number. The FNP tells the gentleman that he cannot confirm or verify any information and turns the patient's husband away. The FNP's action is an example of:

    (A) justice.
    (B) confidentiality.
    (C) fidelity.
    (D) veracity.

74. The National Provider Identifier (NPI) number is a unique identification number for covered health providers. The Health Insurance Portability and Accountability Act (HIPAA) adopted the NPI as a Simplification Standard. This number is used in all administrative and financial transactions adopted by the HIPAA. The NPI number contains:

(A) 10 digits.
(B) 15 digits.
(C) 20 digits.
(D) 25 digits.

75. Which of the following is the code used to bill for outpatient and office procedures?

(A) Common Procedural Terminology
(B) Common Professional Terminology
(C) Current Procedural Terminology
(D) Current Professional Terminology

76. Which of the following is not the role of the Internal Research Board (IRB)?

(A) to protect the researcher's rights and safety
(B) to protect vulnerable populations
(C) to protect the confidentiality of the participants
(D) to review the researcher's application and determine eligibility

77. An FNP is reviewing the efficacy report of a comparison of new drugs in managing the reduction of blood pressure for a certain age group of the population. The baseline of average blood pressure is listed in the "Before" section. Upon one week of taking Drug X, the average blood pressure is listed in the "After" section. The results are stated below:

Age Group	Drug X			
	Before (mm Hg)		After (mm Hg)	
	Systolic	Diastolic	Systolic	Diastolic
30–39 ($n = 1000$)	160 (± 15)	120 (± 5)	120 (± 5)	90 (± 5)
40–49 ($n = 1,000$)	160 (± 15)	120 (± 5)	130 (± 10)	110 (± 5)
50–59 ($n = 1,000$)	160 (± 15)	120 (± 5)	140 (± 25)	110 (± 15)
60–69 ($n = 1,000$)	160 (± 15)	120 (± 5)	155 (± 15)	120 (± 5)
$N = 4,000$				

How many participants are in the age group of 60–69?
(A) 4,000
(B) 3,000
(C) 2,000
(D) 1,000

78. Shared decision-making includes:

(A) presentation of all options to the patient.
(B) clarification of patient values and goals.
(C) discussion of risks versus benefits.
(D) all of the above.

79. To critically evaluate a randomized controlled trial, which of the following should be used?

    (A) SQUIRE
    (B) PRISMA
    (C) STROBE
    (D) CONSORT

80. Which of the following is considered a visual acuity of blindness?

    (A) 20/200
    (B) 20/100
    (C) 20/20
    (D) 20/60

81. Your patient is a six-month-old male who is brought to the clinic by his mother. His mother reports the baby has had a fever for a day or two and does not want to eat. She tells you he only sleeps a couple of hours at a time and wakes up crying. Upon physical examination, you note mild rhinitis, clear oropharynx, and eyes without redness or drainage. An otoscopic exam demonstrates a bright red, bulging, tympanic membrane (TM) in the right ear. The left TM is pearly gray, with fluid noted behind the TM. Based on this presentation, the diagnosis is most likely:

    (A) acute otitis externa (AOE).
    (B) acute otitis media (AOM).
    (C) acute upper respiratory infection (URI).
    (D) none of the above.

82. The definition of sleep apnea is:

    (A) a temporary pause in breathing during sleep lasting 1–5 seconds.
    (B) a temporary pause in breathing during sleep lasting 6–10 seconds.
    (C) a temporary pause in breathing during sleep lasting 11–90 seconds.
    (D) a temporary pause in breathing during sleep where the patient begins to choke.

83. Which electrocardiography (ECG) change is a characteristic finding with cardiac ischemia?

    (A) T-wave inversion
    (B) ST-segment elevation
    (C) deep Q-wave
    (D) presence of a U-wave

84. Which of the following tests may assist the FNP to derive a diagnosis of diabetic mellitus (DM)?
    Select all that apply.

    (A) A1c equal to or greater than 6.5%
    (B) fasting blood glucose level equal to or greater than 126 mg/dL
    (C) a two-hour plasma glucose level equal to or greater than 200 mg/dL following a 75 g oral glucose tolerance test (OGTT)
    (D) a random blood glucose level greater than 200 mg/dL in a patient who presents with polyuria, polydipsia, polyphagia, and weight loss

85. Which of the following is the appropriate drug of choice for the management of urinary incontinence concurrent with benign prostatic hyperplasia (BPH)?

   (A) oxybutynin (Ditropan XL)
   (B) solifenacin (Vesicare)
   (C) tolterodine (Detrol LA)
   (D) doxazosin mesylate (Cardura)

86. An FNP should consider a diagnosis of urinary tract infection in an older adult with:

   (A) fever.
   (B) altered mental status.
   (C) nausea and vomiting.
   (D) abdominal pain.

87. Your adult patient has a chief complaint of malaise and fatigue. An in-office urinalysis reveals dark colored urine with a high level of bilirubin. Which of the following could contribute to these findings?

   (A) biliary obstruction
   (B) hepatic dysfunction
   (C) increased breakdown of RBCs
   (D) all of the above

88. A patient presents with a sudden onset of difficulty speaking, weakness of extremities, and unilateral hemiparesis. These symptoms suggest a diagnosis of:

   (A) hemorrhagic stroke.
   (B) embolic stroke.
   (C) transient ischemic attack.
   (D) Bell's palsy.

89. What is the current recommended daily intake of vitamin D for adults younger than 50?

   (A) 400–800 IU daily
   (B) 800–1,200 IU daily
   (C) 1,200–1,600 IU daily
   (D) 1,600–2,000 IU daily

90. When a baby receives immunity from measles, mumps, and rubella from the mother, this is called:

   (A) artificial passive immunity.
   (B) artificial active immunity.
   (C) natural passive immunity.
   (D) natural active immunity.

91. The chief complaint associated with pediculosis capitis is:

   (A) alopecia.
   (B) pain.
   (C) itching.
   (D) burning.

92. Which of the following is a symptom consistent with a diagnosis of gonorrhea?

    (A) lesion on the penis
    (B) fever
    (C) dysuria
    (D) fatigue

93. Your patient is a 24-year-old female who is in her second trimester of pregnancy. She reports that she has not been feeling well but denies specific complaints. You obtain a urine sample and the dipstick test is positive for bacteria. How should you treat this patient?

    (A) collect urine for culture and call the patient with results
    (B) advise her to increase water intake and report any dysuria
    (C) prescribe oral ciprofloxacin 500 mg PO TID × 3 days
    (D) prescribe oral nitrofurantoin 50 mg PO QID × 7 days

94. Which of the following may be a contributing factor to urinary tract infections in menopausal women?

    (A) the use of spermicidal agents
    (B) obesity
    (C) the use of hormone replacement therapy
    (D) atrophic vaginitis (AV)

95. For an older adult with a new diagnosis of depression, which class of medications is indicated as first-line therapy?

    (A) SSRIs
    (B) TCAs
    (C) MAOIs
    (D) SNRIs

96. Signs of acrocyanosis in a newborn include:

    (A) bluish color of the mucous membranes.
    (B) bluish color of the tongue.
    (C) bluish color of the torso.
    (D) bluish color of the hands and feet.

97. What immunizations are recommended for the 11-year-old well-child visit?

    (A) MMR, hep B, IPV
    (B) TDaP, HPV, MCV4
    (C) DTaP, MCV4, hep B
    (D) no vaccines

98. A patient with a diagnosis of Alzheimer's disease (AD) has increasing agitation and restlessness toward the end of each day. He becomes confused, disoriented, and irritable. This group of symptoms in this context is consistent with:

    (A) delirium.
    (B) sundowning.
    (C) infection.
    (D) polypharmacy.

99. An FNP is attending to a 98-year-old hospice patient who is in stage V non-small cell lung cancer (NSCLC). The patient has dyspnea, and generalized crackles are present. Current hospice medications are as follows: IV hydration 100 cc, furosemide 20 mg, spironolactone 100 mg. What should the FNP consider first?

    (A) reduce the IV fluids
    (B) refer the patient to the emergency department
    (C) refer the patient to a pulmonologist
    (D) increase the furosemide

100. How are malpractice cases determined?
     Select all that apply.

    (A) standard of care
    (B) expert witness
    (C) national guidelines
    (D) consensus opinion

101. To which of the following professional organizations' websites should an FNP refer for the ethical obligations of the profession?

    (A) American Nurses Association (ANA)
    (B) Nurse Practice Act (NPA)
    (C) American Association of Nurse Practitioners (AANP)
    (D) American Academy of Nurse Practitioners (AANP)

102. The purpose of the Agency for Healthcare Research and Quality (AHRQ) is to:

    (A) evaluate and promote cost-effective health care.
    (B) monitor national research studies and report on findings.
    (C) promote evidence-based practice.
    (D) write and disseminate clinical practice algorithms.

103. The FNP reviews four article summaries on four different drugs that may be helpful for her patients. Place the article summaries in sequential order of strength of evidence from *strongest to weakest*:

    (A) In a single trial, Drug A was significantly more effective than placebo in terms of reductions in HAM-D and GDS scores (both, $P < 0.001$).
    (B) In a randomized, multi-center, double-blind trial, Drug A was significantly more effective than a placebo in terms of reductions in HAM-D and GDS scores (both, $P < 0.001$).
    (C) In a randomized, single-center, single trial,, Drug A was significantly more effective than a placebo in terms of reductions in HAM-D and GDS scores (both, $P < 0.001$).
    (D) In a single center, convenience sampling, Drug A was significantly more effective than a placebo in terms of reductions in HAM-D and GDS scores (both, $P < 0.001$).

104. Which of the following databases could be used to find summarized results of evidence-based guidelines?

    (A) Cochrane Database of Systematic Reviews (CDSR)
    (B) National Guideline Clearinghouse (NGC)
    (C) Turning Research into Practice (TRIP)
    (D) Agency for Healthcare Research (AHRQ)

105. The most common pathogen responsible for symptoms of the common cold is:

(A) rhinovirus.

(B) adenovirus.

(C) ribovirus.

(D) parainfluenza virus.

106. A young adult presenting with fever, rhinorrhea, and a high-pitched, whooping cough has a possible diagnosis of:

(A) epiglottitis.

(B) bronchitis.

(C) pertussis.

(D) croup.

107. When monitoring the electrocardiography (ECG) of a patient, you notice a pattern of PR interval lengthening until a beat is dropped and then the pattern repeats. Which type of AV block does this suggest?

(A) first-degree AV block

(B) second-degree Mobitz I AV block

(C) second-degree Mobitz II AV block

(D) third-degree AV block

108. When FNPs use theory to shape their practice, they are:
Select all that apply.

(A) developing patterns of ideas to assist them in looking at their practice in an organized way.

(B) relying on models of practice developed by the theorist to assist them in defining their own work.

(C) learning to recognize their practice as part of larger whole.

(D) using these organizing frameworks to explore clinical questions and research phenomena.

109. A family nurse practitioner is reviewing the efficacy of a new drug in managing the reduction of blood pressure for one of her patients. The report states as follows:

"Following oral administration of Drug X, the onset of diuresis occurs in 15–30 minutes. Peak activity is reached between 1 and 2 hours. The diuretic action lasts for 8–10 hours."

Based on the statement, suppose that the patient takes the medication at 9:00 A.M. What would be the anticipated first need for a bathroom break?

(A) 9:15–10:00 A.M.

(B) 10:00–11:00 A.M.

(C) 5:00–7:00 P.M.

(D) 9:00 P.M.

110. APRN certification serves to:

(A) facilitate licensure.

(B) provide evidence of academic achievement.

(C) protect the public.

(D) document competence and specialty area.

111. According to HIPAA regulations, which of these scenarios does NOT represent a violation of patient privacy?

   (A) A co-worker calls your office to ask about a mutual acquaintance, who is your patient. You give the co-worker a brief synopsis of how the person is doing but do not go into details.

   (B) Your sister-in-law has been admitted to the hospital where you have privileges. She is not your patient; however, you access her medical record while at the hospital.

   (C) A patient's wife calls the office to ask how her husband is doing during his visit with you today. You place the wife on hold, ask the patient if it is okay for you to give her information, and he says "that's fine." You give the information to the wife.

   (D) The sign-in sheet for your clinic asks for patients' first and last names, as well as their birthdays.

112. A patient presenting with tremor at rest, rigidity, flexed posture, and bradykinesia may have a diagnosis of:

   (A) rheumatoid arthritis (RA).
   (B) Parkinson's disease (PD).
   (C) Alzheimer's disease (AD).
   (D) multiple sclerosis (MS).

113. An FNP is reviewing a genogram of a pregnant patient during the first trimester. The FNP notes that there is a diagonal cross drawn on top of the triangle. What does the symbol mean?

   (A) miscarriage
   (B) pregnancy
   (C) abortion
   (D) male stillbirth

114. Which of the following are elements of advance directives?
   Select all that apply.

   (A) living will
   (B) durable power of attorney
   (C) health care proxy
   (D) primary beneficiary on life insurance policy

115. Brain damage caused by Wernicke-Korsakoff dementia is because of:

   (A) thiamine deficiency.
   (B) hyperbilirubinemia.
   (C) alcohol toxicity.
   (D) vitamin C deficiency.

116. Your patient is a seven-year-old male with a diagnosis of pneumonia. He is febrile but not in distress. What is a first-line treatment recommendation for pneumonia in this otherwise healthy child?

(A) supportive measures only
(B) amoxicillin 80–90 mg/kg/day PO
(C) azithromycin PO
(D) doxycycline PO

117. Your patient is an 18-year-old female who is going to college. She is at least 15% under her ideal weight and reports dizziness and bradycardia when she stands up. She tells you she is doing well in her classes and drinks several cups of coffee daily. She usually drinks some alcohol every evening. Based on this information, what additional symptom/sign would you expect to see in this patient?

(A) amenorrhea
(B) migraine headaches
(C) hypothyroidism
(D) mitral regurgitation

118. One risk factor for endometrial cancer in women is high estrogenic states. These include all of the following, EXCEPT:

(A) metabolic syndrome.
(B) polycystic ovarian syndrome (PCOS).
(C) obesity.
(D) oral contraceptive use.

119. Your patient is a 30-year-old female who just learned that she is pregnant. Using Naegle's rule to calculate, what is her estimated date of delivery if her last menstrual period started on June 1, 2021?

(A) March 8, 2022
(B) April 8, 2022
(C) May 15, 2022
(D) June 15, 2022

120. Which of the following is NOT considered a basic right for individuals participating in human research studies?

(A) informed consent
(B) compensation
(C) withdrawal
(D) alternative therapy

121. Which of the following would NOT be considered part of a patient's "individually identifiable health information"?

(A) a list of patient diagnoses
(B) a list of patient medications
(C) a form containing the number of clinic vaccines given per year
(D) a record of patient PMH

122. What are the four essential elements regulating Advanced Practice Nursing practice?

    (A) education, licensure, accreditation, performance

    (B) licensure, education, accreditation, certification

    (C) prescriptive privileges, practice setting, collaborative requirements, practice autonomy

    (D) licensure, practice, collaboration, teams

123. Who should an FNP consult if she plans to conduct a quality improvement study in her clinic?

    (A) local city council

    (B) board of nursing

    (C) institutional review board (IRB)

    (D) better business bureau (BBB)

124. All the following patients meet the hospice criteria, EXCEPT:

    (A) a 23-year-old male who has a life expectancy of five months or less, without a will in place, and is documented with an official written hospice care order created by a physician.

    (B) a 63-year-old female who has a life expectancy of six months or less and is documented with an official written hospice care order created by a physician.

    (C) a 41-year-old male who has a life expectancy of two months or less and is documented with an official written hospice care order created by a physician.

    (D) a 56-year-old female who has a life expectancy of two months or less and is documented with an official written hospice care order created by an FNP.

125. A poorly defined, bluish-black macule, present at birth and present on the trunk and buttocks, is a:

    (A) blue nevus.

    (B) milia.

    (C) Koplik spot.

    (D) Mongolian spot.

126. At what age do the symptoms of bipolar disorder usually present?

    (A) during childhood

    (B) during adolescence

    (C) between 15 and 30 years old

    (D) in the third decade of life

127. Which of the following factors is NOT considered a risk factor in the development of sexually transmitted infections (STI)?

    (A) previous STI

    (B) age younger than 25

    (C) urinary tract infection

    (D) injection drug use

128. A mammogram in a healthy 50-year-old woman is an example of:

(A) primary prevention.

(B) secondary prevention.

(C) tertiary prevention.

(D) none of the above.

129. Vasomotor symptoms, such as hot flashes, are seen during the perimenopausal period and may persist into the menopausal years. Vasomotor symptoms occurring during this time are believed to result from:

(A) low prolactin levels.

(B) fluctuating estrogen levels.

(C) ovarian cyst formation.

(D) low progesterone levels.

130. A 51-year-old female complains of experiencing painful intercourse and vaginal pruritus. The FNP conducts a pelvic exam and notes atrophic changes in the vaginal vestibule and vaginal thinning. Vagina pH: 7.5, whiff test is positive, KOH test is negative. What is the diagnosis?

(A) candidiasis

(B) bacterial vaginosis

(C) trichomoniasis

(D) atrophic vaginitis

131. What must be included on the Medicare, Medicaid, or other insurance claim form for an out-patient visit?

(A) all pertinent diagnoses and level of care

(B) CPT and ICD-10 code

(C) CPT code

(D) ICD-10 code

132. An NP sees a 62-year-old patient suffering from lower extremity edema. The NP increases his diuretic dose but does not evaluate his potassium level during the visit. The same patient returns a week later for routine laboratory testing, and his potassium is found to be low. The NP immediately orders a potassium supplement and informs the patient that he will need to return to the clinic in two weeks to recheck his potassium level. Is the NP guilty of malpractice?

(A) Yes, because her action fell below the NP standard of care.

(B) No, because she resolved the issue by ordering the potassium supplement.

(C) No, because no harm presented to/from the client.

(D) Yes, because she was negligent.

133. What education is appropriate for the parent of a child with fifth disease (erythema infectiosum)?

(A) The rash is extremely pruritic.

(B) The child can return to school after the rash has disappeared.

(C) Avoid acetaminophen with this illness.

(D) The parent may experience joint symptoms and myalgias for several weeks.

134. During pregnancy, a woman may develop inflammation and hyperplasia of the gingiva. This is:

    (A) a common finding.
    (B) extensive periodontal disease.
    (C) evidence of poor nutritional status.
    (D) evidence of anemia.

135. The current age of natural menopause in the United States is:

    (A) 51 years.
    (B) 55 years.
    (C) 60 years.
    (D) 65 years.

136. An FNP's right to practice falls under the regulation of:

    (A) the board of medicine.
    (B) Medicare regulations and guidelines.
    (C) the board of nursing.
    (D) the American Nurses Association.

137. Who started the first nurse practitioner program?

    (A) Florence Nightingale
    (B) Margaret Sanger
    (C) Loretta Ford
    (D) Martha Rogers

138. Which test is most appropriate in evaluating a patient for a meniscal tear?

    (A) Lachman test
    (B) drawer test
    (C) bulge test
    (D) Apley's compression test

139. Your patient is a 60-year-old female who presents with a report of a fall yesterday. She tells you she tried to catch herself and landed on her left arm and wrist. On physical examination, there is tenderness of the "anatomical snuffbox," which may be an indication of:

    (A) a fracture of the radial head.
    (B) a fracture of the ulnar styloid.
    (C) a scaphoid fracture.
    (D) a hamate fracture.

140. A mother brings her five-year-old son into the clinic for evaluation. Her son fell from a swing set and hit his forehead. There was no loss of consciousness. A superficial minor laceration and ecchymosis is noted on the right side of the forehead. No changes with vision. Vital signs are stable. No diagnostic imaging is warranted for this visit. What should the FNP tell the parent?

Select all that apply.

(A) Make sure the child is moving his arms and legs normally.

(B) Wake the child every 2–4 hours for the first 24 hours after injury; the child should be able to wake easily and stay awake for a couple of minutes.

(C) You may use acetaminophen for headache or soft tissue pain.

(D) Trouble with walking is expected for the first 24 hours.

141. What is the role of the Advisory Committee on Immunization Practices (ACIP)?

(A) evaluate the current scientific evidence based on diseases related to immunization through vaccinations

(B) evaluate current scientific evidence focusing on clinical preventative health care services

(C) highlight 79 evidence-based disease and injury prevention programs that have saved lives and improved health

(D) protect the research participants' rights and safety

142. Which of the following refers to failure of a provider to adhere to current standards of practice?

(A) duty of care

(B) proximal cause

(C) injury

(D) breach of standard of care

143. An FNP refers a bedbound patient to hospice care services due to advanced stage IV small cell lung cancer (SCLC). The patient's daughter thinks that he has a very good chance of recovering and does not understand why the patient needs hospice services. The FNP explains to the daughter his poor diagnosis and the role of hospice in palliative care. The FNP's action is an example of:

(A) justice.

(B) confidentiality.

(C) fidelity.

(D) veracity.

144. A 14-year-old basketball player presents with a complaint of itchy and watery eyes occurring intermittently throughout his practice seasons. Exam reveals 20/40 vision bilaterally with corrective lenses, bilateral chemosis, a small amount of rope-like yellow discharge, and papillary hyperplasia. These findings are most consistent with:

(A) bacteria conjunctivitis.

(B) blepharitis.

(C) allergic conjunctivitis.

(D) hordeolum.

145. Which of the following classes of medications is contraindicated as monotherapy in the management of asthma?

    (A) short-acting bronchodilator
    (B) long-acting bronchodilator
    (C) inhaled steroid
    (D) oral steroid

146. A 45-year-old patient presents to the office with a blood sugar of 223 mg/dL. Which of the following is the appropriate intervention?

    (A) reschedule him to return tomorrow to recheck his glucose
    (B) start him on glucophage today
    (C) start him on insulin today
    (D) start him on glucophage and pioglitazone today

147. Your patient presents with palpitations, sweating, tremors, confusion, and hunger. These symptoms are most likely associated with:

    (A) syncope.
    (B) acute cardiac event.
    (C) hypoglycemia.
    (D) postural hypotension.

148. What is the diagnostic gold standard for chronic kidney disease (CKD)?

    (A) renal ultrasound
    (B) computed tomography scan
    (C) duplex doppler ultrasonography
    (D) renal angiography

149. A 25-year-old female presents with complaints of abdominal pain occurring after meals. She reports feeling constipated much of the time and takes laxatives, which are followed by a couple of days of diarrhea. She temporarily feels better after a bowel movement. She reports concern and embarrassment about persistent flatulence and abdominal distention but denies weight loss or blood in her stool. The problem has been ongoing for about six months. What should your next step be in the evaluation of this patient?

    (A) obtain a complete history
    (B) order a barium enema
    (C) prescribe a trial of antispasmodics
    (D) order a CT of the abdomen

150. Under the tumor-node-metastasis (TNM) classification, what does the T2 represent within the context of colorectal cancer?

    (A) The tumor has spread to other organs.
    (B) The tumor invades the submucosa.
    (C) The tumor is spreading to the muscularis.
    (D) The tumor has penetrated through the bowel wall.

151. A patient presents with a chief complaint of gradual onset and progression of numbness and tingling of the thumb, index, and middle finger. Pain and numbness often occur at night and wake the patient from sleep. The patient works as a computer programmer. Based on this presentation, you suspect carpal tunnel syndrome (CTS). You ask the patient to flex both hands to 90 degrees and press the backs of the hands together for 60 seconds. This test is called the:

   (A) Phalen's test.
   (B) Tinel's test.
   (C) Weber test.
   (D) Rinne test.

152. Which of the following statements accurately describes the difference between ulcerative colitis disease and Crohn's disease?

   (A) With ulcerative colitis, the affected area usually presents from the distal to proximal area of the colon. In Crohn's disease, the affected area more commonly presents in a segmental part of the colon with skipped areas.
   (B) Ulcerative colitis causes weight loss, but Crohn's disease does not.
   (C) For ulcerative colitis, an endoscopy report may report noncaseating granulomas located in the inflamed mucosa. However, superficial inflammation of mucosa can be noted with Crohn's disease.
   (D) Ulcerative colitis patients are more prone to uveitis, iritis, and conjunctivitis. Crohn's disease patients are more prone to primary sclerosing cholangitis.

153. Which of the following is considered a risk factor for ectopic pregnancy?

   (A) multiple gestation
   (B) age > 35 years
   (C) obesity
   (D) sexually transmitted infection

154. A 27-year-old female complains of burning sensation during urination. The FNP performs a pelvic exam and notes a homogeneous, thin, grayish-white discharge coating the vaginal walls. Vaginal pH: 5, whiff test is positive, KOH test is positive, clue cells present in the saline microscopy. What is the diagnosis?

   (A) candidiasis
   (B) bacterial vaginosis
   (C) trichomoniasis
   (D) atrophic vaginitis

155. The clinical difference between minor depression and major depressive disorder (MDD) is:

   (A) how long symptoms have lasted.
   (B) the number of symptoms present.
   (C) the presence of suicidal thoughts.
   (D) the severity of symptoms.

156. A common, benign finding seen frequently in young infants is white papules on the gum line that may resemble a tooth. These lesions are called:

   (A) milia.
   (B) Epstein's pearls.
   (C) leukoplakia.
   (D) none of the above.

157. Which immunizations are recommended for the four-to-six-year well-child visit in a child who is up to date on vaccinations?

   (A) DTaP, IPV, MMR, varicella
   (B) TDaP, MMRV
   (C) IPV, Hib, rotavirus
   (D) hepatitis B

158. A patient reporting a gradual, painless, progressive loss of vision, glare at night, and photophobia should be evaluated for:

   (A) glaucoma.
   (B) cataracts.
   (C) macular degeneration.
   (D) retinopathy.

159. The most common causative organism responsible for otitis externa infections associated with swimming is:

   (A) *Moraxella catarrhalis.*
   (B) *Pseudomonas aeruginosa.*
   (C) *S. pneumoniae.*
   (D) *H. influenzae.*

160. There are four stages in rapid eye movement (REM) sleep. Rearrange the following statements to represent stage 1, stage 2, stage 3, and stage 4 for the REM sleep pattern. Select all that apply.

   (A) This stage involves slowing of the eye movements, preceding sleep onset.
   (B) This stage is manifested by low-frequency delta waves with occasional sleep spindles but no slow eye movements.
   (C) This stage involves further slowing the EEG, presence of sleep spindles, and slow eye movements.
   (D) High-voltage delta waves are presented in this stage.

161. A patient presenting with bilateral itching, tearing eyes with a moderate amount of mucopurulent drainage without vision changes or pain most likely has:

   (A) viral conjunctivitis.
   (B) bacterial conjunctivitis.
   (C) allergic conjunctivitis.
   (D) none of the above.

162. A 28-year-old female presents to the clinic with a complaint of urination frequency. The patient has a family history of diabetes mellitus. She read an article on the internet and requests the FNP order an oral glucose tolerance test (OGTT). What should the FNP do next?

   (A) Order the OGTT.
   (B) Order a fasting plasma glucose (FPG) test.
   (C) Order a hemoglobin A1c test.
   (D) Assess the patient for any other symptoms/signs of diabetes mellitus.

163. An FNP (NP) orders a hemoglobin A1c for a patient on March 15. The A1c is 8.5% and the patient is started on monotherapy. When should the NP follow up to evaluate progress and recheck labs?

   (A) April 15
   (B) May 15
   (C) June 15
   (D) March 30

164. Which of the following factors is the most common cause of Cushing's syndrome?

   (A) adrenal insufficiency
   (B) pituitary adenoma
   (C) autoimmune disease
   (D) exogenous corticosteroid use

165. John presents with his 78-year-old father with concerns about episodes of enuresis (in the father) over the past three days. The patient lives in a long-term care nursing home and is unable to communicate. His vitals are within normal range. Focused exam is unremarkable. What should the FNP do next?

   (A) refer patient to neurologist
   (B) send patient's urine for culture
   (C) report for possible elderly abuse
   (D) order a complete metabolic panel (CMP)

166. Which of the following statements is correct about irritable bowel syndrome (IBS)?

   (A) IBS is a nonfunctional gastrointestinal disorder.
   (B) IBS is characterized by abdominal pain with constipation.
   (C) IBS is characterized by change in the frequency and appearance of the stool.
   (D) IBS is an emergency condition and requires IV antibiotics.

167. The principal goal for life-long treatment of Parkinson's disease (PD) is:

   (A) to prevent the progression of the disease.
   (B) to prevent behavioral changes.
   (C) to help the patient function independently for as long as possible.
   (D) to reverse and improve myelination of the neurons.

168. Confirmation test for de Quervain's tenosynovitis is:

    (A) Allen's test.
    (B) Phalen's maneuver.
    (C) Finkelstein's test.
    (D) Tinel's sign.

169. Your patient has a diagnosis of vitamin B12 deficiency. In addition to exogenous vitamin B12, all of the foods below are high in this vitamin, EXCEPT:

    (A) animal kidney and liver.
    (B) clams.
    (C) oatmeal.
    (D) fortified cereal.

170. An adult male with a chief complaint of dysuria without frequency or urgency may have a diagnosis of:

    (A) acute prostatitis.
    (B) constipation.
    (C) cystitis.
    (D) urethritis.

171. Preeclampsia is a pregnancy complication that occurs more often in primigravida women. The goal of management is to prevent development of eclampsia, which has a high mortality rate. The classic triad of symptoms associated with preeclampsia is hypertension, edema, and:

    (A) elevated blood sugar.
    (B) altered mental status.
    (C) seizures.
    (D) proteinuria.

172. Which medication listed below has the longest half-life and may be appropriate for a patient who is likely to skip doses?

    (A) citalopram
    (B) fluoxetine
    (C) bupropion
    (D) escitalopram

173. Newborns may lose up to 7% of their birth weight within the first week; however, they should return to birth weight by:

    (A) two weeks.
    (B) four weeks.
    (C) six weeks.
    (D) eight weeks.

174. The top three leading causes of death in adults over age 65 include heart disease, cancer, and:

    (A) suicide.
    (B) stroke.
    (C) COPD.
    (D) pneumonia.

175. The FNP shared one of her patient encounters with a group of nursing students. She described the patient as "the old fart coming in without a walking cane." The FNP is exhibiting:

    (A) HIPAA violation.
    (B) justice.
    (C) gender bias and ageism.
    (D) veracity.

ANSWER KEY
Practice Test 1

ANCC-Style

1. **(A)**	36. **(A, B)**	71. **(A)**	106. **(C)**	141. **(A)**
2. **(B)**	37. **(B)**	72. **(B)**	107. **(B)**	142. **(D)**
3. **(D)**	38. **(A, B)**	73. **(B)**	108. **(A, B, C, D)**	143. **(D)**
4. **(D)**	39. **(A)**	74. **(A)**	109. **(A)**	144. **(C)**
5. **(B, C)**	40. **(D)**	75. **(C)**	110. **(D)**	145. **(B)**
6. **(D)**	41. **(C)**	76. **(A)**	111. **(C)**	146. **(C)**
7. **(A, A, B, A, B)**	42. **(B)**	77. **(D)**	112. **(B)**	147. **(C)**
8. **(C)**	43. **(B)**	78. **(D)**	113. **(A)**	148. **(D)**
9. **(B)**	44. **(C)**	79. **(D)**	114. **(A, B, C)**	149. **(A)**
10. **(B)**	45. **(C)**	80. **(A)**	115. **(A)**	150. **(C)**
11. **(C)**	46. **(A)**	81. **(B)**	116. **(C)**	151. **(A)**
12. **(C)**	47. **(C)**	82. **(C)**	117. **(A)**	152. **(A)**
13. **(D)**	48. **(B)**	83. **(A)**	118. **(D)**	153. **(B)**
14. **(D)**	49. **(C, D)**	84. **(A, B, C, D)**	119. **(A)**	154. **(B)**
15. **(A)**	50. **(B)**	85. **(D)**	120. **(B)**	155. **(B)**
16. **(A)**	51. **(C)**	86. **(B)**	121. **(C)**	156. **(B)**
17. **(A)**	52. **(D)**	87. **(D)**	122. **(B)**	157. **(A)**
18. **(A)**	53. **(D)**	88. **(B)**	123. **(C)**	158. **(B)**
19. **(C)**	54. **(C)**	89. **(A)**	124. **(D)**	159. **(B)**
20. **(C)**	55. **(C)**	90. **(C)**	125. **(D)**	160. **(A, C, B, D)**
21. **(D)**	56. **(C)**	91. **(C)**	126. **(C)**	161. **(B)**
22. **(A)**	57. **(A, B, D)**	92. **(C)**	127. **(C)**	162. **(D)**
23. **(A)**	58. **(A)**	93. **(D)**	128. **(B)**	163. **(C)**
24. **(B)**	59. **(C)**	94. **(D)**	129. **(B)**	164. **(D)**
25. **(B)**	60. **(C)**	95. **(A)**	130. **(D)**	165. **(B)**
26. **(B)**	61. **(C)**	96. **(D)**	131. **(B)**	166. **(C)**
27. **(D)**	62. **(D)**	97. **(B)**	132. **(C)**	167. **(C)**
28. **(C)**	63. **(A)**	98. **(B)**	133. **(D)**	168. **(C)**
29. **(D)**	64. **(D, A, B, C)**	99. **(A)**	134. **(A)**	169. **(C)**
30. **(B)**	65. **(B)**	100. **(A, B, C, D)**	135. **(A)**	170. **(D)**
31. **(D)**	66. **(B)**	101. **(A)**	136. **(C)**	171. **(D)**
32. **(B)**	67. **(C)**	102. **(C)**	137. **(C)**	172. **(B)**
33. **(D)**	68. **(B)**	103. **(B, C, A, D)**	138. **(D)**	173. **(A)**
34. **(B, C)**	69. **(B)**	104. **(C)**	139. **(C)**	174. **(C)**
35. **(D)**	70. **(B)**	105. **(A)**	140. **(A, B, C)**	175. **(C)**

Answer Explanations

1. **(A)** The patient should be re-treated with different types of antibiotics. In this scenario, the FNP should initiate amoxicillin/clavulanate (Augmentin) and OTC acetaminophen to reduce the pain and fever. The clavulanate component of the antibiotic is effective against pathogens that produce beta-lactam; therefore, it provides broader microbial coverage. Actions that do not include all three of these components (choices (B), (C), and (D)) are not sufficient on their own.

2. **(B)** Infectious mononucleosis is commonly caused by Epstein-Barr virus. Cytomegalovirus (choice (A)) is a possible cause, but it is less commonly seen in infectious mononucleosis. The influenza virus (choice (C)) causes influenza, and varicella zoster virus (choice (D)) causes chicken pox.

3. **(D)** Exercise-induced asthma is an outdated term that suggests exercise causes asthma. Exercise-induced bronchoconstriction (EIB) should be used instead. Sports or activities that use short bursts of exercise are best for people with EIB. Examples include volleyball, baseball, gymnastics, walking, or leisure biking. Swimming in a warm, humid environment is an option too. Sports or activities that will trigger exercise-induced bronchoconstriction include any activity in a cold environment—such as ice hockey (choice (A)), ice skating, snowboarding (choice (B)), and skiing—or any activity that requires constant exertion, such as long distance running (choice (C)) and soccer.

4. **(D)** Supplemental oxygen used for at least 15–18 hours per day has been shown to improve symptoms and quality of life for individuals with COPD.

5. **(B, C)** Per JNC 8 guidelines, in patients 18 years and older with chronic kidney disease and hypertension, the initial or add-on treatment should include an angiotensin-converting enzyme (ACE) inhibitor or an angiotensin receptor blocker (ARB) to improve kidney outcome. The recommendation applies regardless of diabetes or ethnic background.

6. **(D)** A patient who presents with a positive Trousseau's sign or Chvostek's sign accompanied by respiratory distress (stridor, cyanosis) requires immediate referral to the emergency department. Symptoms may be due to the possibility of hyperactivity of the neuromuscular system (from hypocalcemia), which could trigger laryngospasm, seizures, and dysrhythmias. T3, T4, and TSH tests (choice (A)); a 25-hydroxycholecalciferol assay (choice (B)); and an electrocardiography (choice (C)) are appropriate in order to evaluate thyroid function. Emergency treatment of hypocalcemia is IV replacement of calcium.

7. **(A, A, B, A, B)** Growth hormone, estrogen, and corticosteroids stimulate *ductal* growth in the breasts. Progesterone and prolactin stimulate *alveolar lobular* growth of the breasts.

8. **(C)** The major differential diagnoses of weight gain include hypothyroidism, Cushing's syndrome (choice (A)), renal or hepatic disease, premenstrual syndrome (choice (B)), depression (choice (D)), medication, excessive caloric intake, pregnancy, and chronic heart disease, making choices (A), (B), and (D) true and therefore incorrect. Graves' disease, also known as toxic diffuse goiter, is an autoimmune disease that triggers hyperthyroidism. One example of the symptoms associated with Graves' disease is weight loss (despite normal eating habits), making choice (C) false and therefore the correct answer.

9. **(B)** Metformin (Glucophage) is a biguanide agent that decreases hepatic production of glucose and increases peripheral tissue use of glucose. This medication does not stimulate the pancreas to make more insulin. The American Diabetic Association recommends metformin

as first-line therapy for patients with T2DM. This medication should not be used in patients with decreased renal function (those with an elevated serum creatinine or decreased creatinine clearance). Metformin may cause lactic acidosis (choice (B)), so it should not be used in patients with liver disease, alcoholics, or patients with cardiopulmonary insufficiency. The risk for lactic acidosis is increased with the use of contrast dyes for imaging as well as with surgery (which also decreases renal function); therefore, the medication must be discontinued prior to and for some time after these procedures. The most common side effects of metformin are nausea and vomiting (choice (A)); however, these symptoms usually resolve with slow dose titration. Because of the mechanism of action, metformin does not cause hypoglycemia (choice (C)).

10. **(B)** The term used to describe an enlarged thyroid gland is goiter. With a physical finding of goiter, thyroid gland function may be normal, increased, or decreased. Exophthalmos (choice (A)) is a term used to indicate an abnormal protrusion of the eyes (bilateral) seen with thyroid disease. This condition may not be reversible with disease management. Acromegaly (choice (C)) is a condition characterized by bone overgrowth. Organomegaly (choice (D)) is a general term used to indicate organ enlargement.

11. **(C)** The drug pioglitazone lowers glucose levels by decreasing insulin resistance and liver production of glucose. Patients taking pioglitazone should have liver function testing when the medication is prescribed and periodically thereafter, as there is a risk for liver dysfunction in patients taking this medication.

12. **(C)** There are no recommendations involving the screening and management of asymptomatic bacteriuria among men and women, except for pregnant women (choice (D)), who should be treated. If left untreated in a pregnant woman, bacteria have a strong propensity to develop into a systemic urinary tract infection, including pyelonephritis, which is a serious illness in this population.

13. **(D)** Ampicillin, nitrofurantoin, and cephalexin are appropriate treatments for a urinary tract infection and are safe to use during pregnancy, making choices (A), (B), and (C) true. Tetracycline is a category D drug, which means that this drug will cause harmful effects to the human fetus or neonate. This drug should not be used during pregnancy, making choice (D) false and therefore the correct answer.

14. **(D)** Third National Health and Nutrition Examination Survey defined the five stages of chronic kidney disease. Stage 1 is persistent albuminuria with a normal GFR > 90 mL/min, making choice (A) incorrect. Stage 2 is persistent albuminuria with a GFR 60–89 mL/min, making choice (B) incorrect. Stage 3 is GFR 30–59 mL/min, making choice (C) incorrect. Stage 4 is GFR 15–29 mL/min, making choice (D) the correct answer. Stage 5 is GFR < 15 mL/min.

15. **(A)** CVA tenderness is a characteristic finding in pyelonephritis and is associated with visceral irritation and organ sensitivity in the setting of an upper urinary tract infection. Dysuria (choice (B)) is not associated with pyelonephritis unless there is a concomitant cystitis present. A positive Murphy's sign (choice (C)) is usually seen in patients with acute cholecystitis. Intermittent abdominal pain (choice (D)) could be due to early appendicitis, inflammatory bowel disease, or gastroenteritis, among others.

16. **(A)** The lab report confirms a diagnosis of acute hepatitis B, as shown in the first row of the chart that follows. Review the rest of the chart for explanation of why choices (B), (C), and (D) are incorrect.

HBsAg	Anti-HBs	HBeAg	Anti-HBe	Anti-HBc	Interpretation
(+)	(−)	(+)	(−)	(IgM)	Confirms diagnosis of acute hepatitis B
(−)	(−)	(+) or (−)	(−)	(IgM)	Acute hepatitis B
(−)	(+)	(−)	(+) or (−)	(IgG)	Body developed immunity or recovery from hepatitis B infection (choice (B))
(−)	(+)	(−)	(−)	(IgG)	Body developed immunity via vaccination
(+)	(−)	(+)	(−)	(IgG)	Chronic hepatitis B infection with high viral replication (high risk for transmission) (choice (C))
(−)	(−)	(−)	(+)	(IgG)	Chronic hepatitis B infection with low viral replication activity (low risk for transmission) (choice (D))

17. **(A)** Intussusception most commonly occurs in infants between 5 and 10 months old. The physical examination may show glassy eyes, lethargy, sleepiness, and a sausage-like mass palpated within the right upper quadrant region with emptiness (retraction in the area of the right iliac fossa, commonly known as Dance sign). The abdomen is usually distended and tender to palpation. Jelly-colored stools may be seen as well. This is an emergency, and the FNP should refer the patient to the emergency department as soon as possible.

18. **(A)** Dementia presents slowly over months or years. It may last months to years and is caused by neurologic disease (Alzheimer's, Parkinson's), trauma, or infections. There is no subjective data to support the diagnosis of depression (choice (B)) or stroke (choice (D)). Delirium (choice (C)), or acute delusional state, has an abrupt onset over a short period, with confusion fluctuations throughout the day, and could be caused by an acute medical condition, polypharmacy, or abrupt withdrawal of a medication.

19. **(C)** The FNP should use the Mini-Mental State Exam, which is the most widely used tool to assess dementia via cognitive function evaluation. The Delirium Rating Scale (choice (A)) assesses a range of symptoms associated with delirium and is useful in distinguishing delirium from other disorders. The Confusion Assessment Method (choice (B)), a screening tool for delirium, is quick and easy to use and provides data relevant to bedside care. The PHQ 9 (choice (D)) is a screening tool for major depressive disorder.

20. **(C)** Cluster headaches are excruciatingly painful headaches that occur in "clusters" over weeks or months. Some patients become suicidal due to the unrelenting pain. A primary treatment measure is administration of 100% oxygen at 12 L/min via mask, along with 4% lidocaine given intranasally. This treatment may lead to spontaneous remission of symptoms.

21. **(D)** An alternate name for osteoarthritis is degenerative joint disease. The most common symptom of osteoarthritis is joint pain. The pain tends to worsen with activities, making

choice (A) true, and usually affects asymmetrical joints, making choice (B) true. Commonly affected joints include the hands, knees, hips, and spine, making choice (C) true as well. Patients with osteoarthritis usually have morning stiffness with symptoms lasting less than 30 minutes, making choice (D) false and therefore the correct answer.

22. **(A)** There are 18 "tender points" for the diagnosis of fibromyalgia. To diagnose a patient with fibromyalgia, the patient needs to report tenderness in a minimum of 11 out of the 18 tender points.

Front	Back
Neck (under the lower sternomastoid muscle)	Head (insertion of the suboccipital muscle)
Chest (near the second costochondral junction)	Shoulders (mid upper trapezius muscle, choice (C))
Elbow (distal to the lateral epicondyle, choice (B))	Mid upper back (origin of the supraspinatus muscle)
Waist (at the prominence of the greater trochanter)	Hip (upper outer quadrant of the buttock, choice (D))
Knee (at the medial fat pad of the knee)	

23. **(A)** Epicondylitis is an inflammation of the epicondyle due to repetitive movement and/or overuse. Tennis elbow is the inflammation of the *lateral* side of epicondylitis. Golfer's elbow is the inflammation of the *medial* epicondylitis. Osteochondritis dissecans (choice (B)) is a joint disorder, which usually reveals cracking sounds, effusions, and tenderness with joint movement. Typical locations are the knee (75%), elbow (6%), ankle (4%), and other joints (15%). There is no evidence to support the diagnosis of radial head subluxation (nursemaid's elbow) (choice (C)) or carpal tunnel syndrome (choice (D)).

24. **(B)** Anti-CCP antibodies are primarily specific for a certain type of protein seen with rheumatoid arthritis. Presence of these antibodies is useful in recognizing early RA. Although used for detection, anti-CCP antibodies do not play a major role in joint destruction as does RF. Historically, the serum RF titer (choice (A)) was used in the early recognition of RA. Currently, the titer level, if present, does correspond to disease severity; however, RF is also found in patients with scleroderma, SLE, and viral infections, thus is not particularly specific for RA. TNF-alpha (choice (C)) is a central cytokine responsive for triggering synovial proliferation with RA, and therapies targeting this cytokine are proving effective in slowing disease progression. ANA (choice (D)) is a useful marker for some autoimmune disorders and is consistently found in SLE, thus assisting in differentiating SLE from RA.

25. **(B)** The low MCV prompts further testing of TIBC, ferritin, and serum iron levels. If these tests are within normal limits, the patient probably has thalassemia trait.

26. **(B)** Cryptosporidium is the most common cause of massive diarrheal illness in patients with HIV. This organism attacks the small intestine, producing large amounts of diarrhea, sometimes more than 4 L/day. Patients also report nausea and extreme fatigue. Toxoplasmosis infection (choice (A)) is very common in patients with HIV. Presenting symptoms include headache, seizures, altered mental status, and focal neurologic deficits. Progressive multifocal leukoencephalopathy (choice (C)) is a viral infection affecting the white matter of the brain and is seen in patients with advanced disease. This infection results in focal deficits such as aphasia, cortical blindness, and hemiparesis. Cryptococcal meningitis (choice (D)) presents with fever and headache.

27. **(D)** Chronic renal failure produces xerosis (dry skin), pruritus, pallor, hyperpigmentation, and uremic frost. Because the kidneys are unable to clear toxins well, waste products accumulate on the skin. Poorly controlled diabetes mellitus (choice (A)) causes poor wound healing and peripheral neuropathy. Hyperthyroidism (choice (B)) causes the skin to be smooth, velvety in texture, and warm to the touch. Hepatic dysfunction and disease (choice (C)) may cause jaundice, ascites, bleeding, and peripheral edema.

28. **(C)** The chief complaint associated with pediculosis capitis is itching. Pediculosis is also known as louse infestation. During the infestation, the body releases histamine which results in an itching sensation. Alopecia is the loss of one's hair. Pain and burning symptoms are not part of the chief complaint for pediculosis capitis.

29. **(D)** A varicocele occurs when blood backs up in the main veins that drain the scrotum. No treatment is indicated. However, some studies have reported the association between varicocele and infertility. Hydrocele is fluid build-up around the testicle(s).

30. **(B)** Acyclovir is the current medication used to treat herpes simplex virus. However, the dosage varies based on the acuity of the infections (primary, recurrent, and suppression treatment). Abacavir (choice (A)), raltegravir (choice (C)), and darunavir (choice (D)) are antiretroviral medications used to prevent and treat HIV/AIDS.

31. **(D)** A distinct hard nodule altering the contour of the gland is suggestive of carcinoma of the prostate. As the cancer grows, the gland begins to feel irregular throughout and may extend beyond the prostate. The normal prostate gland (choice (A)) is a rounded, heart-shaped organ that is somewhat rubbery in texture and should be nontender. During acute bacterial prostatitis (choice (B)), the gland feels boggy, tender, and swollen. Benign prostatic hyperplasia (choice (C)) presents as a markedly enlarged gland and is present in more than 50% of men by age 50.

32. **(B)** Chronic prostatitis is a condition of long-term prostate irritation. It may occur following an episode of acute prostatitis. Chronic pelvic pain that originates from the prostate and urethral irritation after voiding are usually seen. Epididymitis (choice (A)) is an acute infection of the epididymis that causes unilateral pain and swelling. Bladder cancer (choice (C)) most often presents as painless hematuria. Asymptomatic bacteriuria (choice (D)) would, by definition, produce no symptoms (and the urinalysis would reveal bacteria).

33. **(D)** Research indicates that neural tube deficiency can be prevented with appropriate folic acid intake during pregnancy. The American College of Obstetricians and Gynecologists (ACOG) and the March of Dimes recommend 400 mcg per day for all healthy pregnant women. Additional folic acid dosage (choices (A), (B), and (C)) may be required for at-risk patients.

34. **(B, C)** Amenorrhea is the absence of menses. Normally, menarche (the onset of menses) occurs between the ages of 11 and 15. Primary amenorrhea is defined as no menses by age 14 in girls who have not developed any secondary sexual characteristics (breast buds) or by age 16 in girls who may or may not have developed secondary sexual characteristics.

35. **(D)** The FNP should document the GTPAL as G: 2, T: 1, P: 0, A: 0, L: 1, because the patient has not yet delivered her second baby. GTPAL is an acronym commonly documented in a woman's obstetrical health history. FNPs need to be comfortable interpreting the acronym. **G:** gravidity, or the number of pregnancies conceived. For example, the gravidity of a woman with three pregnancies would be G: 3. A nulligravida is someone that has never been pregnant (G: 0). **T:** the number of full-term infants. **P:** the number of preterm infants. **A:** the number of abortions. **L:** the number of living children delivered.

36. **(A, B)** The male-to-female patient is on HRT; however, she has not had gender confirmation surgery. Thus, she still has male sexual anatomy, not female sexual anatomy; therefore, there is no need to initiate a pap test (choice (D)). The patient needs a PSA screening and a breast examination.

37. **(B)** Bupropion is an SNRI that is used in the treatment of major depressive and other mood disorders. This agent should not be used in patients with bulimia nervosa because of the risk of increasing binging behavior and inducing seizures.

38. **(A, B)** Health care providers are one of the groups that are required by law to report suspected or known child abuse to authorities. The FNP should accurately document his or her findings (choice (A)) as well as the fact that a report was filed (choice (B)).

39. **(A)** Opioid intoxication may cause euphoria, constricted pupils, drowsiness, slurred speech, and impaired judgment. These symptoms indicate central nervous system (CNS) depression. Barbiturates, alcohol, and benzodiazepines (choice (B)) are all CNS depressants. Marijuana intoxication (choice (C)) produces relaxation, euphoria, detachment, slowed perception of time, and talkativeness. Amphetamines (choice (D)) are CNS stimulants and produce symptoms such as ataxia, seizures, respiratory distress, coma, or death.

40. **(D)** The pneumococcal conjugate vaccine (PCV 13) protects children from the most common strains of *S. pneumoniae*. It has dramatically reduced the incidence of primary and recurrent cases of acute otitis media. The pathogenesis of AOM has now shifted toward more cases of *H. influenzae*, which is less likely to become resistant to antibiotics than *S. pneumoniae*.

41. **(C)** Medicare Part A and Part B (choices (A) and (B)) do not cover the shingles vaccination. Medicare Part C, also known as the Medicare Advantage Program, will cover the shingles vaccination. Beneficiaries may enroll in private health plans and have the same access to the Medicare health benefits, in addition to Medicare Part D, prescription drug coverage. Examples of these plans include health maintenance organization (HMOs), preferred provider organizations (PPOs), provider-sponsored organizations (PSOs), and private fee-for-service (PFFS) plans.

42. **(B)** A state board of nursing is responsible for ensuring public safety by requiring all advanced practice nurses to meet minimum requirement qualifications. The board of nursing has no role in the evaluation of the outcome of the family nurse practitioner certification exam (choice (A)). The board of nursing does not set universal requirements (choice (C)); rather, every state sets their own requirements. The board of nursing is not responsible for ensuring the job satisfaction outcomes for advanced practice nurses (choice (D)).

43. **(B)** Transformational nursing leaders are able to effectively share their vision with peers and staff members. This type of leader is often charismatic, a good communicator, and someone who promotes higher job satisfaction. Situational leadership (choice (A)) involves flexibility on the part of the leader to continue to adjust to organizational needs. This type of leadership fosters rapport and strong relationships with improved teamwork and job satisfaction. Authoritarian leaders (choice (C)) like structure and control and are comfortable giving directions to others. These leaders often have a lot of rules and desire minimal staff input in decisions. This type of leader is often motivated, independent, and self-directed. Staff may not enjoy working in this type of environment. Democratic leaders (choice (D)) value frequent staff input into decisions and goals. Teams share in decision-making and the leader values work relationships.

44. **(C)** For established patients, the common service codes are 99212 (10 minutes), 99213 (15 minutes) (choice (B)), 99214 (25 minutes) (choice (D)), and 99215 (40 minutes). In this scenario, the FNP does not need additional workup. Evaluation of the left ear shows no sign of infection, and the patient has no new symptoms. Thus, 99212 is the appropriate choice.

45. **(C)** A researcher reviewing de-identified data is an example of the collection of secondary data, as there is no mechanism to verify the accuracy of the presented data. Other options (choices (A), (B), and (D)) are primary data, as they come directly from the actual source. Primary data is usually verifiable.

46. **(A)** The first-line therapy for acute bacterial sinusitis in patients who are penicillin-allergic or cephalosporin-allergic is trimethoprim/sulfamethoxazole or a quinolone drug. Amoxicillin/clavulanate (choice (B)) and amoxicillin (choice (C)) are not correct because the patient has a penicillin allergy. Clarithromycin (choice (D)) is appropriate for treating anaerobic organisms such as *Peptostreptococcus* and *Bacteroides*.

47. **(C)** These are classic signs of acute angle-closure glaucoma that require immediate urgent referral to ophthalmology. The patient presents as ill-appearing, with onset of vision changes, nausea and vomiting, elevated blood pressure, and a fixed pupil (nonreactive to light). Retinal detachment (choice (A)) may cause changes in vision; however, the pupils should be able to respond to light. Patients with retinal detachment report a "curtain" coming down in one eye. Patients with cataracts (choice (B)) may complain of night vision problems (unable to drive at night), sensitivity to sunlight, seeing halos or double vision, and cloudy lenses. Conjunctivitis (choice (D)) is also known as pink eye and does not cause pain, onset of elevated blood pressure, or vision changes.

48. **(B)** The Weber test is performed by placing a vibrating tuning fork in the midline of the skull. With normal hearing, the sound is heard equally in both ears. With sensorineural hearing loss, the sound in the unaffected ear is louder. The opposite is true with conductive hearing loss (choice (A)); sound in the affected ear is louder.

49. **(C, D)** Tuberculin skin testing (TST) must be read 72 hours after the intradermal test is placed. Since the operating business days are from Monday to Thursday, the patient may only receive the tuberculin skin testing services on Monday and Tuesday. Patients receiving the tuberculin skin test on Wednesday and Thursday will not be able to have the test interpreted within the appropriate time frame and will need to have it redone.

50. **(B)** One daily controller medication. There are four classifications of asthma severity. **Mild intermittent:** Intermittent reliever medication taken as needed (choice (A)): inhaled short acting beta-2-agonist or cromolyn before exercise or allergen exposure. **Mild persistent:** One daily controller medication: low dose inhaled corticosteroids; cromolyn/nedocromil; leukotriene modifiers. **Moderate persistent:** Daily controller medications: *combination* inhaled medium-dose corticosteroids (choice (C)) and long-acting bronchodilator; cromolyn/nedocromil; leukotriene modifiers. **Severe persistent:** Multiple daily controller medications: *high*-dose inhaled corticosteroids (choice (D)) and long-acting bronchodilator; cromolyn/nedocromil; leukotriene modifiers; inhaled beta-2 agonists as needed.

51. **(C)** A patient with dilated cardiomyopathy will likely demonstrate jugular venous distention (choice (A)), right upper quadrant abdominal tenderness (choice (B)), and peripheral edema (choice (D)). An FNP would not expect to find a point of maximal impulse at the fifth intercostal space midclavicular line on the left. This is a normal finding. With dilated cardiomyopathy, the PMI may be shifted to the right.

52. **(D)** An optimal level of HDL is greater than 60 mg/dL. This level is considered to be a cardio protective factor because HDL is excreted from the body instead of deposited on arterial walls. HDL removes excess cholesterol from the vasculature and returns it to the liver to be excreted through the intestines.

53. **(D)** A decrease in the glomerular filtration rate may be seen prior to any physical symptoms and is a good reflection of renal function. The urinalysis (choice (A)) may demonstrate proteinuria; however, the GFR is a better measurement of function. Because renal cells (the nephrons) have the ability to adapt to declining function (for a time), the patient's serum creatinine level (choice (B)) may remain normal. Urine quantity (choice (C)) is not a helpful measure of renal function.

54. **(C)** Individuals with a bladder tumor are usually asymptomatic until late in the disease, at which time painless hematuria may be noted. This hematuria varies from microscopic amounts of blood to gross bleeding. Other presenting symptoms include weight loss (choice (A)), uremia (choice (B)), dysuria, urinary frequency, lower abdominal pain, and low-grade fever (choice (D)).

55. **(C)** Positive anti-HBs indicated immune due to hepatitis B vaccination. Positive HBsAg, positive anti-HBc, and positive IgM anti-HBc indicate a current acute hepatitis B infection

HBsAg: (choice (A))	Detection of the hepatitis B surface antigen
	Positive of HBsAg confirms acute hepatitis B
Anti-HBs: (choice (C))	Detection of antibody to the hepatitis B surface antigen
HBeAg:	An antigen of hepatitis B virus sometimes present in the blood during acute infection
Anti-HBe: (choice (D))	An antibody to the e antigen of the hepatitis B virus
	Someone who has been exposed to or recovered from hepatitis B, or initiated hepatitis B vaccination
Anti-HBc (choice (B)):	Antibody to hepatitis B core antigen
	The presence of anti-HBc in a sample of serum provides information of infection (past or present) with hepatitis B virus
	For example: IgM = acute cases, IgG = recovery stage or chronic stage

56. **(C)** Most adenocarcinomas occur at the junction of the esophagus and the stomach.

57. **(A, B, D)** A focused assessment for this scenario includes an evaluation of the ear, eyes, throat (peripheral vestibular system), the cardiovascular system, and the neurological system (central nervous system). The integumentary system (choice (C)) is not part of the focused assessment for this patient, as there is no relationship between the integumentary system and dizziness.

58. **(A)** Carbamazepine (Tegretol) (choice (A)), clonazepam (Klonopin), and primidone (Mysoline) may help with tremors. Tizanidine (Zanaflex) (choice (B)), dantrolene (Dantrium) (choice (C)), and diazepam (Valium) (choice (D)) may help with spasticity.

59. **(C)** According to the World Health Organization, diagnostic criteria for osteoporosis:
Normal (choice (A)): BMD within 1 SD of young adult reference mean
Osteopenia (choice (B)): BMD > 1 SD below young adult reference mean (21)

Osteoporosis: BMD > 2.5 SD below young adult reference mean (22.5)

Osteoporosis (severe) (choice (D)): BMD > 2.5 SD below young adult reference mean (22.5) *and* presence of osteoporotic fractures.

60. **(C)** If the MCV is elevated, the anemia is macrocytic. The FNP should order a test of vitamin B12 levels and a folate level, even in the absence of clinical neurologic symptoms.

61. **(C)** The "A" represents asymmetry of the lesion; the "B" is for border (irregular); the "C" is color (varied colors are suspicious); the "D" is for diameter (larger than a pencil eraser); and the "E" is for elevation or enlarging (both are concerning).

62. **(D)** Ceftriaxone 250 mg IM as a single dose plus a single dose of oral azithromycin 1 g PO is the preferred treatment for uncomplicated gonococcal infection for a 44-year-old female patient. The treatment regimen is simple. Ceftriaxone IM is given at the clinic, and the patient only needs to take one pill at home. Thus, medication adherence is higher. Amoxicillin (choice (A)), TMP-SMX (choice (B)), and metronidazole (choice (C)) are not the recommended treatments for uncomplicated gonococcal infection.

63. **(A)** In most cases, epididymitis will improve over time. In children, it usually develops due to inflammation from a direct trauma, torsion of the appendix epididymis, or reflux of urine into the epididymis. Rest and ibuprofen can help decrease the inflammation and improve the pain.

64. **(D, A, B, C)** Postcoital control (chance withdrawal 85%), barrier methods (vaginal contraceptive sponge 18–29%), regulated abstinence (calendar calculation 9%), hormonal methods (combination oral contraceptives 0.1%)

65. **(B)** **Transgender:** broad term for individuals whose gender identity is different from natal gender. Address individuals based on gender identity (the gender they identify with), rather than natal gender. For example, a transgender woman living as a woman at the present time should be referred to as "she" or "her." Likewise, a transgender man currently living as a man should be referred to as "he" or "him." This is the first time the FNP has seen the patient. It is important for the FNP to be respectful, introduce herself/himself, and ask the patient how they would like to be addressed. In clinical practice, the medical chart may not reflect the patient's preferred name.

66. **(B)** Weight gain is a commonly reported finding in patients who take SSRIs and TCAs for management of depression. These medications stimulate appetite. Decreased libido, not increased (choice (A)), is an extremely common finding that occurs after several weeks of starting the medication and may persist as long as the individual is taking the drug. Improved sleep is often noted, as opposed to sleep disorders (choice (C)), while hyperglycemia (choice (D)) is not associated with SSRI or TCA use.

67. **(C)** Erosion of the nasal septum is a classic presentation of cocaine abuse. Other causes include "huffing" substances such as glue or other toxic agents.

68. **(B)** The presentation of a bright red rash with satellite lesions in the diaper area is consistent with candidiasis, which should be treated with a topical antifungal cream. Leaving the diaper off and allowing the area to dry out will also assist in clearing the rash.

69. **(B)** Osgood-Schlatter is a disease affecting adolescents, usually during a growth spurt. Overuse of the knee places stress on the patellar tendon with pain, swelling, and tenderness at the tendon insertion site into the quadriceps muscle. The condition improves when growth

stops. NSAIDs and rest are used to manage symptoms. Klinefelter syndrome (choice (A)) is a genetic condition in which there is an extra X chromosome. The condition affects males and presents with tall stature, wider hips, reduced facial and body hair, small testicles and penis. Treatment includes fertility measures and testosterone replacement. Meniscal tears (choice (C)) and ligamentous injuries (choice (D)) occur during an active traumatic event.

70. **(B)** Based on the patient's age and the provided options, there is no recommended screening. Note the criteria for lung cancer screening (low dose CT): ages 55–77, tobacco smoking history of at least 30 packs per year, current smoker or one who has quit smoking within the last 15 years.

71. **(A)** The Mini-Mental State Exam is a brief screening test for cognitive impairment. Within the exam, the patient is asked about the season, date, time, year, and location. Short-term memory, attention, and calculation are evaluated. Recall is assessed, along with the ability to write a sentence and copy a design. The maximum score is 30, with a higher score indicating less impairment. A score from 0–10 indicates severe impairment, 10–20 moderate impairment, and 20–25 mild impairment. Delirium (choice (B)) is an acute disorder of cognition that is secondary to another condition, such as infection. Depression (choice (C)) screening tools include the PHQ 2 and PHQ 9. Parkinson's disease (choice (D)) presents with rigidity and bradykinesia, along with tremors and a shuffling gait.

72. **(B)** The FNPs legal right to practice in a state is derived from the state board of nursing. While certification is a requirement in most states, becoming certified does not meet all the requirements for practice. The Institute of Medicine (choice (A)) is a national organization that has long advocated for removal of practice barriers for nurse practitioners, and the U.S. Department of Health and Human Services (choice (D)) is a governmental agency overseeing health organizations throughout the nation.

73. **(B)** The principle of confidentiality is the obligation to respect a patient's privileged information through the protection of the patient's identity, personal information, medical history, and medical records. The FNP is protecting the confidentiality of his patient by not confirming or providing any information about the patient. Note that patient rights are also protected under the Health Insurance Portability and Accountability Act (HIPAA). Justice (choice (A)) is the concept of fair and equal treatment for everyone. Fidelity (choice (C)) is about keeping promises. Veracity (choice (D)) refers to telling the whole truth.

74. **(A)** The NPI is a 10-digit number that must be used in lieu of identifying information for all HIPAA standard transactions.

75. **(C)** CPT stands for Current Procedural Terminology and is published by the American Medical Association. CPT is used to document the procedures and services conducted. For example, when removing a marble from the nose of a three-year-old child, the CPT code is 30300 (removal of foreign body).

76. **(A)** The role of the IRB is to protect the research participants' rights and safety. The IRB is not responsible for protecting the validity of research, nor the researcher's findings. It is the researcher's responsibility to contact the IRB and initiate any IRB application prior to conducting research.

77. **(D)** $n = 1,000$. There are 1,000 participants in the age group of 60–69. The capital $N =$ sum of *all* participants $= 4,000$ (choice (A)).

78. **(D)** Shared decision-making is a partnership with the patient as the center of care. Decisions are shared and based on clarification of patient goals and values.

79. **(D)** CONSORT is useful in assessing the quality of a randomized control trial. SQUIRE (choice (A)) is useful in the evaluation of a quality improvement study. PRISMA (choice (B)) is used to look at meta-analyses and systematic reviews, while STROBE (choice (C)) analyzes observational studies.

80. **(A)** 20/200 vision is considered legally blind by most standards. There are two components of the result when testing visual acuity using a Snellen chart. The upper number represents the distance from the visual chart to the patient (in feet). The lower number represents the *distance vision* (not near vision) at which the eye can read the value on the chart. For example, 20/40 means that the patient can see at 20 feet what the average person (20/20) can see at 40 feet. Likewise, 20/200 (choice (A)) means the patient can see at 20 feet what the average person (20/20) can see at 200 feet. Note that the U.S. Social Security Administration (SSA) defines legal blindness as follows: 1) reduced visual acuity of 20/200 or less with use of eyeglass lens, or 2) limitation of widest visual field in better eye no greater than 20 degrees.

81. **(B)** This presentation is suggestive of acute otitis media, which is an infection of the middle ear space and is a common complication of upper respiratory infection (choice (C)). Environmental risk factors for AOM include daycare attendance, exposure to tobacco smoke, exposure to older siblings, bottle feeding in a supine position, and pacifier use. The most common pathogens associated with AOM include *Streptococcus pneumoniae*, *Haemophilus influenzae*, and *Moraxella catarrhalis*.

82. **(C)** Sleep apnea is defined as a temporary pause in breathing during sleep that ranges from 11 seconds to 90 seconds. For a confirmed diagnosis, the pauses in breathing should occur a minimum of five times within an hour.

83. **(A)** T-wave inversion is seen in the presence of cardiac ischemia. ST-segment elevation (choice (B)) indicates tissue injury. A deep Q-wave (choice (C)) is present with a history of infarction. These Q-waves appear about one to three days after an MI. ST-segment elevation indicates subepicardial injury, while ST-segment depression represents subendocardial injury. A U-wave (choice (D)) follows the T-wave and may not be visible because of its small size. The presence of the U-wave is believed to represent repolarization of the Purkinje fibers.

84. **(A, B, C, D)** All of the choices are diagnosis criteria for diabetes mellitus. Any positive test results should be confirmed by repeating the fasting plasma glucose (FPG) test or the oral glucose tolerance test on a different day. Note that FPG is most reliable when performed in the morning. OGTT is more sensitive than FPG, but it is less convenient to perform.

85. **(D)** All of the options are appropriate treatment in the management of urinary incontinence. However, doxazosin mesylate (Cardura) is an alpha-1-adrenergic blocking agent commonly used in men for treatment of benign prostatic hyperplasia and urinary incontinence concurrently. Note that Cardura can also be used to help treat bladder problems in women.

86. **(B)** In older adults, there is often an atypical presentation with a urinary tract infection. Mental status changes, such as confusion or delirium, may be the only presenting symptom in this age group.

87. **(D)** Dark-colored urine with elevated urobilinogen indicates a problem or dysfunction of the biliary system or the hematologic system. Jaundice (a yellow coloring of the skin and mucous membranes) results from accumulation of bilirubin in body tissues. The cause may be

hepatic or non-hepatic. Hepatic causes include an obstruction in the biliary system (choice (A)) and liver disease (choice (B)). A non-hepatic cause includes hemolysis with excessive RBC breakdown (choice (C)).

88. **(B)** An embolic stroke results from cerebral ischemia caused by an embolus lodged in a cranial artery. The area of ischemia will determine the presenting symptoms and severity. A hemorrhagic stroke (choice (A)) presents with acute onset of a severe "worst headache of my life." There is a rapid decrease in the level of consciousness, and death may occur quickly. A transient ischemic attack (choice (C)) occurs when there is a brief interruption of blood flow to an area of the brain, and it is a strong predictor for a later CVA. Bell's palsy (choice (D)) presents as rapid development of painless paralysis of one side of the face. Sensation remains intact; however, eyelid movement is usually impaired.

89. **(A)** The National Osteoporosis Foundation recommends that adults younger than 50 should have an intake of 400–800 IU vitamin D daily. Adults older than 50 should have an intake of 800–1,000 IU vitamin D daily.

90. **(C)** A baby receiving immune protection from its mother is an example of natural passive immunity. Maternal antibodies are transferred passively to the baby through the placenta or breast milk. Receiving gamma globulin after exposure to an illness is a type of artificial passive immunity (choice (A)). Vaccines such as MMR, hep B, and pertussis are examples of artificial active immunity (choice (B)). When a child has chickenpox, he develops natural active immunity (choice (D)), because he develops his own antibodies as a result of natural disease.

91. **(C)** Pediculosis capitis is head lice, which produces severe itching. The itching results from an allergic response to the saliva of the lice deposited on the skin. Alopecia (choice (A)) may be seen with tinea capitis but is not associated with lice. The infestation usually does not cause pain (choice (B)) or burning (choice (D)), unless a secondary infection is present.

92. **(C)** Gonorrhea in men has a varied presentation and may even be asymptomatic. Dysuria, however, is fairly common. A lesion on the penis (choice (A)) would suggest herpes simplex 2 or syphilis. Fever (choice (B)) and fatigue (choice (D)) are not associated with gonorrheal infection.

93. **(D)** Asymptomatic bacteriuria is the presence of bacteria in the urine without clinical signs of illness or infection. In healthy adult women, treatment is not needed because the bacteria clear on their own. However, pregnant women are at higher risk for pyelonephritis, which is a serious illness during pregnancy. Therefore, asymptomatic bacteria discovered in a woman who is pregnant should be treated to prevent the illness from progressing. Nitrofurantoin is specifically indicated for urinary tract infections, as it concentrates in urine. Ciprofloxacin (choice (C)) is contraindicated during pregnancy. Antibiotic therapy should begin immediately and change later if indicated by urine culture and sensitivity results.

94. **(D)** Atrophic vaginitis (AV) occurs in states of decreased estrogen production. The condition is commonly seen in menopausal women and develops as a result of atrophy of vaginal tissue. Untreated AV is a progressive condition that may adversely affect quality of life. This alteration in vaginal membranes predisposes the woman to development of infections, such as urinary tract infection. Spermicidal agents (choice (A)), when used with a diaphragm for contraception, have been implicated as a vaginal irritant, possibly predisposing to UTIs. However, this occurs in women of reproductive age, not menopausal. Obesity (choice (B)) may predispose a woman to overgrowth of candida but does not contribute to UTI develop-

ment. The use of hormone replacement therapy (choice (C)) to treat vasomotor symptoms associated with menopause may actually decrease the risk for UTI.

95. **(A)** SSRIs are a good choice for initial therapy for depression in an older adult. TCAs (choice (B)) have significant side effects and are lethal in overdose. MAOIs (choice (C)) have multiple food and drug interactions and should be considered only if nothing else is effective. SNRIs (choice (D)) are a treatment option; however, they are more likely to produce activating symptoms, which may affect sleep in older adults.

96. **(D)** Acrocyanosis is a blue color seen in the hands and feet of a newborn and is benign. Bluish color of the mucous membranes (choice (A)), the tongue (choice (B)), or the torso (choice (C)) may be normal shortly after birth but should resolve rapidly. Seen later, this may indicate hypoxia.

97. **(B)** During the 11-to-12-year-old well-child visit, the child should receive a TDaP vaccine booster, HPV vaccine (series of three), and MCV4 to protect against meningococcal disease. This vaccine should be repeated around age 18–19. MMR is given at 12–15 months, with a second dose at 4–6 years. Hepatitis B vaccine is started at birth, with the series completed by 18 months; and IPV is given at 2 months, 4 months, and between 6 and 18 months, with a booster between 4 and 6 years, making choice (A) incorrect. DTaP is the combination given to infants and children younger than 7, while TDaP is given thereafter, making choice (C) incorrect. Vaccines are recommended at age 11–12, making choice (D) incorrect as well.

98. **(B)** Sundowning is a phenomenon seen commonly in patients with Alzheimer's disease. The cause is unknown; however, symptoms seem to be triggered by fading light at the end of the day. Patients become agitated, confused, and angry and may pace or move continuously. Caregivers are instructed to remain calm and keep the patient safe. Delirium (choice (A)) is an acute change in level of consciousness secondary to an infection or some other cause. Delirium resolves when the underlying condition is managed. Older adults often present with atypical symptoms in the setting of infection. A change in the level of consciousness may be the only sign of an infectious process (choice (C)) in this age group. Polypharmacy (choice (D)) can certainly cause the symptoms described but should be linked to medication dosing with resolution when medications are reduced.

99. **(A)** The FNP should reduce or stop the IV fluids, then increase the furosemide to 40 mg. The patient is in hospice care, so referral to the emergency department (choice (B)) is not a correct choice. Increasing the furosemide doses (choice (D)) without reducing/stopping the IV fluids may not provide the optimum outcome. Note that an FNP must have a face-to-face encounter with every hospice patient whose total stay across all hospices is anticipated to reach the third benefit.

100. **(A, B, C, D)** A malpractice case is established once it meets all four required components. The case will be further evaluated based on the current nursing standard of care, expert witness or witnesses, the current national guidelines, and the consensus opinion of the jury.

101. **(A)** The American Nurses Association established a set of ethical principles titled "The Code of Ethics for Nurses with Interpretive Statements," and it is accessible to anyone, without the requirement of membership affiliation.

102. **(C)** The AHRQ was established to develop large-scale databases for clinical guidelines and research and thereby promote evidence-based practice.

103. **(B, C, A, D)** Single trial research is conducted in only one setting. Multi-center research is conducted in different sites using the same protocol. Convenience sampling is a type of non-probability sampling that is recruited from the population and is easily accessible (close to hand). This type of sampling is useful for pilot testing. In double-blind trials, the researcher and participants have no prior knowledge about the outcome of the study. This is to eliminate any biases. In randomized trials, the participants are randomly selected and assigned to different groups.

104. **(C)** Turning Research into Practice is a free resource that provides a comprehensive search engine for clinicians who are looking for synopses of evidence-based guidelines. The Cochrane Database of Systematic Reviews (choice (A)) looks at primary research in human health care and health policy. National Guideline Clearinghouse (choice (B)) and the Agency for Healthcare Research (choice (D)) are both collections of databases for health-related research and topics. (Both NGC and AHRQ suspended online operations in July 2018.)

105. **(A)** Rhinoviruses are responsible for most cases of the common cold. This illness presents with nasal congestion, clear rhinorrhea, and erythematous, engorged nasal mucosa. This self-limiting illness usually resolves within 10 days. Adenovirus (choice (B)) causes conjunctivitis, upper respiratory tract infections, GI infection, and cystitis. After the acute phase of the illness, adenovirus may persist in a latent state in lymphoid tissues of the body, such as the tonsils and adenoids. Ribovirus (choice (C)) is an RNA virus that is also implicated in URIs, though it is not as common as rhinovirus. Parainfluenza virus (choice (D)) is a myxovirus causing respiratory illnesses such as laryngotracheobronchitis or croup in infants and young children.

106. **(C)** Pertussis is a highly contagious respiratory illness caused by *Bordetella pertussis* bacteria. The illness is often called "whooping cough" because of the characteristic cough. Pertussis has three stages: a catarrhal stage, a paroxysmal stage, and the stage of recovery or convalescence. The illness causes severe illness in young infants and may be fatal in this population. Several years ago, an outbreak of pertussis in Iowa led to the finding that antibody titers were low in adulthood. A new recommendation is for all adults living in a household with an infant to receive the TDaP vaccine one time only. It is offered now to all adults.

107. **(B)** Mobitz I AV block is represented on ECG. AV block itself is a disturbance of the electrical signal between the atria and ventricles. Blocks are labeled based on the degree of this disturbance. First-degree AV block (choice (A)) is seen as a regular rhythm with only a prolonged PR interval on ECG. Mobitz II block (choice (C)) occurs at the level of or below the bundle of His and appears as a normal or lengthened PR interval with an occasional dropped beat. A third-degree AV block (choice (D)) occurs when there is no communication between the atria and ventricles, and these structures are contracting independently of each other.

108. **(A, B, C, D)** Theory is a way for FNPs to organize their thinking around and see patterns in their practice. These patterns will help the FNP to develop novel ways of providing care while maintaining an overall sense of coherence.

109. **(A)** The onset of diuresis occurs in 15–30 minutes. Thus, if the patient took the drug at 9:00 A.M., the anticipated first use of the bathroom could be as early as 9:15–10:00 A.M.

110. **(D)** Certification is a voluntary process through which individuals receive documentation of competence and specialization from a nongovernmental agency.

111. **(C)** A family member requesting information about a patient may receive that information if the patient is present and agrees that information may be shared. The other three scenarios represent violation of HIPAA.

112. **(B)** Although presentation of PD is highly variable, six cardinal features are often present: resting tremor, rigidity, bradykinesia, flexed posture, loss of postural reflexes, and the freezing phenomenon. PD is a progressive, degenerative disease of the motor systems of the brain. Pathophysiology includes progressive loss of cells from the substantia nigra and basal ganglia. PD also destroys dopaminergic neurons producing Lewy bodies (characteristic of PD). Rheumatoid arthritis is a progressive, chronic, systemic disorder of the synovial joints, although many other organ systems may be involved. A patient with RA (choice (A)) presents with increasing pain in the extremities. RA produces early morning stiffness and joint pain that gradually improves as the day progresses. AD (choice (C)) is the most common cause of dementia, with a long asymptomatic period. This progressive, neurodegenerative condition usually presents when the patient or family members notice problems with memory. As the disease progresses, the patient loses all memory and eventually requires care for all activities of daily living. MS (choice (D)) is an autoimmune disorder that causes demyelination of the CNS. MS is seen more often in females and diagnosed between age 20 and 50. MS presents with sensory disturbances affecting the extremities, bowel and bladder dysfunction, optic neuritis, and severe fatigue.

113. **(A)** A triangle is used to represent a pregnancy (choice (B)). In the case of a miscarriage (choice (A)), there is a diagonal cross drawn on top of the triangle to indicate death. In the case of an abortion (choice (C)), there is an additional horizontal line on top of the diagonal cross drawn on top of the triangle to indicate abortion. In the case of a male stillbirth (choice (D)), it is the same as the representation of a deceased male.

114. **(A, B, C)** Elements of advance directives can include a living will, a health care proxy, and a durable power of attorney for health care (DPAHC). This is separate and distinct from a durable power of attorney relating to financial and monetary decisions (such as a beneficiary) and the decision to donate some or all body organs, according to the U.S. Uniform Anatomical Gift Act.

115. **(A)** Wernicke-Korsakoff syndrome (WKS) is a neurodegenerative disorder caused by thiamine deficiency, usually caused by alcoholism. The syndrome encompasses two different disorders with Wernicke's disease (WD) usually occurring first. WD often produces double vision, ptosis, nystagmus, ataxia, and confusion. Management includes thiamine replacement, among other interventions to improve overall nutritional state. Hyperbilirubinemia causes jaundice, a yellowish color of the skin and mucous membranes. The condition may be caused by excessive breakdown of red blood cells or an obstruction within the biliary system. Hyperbilirubinemia (choice (B)) is seen most often in newborns, with the cause usually related to physiologic jaundice, breast milk jaundice, or hemolysis. Bilirubin is toxic to the brain and may cause kernicterus, which may lead to seizures and brain damage. Alcohol toxicity (choice (C)) results from consumption of large amounts of alcohol in a short time. Symptoms include confusion, hypothermia, respiratory depression or arrest, vomiting, coma, and death. Vitamin C deficiency (choice (D)) is associated with persistent IDA, decreased immunity, slowed healing, bright red hair follicles, and corkscrew-shaped body hair because of defective protein structure.

116. **(C)** In children over age five, the most common pathogen is an atypical bacteria such as mycoplasma or chlamydia. A macrolide is the preferred agent and is usually selected because of its coverage of atypical pathogens. Doxycycline (choice (D)) is contraindicated in children younger than eight years. Amoxicillin (choice (B)) has no coverage against atypical pathogens.

117. **(A)** This patient probably has anorexia nervosa (AN), based on this presentation. More than 90% of individuals with AN have anemia, demonstrating evidence of poor nutrition. Amenorrhea is a common finding and is related to hypoestrogenic state and low levels of luteinizing hormone and follicle stimulating hormone. Migraine headaches (choice (B)) and hypothyroidism (choice (C)) are not associated with a diagnosis of AN. Patients with AN often have mitral valve prolapse, not mitral regurgitation (choice (D)).

118. **(D)** Combined oral contraceptive use, controlling ovulation and the menstrual cycle, provides for times of relatively low estrogen each month. Metabolic syndrome (choice (A)) is a group of disorders associated with CVD and diabetes. The underlying pathophysiology is insulin resistance. Patients with metabolic syndrome usually have an increased body mass index, elevated blood pressure, and dyslipidemia. Obesity (choice (C)) is associated with high estrogenic states and, in fact, adipose tissue produces small amounts of estrogen. Therefore, both metabolic syndrome and obesity are high estrogenic states. Polycystic ovarian syndrome (PCOS) (choice (B)) is an endocrine disorder characterized by high androgenic states. Ovulatory dysfunction occurs, often leading to polycystic ovarian morphology. This disorder also produces high levels of estrogen.

119. **(A)** To determine the estimated date of delivery, take the first day of the last normal menstrual period and add seven days to this date. Then, subtract three months. Next, add one year. Naegle's rule is more accurate for women with regular 28-day cycles but can be helpful for women who just found out they are pregnant to estimate when their baby will be born.

120. **(B)** Although some researchers offer compensation to human subjects, this is not considered a basic right relating to research participation.

121. **(C)** Patient diagnoses (choice (A)), medications (choice (B)), and past medical and surgical history (choice (D)) are all included in "individually identifiable information" protected by HIPAA. The number of vaccines provided by a clinic per year does not qualify as protected information.

122. **(B)** The acronym LACE is used to describe the four essential elements for advanced practice nursing: licensure, accreditation, certification, and education.

123. **(C)** Institutional review board, also known as an independent ethics committee, ethical review board, or research ethics board, is a type of committee that applies research ethics by reviewing the methods proposed for research to ensure that they are ethical.

124. **(D)** The documented official written hospice care order must be created by a physician, *not* an FNP. Other criteria include that life sustaining equipment during an emergency is not part of hospice service, that patients consent to begin and receive hospice care services, and that patients have a life expectancy of six months or less.

125. **(D)** A Mongolian spot is a poorly-defined, bluish-black macule seen on the trunk and buttocks of infants. These lesions are common in people of Asian and African descent. These areas are asymptomatic and may fade with time. A blue nevus (choice (A)) is a mole that is

blue in appearance. Milia (choice (B)) are tiny, pearl-like bumps present on the nose and face of newborns. They are benign and resolve spontaneously. Koplik spots (choice (C)) are white spots seen inside the mouth and are associated with measles.

126. **(C)** Symptoms of bipolar disorder usually present between the ages of 15 and 30, and onset is rare in individuals younger than 15 or older than 65.

127. **(C)** Sexually transmitted infections are the most common communicable diseases in the United States, and risk factors include a history of a previous STI (choice (A)), age under 25 years (choice (B)), and injection drug use (due to lifestyle factors surrounding injection drug use) (choice (D)). Having a urinary tract infection is not a specific risk factor for development of an STI but may be a comorbid illness.

128. **(B)** Secondary prevention measures aim to detect the presence of a condition or disease during an early, asymptomatic period. During this time, if a condition is recognized, treatment will likely be more effective. Primary prevention (choice (A)) activities work to prevent the occurrence or onset of a disease or condition. An example of primary prevention is immunization. Tertiary prevention (choice (C)) measures are designed to slow disease progression and improve quality of life for individuals with chronic illness.

129. **(B)** Vasomotor symptoms are believed to result from fluctuating estrogen levels that occur during the perimenopausal period. These hormone changes trigger the body's temperature control system and induce symptoms of hot flashes and sweating. Prolactin hormone (choice (A)) is secreted in response to pregnancy hormones and works to prepare the breast for milk production. Ovarian cysts (choice (C)) are common occurrences among women and most are benign and asymptomatic. Some women, however, experience transient sharp lower abdominal pain coinciding with ovulation that may be related to ovarian cysts. Progesterone (choice (D)) works with estrogen to promote a favorable environment for fertilization and implantation to occur. Low levels would not produce vasomotor symptoms.

130. **(D)** A patient diagnosed with atrophic vaginitis complains of pruritus, bleeding, dyspareunia, vaginal dryness, and no vaginal discharge. Examination findings: vestibular and vaginal thinning, pH: > 6, amine (whiff) test: presence of amine odor, and KOH exam: negative.

131. **(B)** Both CPT code and ICD-10 code are required for submitting a claim for reimbursement. The correct diagnosis: ICD-10 code. The care performed: CPT code.

132. **(C)** All four of these elements must be proven for malpractice to be established. 1) The NP owes the plaintiff a duty. (There is an established provider-patient relationship in any setting: text messaging, phone conversations, social events, providing advice, or giving samples.) 2) The NP's treatment action fell below the NP standard of care (breach of standard of care) (choice (A)). 3) The NP's action caused the plaintiff's injury (proximate cause). 4) The plaintiff was injured (actual injury must have occurred).

133. **(D)** Erythema infectiosum, fifth disease, is a mildly to moderately contagious viral illness common in childhood. The rash begins on the cheeks, producing the characteristic "slapped cheek" appearance. The virus is self-limiting, and children may attend school as long as they have been febrile for 24 hours. Fever and discomfort may be treated with acetaminophen or ibuprofen. Adults who have been exposed to children with fifth disease may experience joint symptoms such as arthralgias and myalgias for weeks.

134. **(A)** Gingival hyperplasia and inflammation are common findings during pregnancy and are caused by hormonal changes. Even though this is common, more severe gingival disease and tooth loss may occur unless meticulous oral hygiene is carried out through pregnancy. Extensive periodontal disease (choice (B)) may result from inflammation in the setting of poor oral hygiene. Bleeding, receding gums, loose teeth, and halitosis are commonly seen with periodontal disease. Poor nutritional status (choice (C)) may be suspected with a bright red, smooth tongue, and anemia (choice (D)) may cause pale mucous membranes.

135. **(A)** In the United States, most women enter menopause at age 51.

136. **(C)** Practice in each state is defined by the Nurse Practice Act and regulated by the board of nursing in that state.

137. **(C)** Loretta Ford, PhD, RN, FAAN is the historical founder of the nurse practitioner movement in the United States. Ford saw a regional shortage of physicians to provide care to rural and underserved families and used a small grant to begin using advanced practice nurses to care for this population.

138. **(D)** The Apley's test is done with the patient lying prone while the injured knee is flexed to 90 degrees. Firm downward pressure is then applied to the foot, pushing the tibia firmly against the femur. The leg is then rotated internally and externally. If there is pain, locking, or clicking with this maneuver, the test is positive and indicates torn tissue trapped in the joint space. The Lachman test (choice (A)) assesses for anterior cruciate ligament injury. The drawer test (choice (B)) assesses anterior and posterior cruciate ligament stability, and the bulge test (choice (C)) evaluates for effusion of the knee.

139. **(C)** The "anatomical snuffbox" is tender in the setting of a scaphoid fracture. This is the most commonly occurring injury of the carpal bones. Because of poor blood supply, this area is prone to avascular necrosis. Because of this risk, the tenderness, even without a history of trauma, warrants an X-ray of the wrist. Hamate fractures (choice (D)) are uncommon and are sometimes seen in golfers. These fractures present as pain and tenderness on the ulnar side of the palm. An ulnar styloid fracture (choice (B)) is associated with tenderness of the distal ulna. A radial head fracture (choice (A)) produces pain at the elbow.

140. **(A, B, C)** If a patient presented with clumsiness, or was unable to walk steadily, he should be referred to the emergency room. Other options are appropriate topics to discuss with parents.

141. **(A)** Advisory Committee on Immunization Practices is composed of medical and public health experts who evaluate the current scientific evidence based on diseases related to immunization through vaccinations. The United States Preventive Services Task Force (USPSTF) is an independent non-federal expert's panel that evaluates current scientific evidence focusing on the clinical preventative health care services. USPSTF develops recommendations for primary care providers in clinical and health care systems. A Compendium of Proven Community-Based Prevention Programs was released by the Trust for America's Health (TFAH) and New York Academy of Medicine (NYAM). The program highlights 79 evidence-based disease and injury prevention programs that have saved lives and improved health. Prevention Status Reports: This website highlights the top 10 public health problems and concerns for all 50 states and the District of Columbia. The role of the IRB is to protect the research participants' rights and safety (choice (D)). The IRB is not responsible for protecting the validity of research, nor the researcher's findings. It is the researcher's responsibility to contact IRB and initiate any IRB application prior to conducting research.

142. **(D)** The four components needed to prove a malpractice case include duty of care (choice (A)), proximal cause (choice (B)), breach of standard of care, and injury to patient (choice (C)).

143. **(D)** Veracity: Telling the whole truth. Advanced small cell lung cancer tends to spread quickly. Stage IV SCLC has a relative five-year survival rate of about 2%. The FNP is being honest and truthful about the patient's prognosis. Justice (choice (A)): Weighing an individual's right without bias. Confidentiality (choice (B)): The obligation to respect the privileged information through the protection of a patient's identity, personal information, medical history, and medical records. Fidelity (choice (C)): Keeping promises.

144. **(C)** Allergic conjunctivitis presents with bilateral symptoms of itching, increased tearing, edema of the eyelid, and bilateral hyperemia with no changes in vision and is often seen with other atopic disorders. Bacterial conjunctivitis (choice (A)) may present with mild lid discomfort with copious purulent discharge without blurring of vision; the eyes are "stuck together" upon awakening. Severe symptoms suggest gonococcal etiology. Blepharitis (choice (B)) is a chronic, bilateral, inflammatory condition that affects the eyelid margins. It may be anterior (eyelids, eyelashes) or posterior (obstruction of the meibomian gland). There is often dryness and flaking involving the eyelashes and eyelid margins. Hordeolum (choice (D)) is also known as a "stye" and usually forms along the border of the eyelid. Causative organism: *Staphylococcus aureus* (90–95% of cases), *Staphylococcus epidermidis*.

145. **(B)** A long-acting bronchodilator may be used in conjunction with an inhaled steroid but should not be used as monotherapy. These medications are associated with an increased risk of death when used alone. Short-acting bronchodilators (choice (A)), inhaled steroid (choice (C)), and oral steroid medications (choice (D)) may be used as monotherapy, depending on patient presentation.

146. **(C)** Because this patient's blood glucose is above 200 mg/dL, he is diagnosed as having diabetes mellitus. Oral agents would have little effect on lowering his blood glucose level. He should be started on insulin today and should return tomorrow for a recheck and assessment of his response to insulin.

147. **(C)** This symptom cluster is commonly associated with hypoglycemia. Patients with syncope (choice (A)) often faint with no prodromal symptoms. An acute cardiac event (choice (B)) USUALLY presents with some chest pain or discomfort or with abdominal or mid epigastric distress. Postural hypotension (choice (D)) is usually asymptomatic but may lead to syncopal episodes if the patient stands up from lying or sitting too quickly.

148. **(D)** Renal angiography is the diagnostic gold standard for chronic kidney disease. Renal ultrasound (choice (A)) is performed as a baseline. Renal computed tomography scan (choice (B)) may detect stenosis or parenchymal disease. Duplex doppler ultrasonography (choice (C)) may be used to assess renal vascular flow.

149. **(A)** The next step in the evaluation of this patient should be to obtain a complete history. Information about past medical history, family history, diet, and lifestyle will assist in the diagnosis. A physical examination should then be performed based on information obtained in the history. A barium enema (choice (B)), trial of antispasmodics (choice (C)), or a CT of the abdomen (choice (D)) may or may not be indicated based on findings obtained during the history and physical.

150. **(C)** T1: tumor invades the submucosa (choice (B)), T2: tumor is spreading to the muscularis (choice (C)), T3: tumor has penetrated through the bowel wall (choice (D)), T4: tumor has spread to other organs (choice (A)).

151. **(A)** The test described is the Phalen's test and is positive if the patient experiences numbness and tingling with the maneuver. This indicates symptoms are produced by compression of the median nerve. CTS may be unilateral or bilateral. Tinel's test (choice (B)) involves using a reflex hammer to briskly tap the anterior wrist. A test is positive if the patient experiences a "pins and needles" sensation. The Weber (choice (C)) and Rinne (choice (D)) tests are used to differentiate conductive and neurosensory hearing loss.

152. **(A)** In ulcerative colitis, the affected area usually presents from the distal to proximal area of the colon. In Crohn's disease, the affected area more commonly presents in a segmental part of the colon. Crohn's disease causes weight loss (choice (B)), but not ulcerative colitis. For Crohn's disease, an endoscopy report may report noncaseating granulomas located in the inflamed mucosa (choice (C)). However, superficial inflammation of mucosa can be noted on ulcerative colitis. Crohn's disease patients are more prone to have uveitis, iritis, and conjunctivitis. Ulcerative colitis patients are more prone to have primary sclerosing cholangitis (choice (D)). Note that ulcerative colitis has a high correlation with the development of colorectal cancer.

153. **(B)** Ectopic pregnancy is a complication resulting from implantation of the fertilized ovum into the fallopian tube, instead of the uterus. This potentially life-threatening condition presents with acute onset of severe lower abdominal pain and possibly vaginal bleeding. Risk factors include maternal age between 15 and 19 or over 35. A history of a previous ectopic pregnancy, previous tubal surgery, history of pelvic inflammatory disease, history of infertility, use of an intrauterine device, history of therapeutic abortion, or use of low-dose progestin or postcoital estrogens for contraception are other risk factors.

154. **(B)** A patient diagnosed with bacterial vaginosis (Gardnerella) may complain of dysuria and malodorous, gray-yellow-green watery, thick adherent vaginal discharge, usually without dyspareunia. Examination findings: Homogeneous, thin, grayish-white discharge that smoothly coats the vaginal walls, vaginal pH: > 4.5, amine (whiff) test: presence of amine odor, clue cells present in saline microscopy, and KOH exam: positive. Note that, per Amsel criteria, a minimum of three criteria must be present for a diagnosis of BV.

155. **(B)** MDD may be diagnosed when at least five of nine characteristic symptoms are present. Depression involves two to four symptoms being present. These symptoms must have been present for at least two weeks and must be pervasive and persistent. The duration of symptoms (choice (A)) must be at least two weeks for both disorders. The presence of suicidal thoughts (choice (C)) may be seen in both disorders. The severity of symptoms (choice (D)) is not used to differentiate MDD from depression.

156. **(B)** Epstein's pearls are common findings that are benign. These small lesions are not painful, do not interfere with nursing, and resolve on their own. Milia (choice (A)) are small white pustules seen on the face of young infants. This, too, is a benign finding and requires no treatment. Leukoplakia (choice (C)) is a whitish lesion within the oral mucosa, most often seen in older adults.

157. **(A)** Recommended immunizations for the four to six-year well-child visit include a fifth dose of DTaP, a fourth dose of IPV (if needed), a second dose of MMR, and a varicella vaccine.

158. **(B)** A cataract is an opacity of the lens of the eye that commonly develops with aging. Other causes or risk factors for cataract development include congenital lens dysphoria, excessive exposure to UVB light, and trauma. Cataracts may be unilateral; however, most progress to bilateral involvement. Cataract surgery is the most common surgery covered by Medicare in the United States. Open-angle glaucoma (choice (A)) presents with slow, painless vision loss, usually beginning with peripheral vision and often with increased intraocular pressure. Macular degeneration (choice (C)) is an age-related progressive loss of central vision. The disorder may present with gradual vision loss or acutely as a result of the leaking of retinal vessels. Retinopathy (choice (D)) associated with diabetes also contributes to vision loss over time. On fundoscopic exam, diabetic retinopathy appears as microaneurysms, exudates, dilated and tortuous vessels, and neovascularization of the retina and optic disc.

159. **(B)** Acute otitis externa (AOE) is most often caused by *Pseudomonas* or *Staphylococcus*. AOE presents with acute onset of severe ear pain, tenderness, aural fullness, itching, and hearing loss. A malignant form of the disease occurs most often in the elderly or those with compromised immune systems. *Moraxella* (choice (A)), *S. pneumoniae* (choice (C)), *and H. influenzae* (choice (D)) are common causes of acute otitis media (AOM).

160. **(A, C, B, D).** REM has four stages. Stage 1 involves slow eye movements, preceding sleep onset. Stage 2 involves further slowing the EEG, presence of sleep spindles, and slow eye movements. Stage 3 is manifested by low-frequency delta waves with occasional sleep spindles but no slow eye movements. Stage 4 presents high-voltage delta waves.

161. **(B)** Bacterial conjunctivitis presents with itching, tearing, and a mucopurulent discharge. Patients often report eyes being "stuck together" in the morning on awakening. The most common cause of bacterial conjunctivitis in children younger than seven is *H. influenzae*, while other common pathogens include *S. pneumoniae*, and *M. catarrhalis*. Viral conjunctivitis (choice (A)) presents as itching, burning eyes, with increased tearing. There is often a watery, mucoid discharge and the conjunctiva appears bright red. Preauricular lymphadenopathy may be present. Allergic conjunctivitis (choice (C)) presents with bilateral itching and a watery discharge. The lids and conjunctiva are swollen and red. This type of conjunctivitis is often accompanied by sneezing, itchy throat, and rhinorrhea.

162. **(D)** The FNP should further assess the patient, including asking about lifestyle, health history, and any other signs and symptoms that would support the need for a diabetes screening test.

163. **(C)** In primary care settings, the hemoglobin A1c are usually ordered two to four times a year. The hemoglobin A1c I is an index of average blood glucose over the previous approximately 120 days. (Human red blood cells live for about 120 days.) Note that each 1% change in A1c represents a change of approximately 35 mg/dL in average blood glucose.

164. **(D)** Cushing's syndrome is a disease caused by elevated cortisol levels, most commonly due to exogenous corticosteroid administration or use. Benign ACTH-secreting pituitary adenoma (choice (B)) is a possible cause. Neuroendocrine neoplasms can also secrete ACTH and lead to elevated cortisol levels. Patients often present with fatigue, malaise, and reduced energy. The classic picture of an individual with central body wasting, "moon face," protuber-

ant abdomen, and supraclavicular fat pads eventually develops as the disease progresses. These patients will have an elevated serum cortisol level, osteoporosis, and poor wound healing. Adrenal insufficiency (choice (A)) would entail a lack of or decreased cortisol production. Autoimmune disease (choice (C)) has not been associated with Cushing's as a cause; however, some individuals with Cushing's may have a comorbid autoimmune disease.

165. **(B)** The patient is unable to communicate, and he lives in a long-term nursing home. There are high incidences of *E. coli* infection in nursing homes. Sending the patient's urine for culture is the appropriate choice at this time. Assessment and vital signs are within normal limits. There is no reason to report possible elderly abuse (choice (C)). Ordering a complete metabolic panel (choice (D)) will not address the concerns for enuresis.

166. **(C)** Irritable bowel syndrome is a functional gastrointestinal disorder that is characterized by abdominal pain and discomfort. To be considered IBS, the patient must present with two of the following elements: abdominal pain and discomfort that is relieved by defecation, change in the frequency of stool, or change in the appearance of the stool. IBS is not an emergency presentation and can be managed in a primary care setting.

167. **(C)** Parkinson's disease is a degenerative disease of the motor system in the brain. Presently, there is no treatment available to prevent the progression of the disease (choice (A)). Most patients with PD exhibit behavioral changes (choice (B)), including changes in handwriting, and more than 50% experience depression. The goal of life-long treatment for PD is to help patients to function independently for as long as possible.

168. **(C)** De Quervain's tenosynovitis (stenosing tenosynovitis) is characterized by tenderness at the base of the thumb. Finkelstein's test is used to assess for de Quervain's disease in people with wrist pain. The patient is instructed to touch the thumb to the palm of the hand and make a fist. The test is positive if moving the wrist into ulnar deviation causes pain. Allen's test (choice (A)), or Allen's sign, is used to assess patency of the radial and ulnar arteries into the hand. To perform this test, the clinician compresses the radial artery at the wrist and has the patient rapidly open and close the hand several times. The patient then opens the hand, which should be pale in color or white. When the clinician relieves the pressure on the artery, the hand should flush, which indicates the artery is patent. Phalen's maneuver (choice (B)) assesses for median nerve inflammation or impingement. The test is performed by instructing the patient to hold both hands back-to-back while flexing the wrists to a 90-degree angle. This position is maintained for 60 seconds. Acute flexion of the wrist should produce no symptoms unless there is impingement or inflammation of the median nerve. A positive Phalen's is consistent with a diagnosis of carpal tunnel syndrome. Another test is Tinel's sign (choice (D)), which is done by light percussion of the palmar surface of the wrist with a percussion hammer. If the patient reports a shock-like or tingling sensation, the test is positive and is suggestive of carpal tunnel syndrome.

169. **(C)** Of the foods listed, all have high amounts of vitamin B12 except oatmeal, which contains no vitamin B12.

170. **(D)** Urethritis is a sexually transmitted infection. Urethritis in men may present without frequency or urgency. The characteristic presentation of urethritis is an acute discharge and dysuria after unprotected sex. It is usually caused by chlamydia and gonorrhea. Risk factors include new sexual partners, multiple partners, and age under 25. Untreated illness may disseminate with resultant arthritis, meningitis, and endocarditis. Acute prostatitis (choice (A)) presents with frequency, dysuria, and urgency. Constipation (choice (B)) should not produce urinary symptoms. Cystitis (choice (C)) presents with dysuria, frequency, and urgency.

171. **(D)** Around 6–10% of pregnancies may be associated with a diagnosis of preeclampsia. The disorder is characterized by the presence of hypertension, edema (often of the face and hands), and proteinuria. Risk factors for preeclampsia include age > 35 years, African American, family or personal history of preeclampsia, obesity, history of vascular disease, and lower socioeconomic status. Preeclampsia is a precursor to eclampsia, which is a serious condition associated with the development of seizures with a high maternal mortality rate.

172. **(B)** Fluoxetine, an SSRI, has a half-life with acute administration of two to three days. With long-term administration, the half-life is four to six days. The half-life of citalopram (choice (A)) is 35 hours, bupropion (choice (C)) 8–24 hours, and escitalopram (choice (D)) 27–32 hours.

173. **(A)** Fairly significant weight loss is expected within the first few days after birth; however, with proper nutrition, the infant should return to birth weight by two weeks with continued weight gain. A baby who has not returned to birth weight should be evaluated for feeding patterns, feeding problems, and possible failure to thrive.

174. **(C)** Although suicide (choice (A)), stroke (choice (B)), and pneumonia (choice (D)) cause a significant number of deaths in this age group, the top three causes are heart disease, cancer, and COPD.

175. **(C)** The FNP is verbalizing a negative descriptor of her patient. She also stereotyped the patient with her language, showing gender bias and ageism.

ANSWER SHEET
Practice Test 2

1. Ⓐ Ⓑ Ⓒ Ⓓ   31. Ⓐ Ⓑ Ⓒ Ⓓ   61. Ⓐ Ⓑ Ⓒ Ⓓ   91. Ⓐ Ⓑ Ⓒ Ⓓ
2. Ⓐ Ⓑ Ⓒ Ⓓ   32. Ⓐ Ⓑ Ⓒ Ⓓ   62. Ⓐ Ⓑ Ⓒ Ⓓ   92. Ⓐ Ⓑ Ⓒ Ⓓ
3. Ⓐ Ⓑ Ⓒ Ⓓ   33. Ⓐ Ⓑ Ⓒ Ⓓ   63. Ⓐ Ⓑ Ⓒ Ⓓ   93. Ⓐ Ⓑ Ⓒ Ⓓ
4. Ⓐ Ⓑ Ⓒ Ⓓ   34. Ⓐ Ⓑ Ⓒ Ⓓ   64. Ⓐ Ⓑ Ⓒ Ⓓ   94. Ⓐ Ⓑ Ⓒ Ⓓ
5. Ⓐ Ⓑ Ⓒ Ⓓ   35. Ⓐ Ⓑ Ⓒ Ⓓ   65. Ⓐ Ⓑ Ⓒ Ⓓ   95. Ⓐ Ⓑ Ⓒ Ⓓ
6. Ⓐ Ⓑ Ⓒ Ⓓ   36. Ⓐ Ⓑ Ⓒ Ⓓ   66. Ⓐ Ⓑ Ⓒ Ⓓ   96. Ⓐ Ⓑ Ⓒ Ⓓ
7. Ⓐ Ⓑ Ⓒ Ⓓ   37. Ⓐ Ⓑ Ⓒ Ⓓ   67. Ⓐ Ⓑ Ⓒ Ⓓ   97. Ⓐ Ⓑ Ⓒ Ⓓ
8. Ⓐ Ⓑ Ⓒ Ⓓ   38. Ⓐ Ⓑ Ⓒ Ⓓ   68. Ⓐ Ⓑ Ⓒ Ⓓ   98. Ⓐ Ⓑ Ⓒ Ⓓ
9. Ⓐ Ⓑ Ⓒ Ⓓ   39. Ⓐ Ⓑ Ⓒ Ⓓ   69. Ⓐ Ⓑ Ⓒ Ⓓ   99. Ⓐ Ⓑ Ⓒ Ⓓ
10. Ⓐ Ⓑ Ⓒ Ⓓ   40. Ⓐ Ⓑ Ⓒ Ⓓ   70. Ⓐ Ⓑ Ⓒ Ⓓ   100. Ⓐ Ⓑ Ⓒ Ⓓ
11. Ⓐ Ⓑ Ⓒ Ⓓ   41. Ⓐ Ⓑ Ⓒ Ⓓ   71. Ⓐ Ⓑ Ⓒ Ⓓ   101. Ⓐ Ⓑ Ⓒ Ⓓ
12. Ⓐ Ⓑ Ⓒ Ⓓ   42. Ⓐ Ⓑ Ⓒ Ⓓ   72. Ⓐ Ⓑ Ⓒ Ⓓ   102. Ⓐ Ⓑ Ⓒ Ⓓ
13. Ⓐ Ⓑ Ⓒ Ⓓ   43. Ⓐ Ⓑ Ⓒ Ⓓ   73. Ⓐ Ⓑ Ⓒ Ⓓ   103. Ⓐ Ⓑ Ⓒ Ⓓ
14. Ⓐ Ⓑ Ⓒ Ⓓ   44. Ⓐ Ⓑ Ⓒ Ⓓ   74. Ⓐ Ⓑ Ⓒ Ⓓ   104. Ⓐ Ⓑ Ⓒ Ⓓ
15. Ⓐ Ⓑ Ⓒ Ⓓ   45. Ⓐ Ⓑ Ⓒ Ⓓ   75. Ⓐ Ⓑ Ⓒ Ⓓ   105. Ⓐ Ⓑ Ⓒ Ⓓ
16. Ⓐ Ⓑ Ⓒ Ⓓ   46. Ⓐ Ⓑ Ⓒ Ⓓ   76. Ⓐ Ⓑ Ⓒ Ⓓ   106. Ⓐ Ⓑ Ⓒ Ⓓ
17. Ⓐ Ⓑ Ⓒ Ⓓ   47. Ⓐ Ⓑ Ⓒ Ⓓ   77. Ⓐ Ⓑ Ⓒ Ⓓ   107. Ⓐ Ⓑ Ⓒ Ⓓ
18. Ⓐ Ⓑ Ⓒ Ⓓ   48. Ⓐ Ⓑ Ⓒ Ⓓ   78. Ⓐ Ⓑ Ⓒ Ⓓ   108. Ⓐ Ⓑ Ⓒ Ⓓ
19. Ⓐ Ⓑ Ⓒ Ⓓ   49. Ⓐ Ⓑ Ⓒ Ⓓ   79. Ⓐ Ⓑ Ⓒ Ⓓ   109. Ⓐ Ⓑ Ⓒ Ⓓ
20. Ⓐ Ⓑ Ⓒ Ⓓ   50. Ⓐ Ⓑ Ⓒ Ⓓ   80. Ⓐ Ⓑ Ⓒ Ⓓ   110. Ⓐ Ⓑ Ⓒ Ⓓ
21. Ⓐ Ⓑ Ⓒ Ⓓ   51. Ⓐ Ⓑ Ⓒ Ⓓ   81. Ⓐ Ⓑ Ⓒ Ⓓ   111. Ⓐ Ⓑ Ⓒ Ⓓ
22. Ⓐ Ⓑ Ⓒ Ⓓ   52. Ⓐ Ⓑ Ⓒ Ⓓ   82. Ⓐ Ⓑ Ⓒ Ⓓ   112. Ⓐ Ⓑ Ⓒ Ⓓ
23. Ⓐ Ⓑ Ⓒ Ⓓ   53. Ⓐ Ⓑ Ⓒ Ⓓ   83. Ⓐ Ⓑ Ⓒ Ⓓ   113. Ⓐ Ⓑ Ⓒ Ⓓ
24. Ⓐ Ⓑ Ⓒ Ⓓ   54. Ⓐ Ⓑ Ⓒ Ⓓ   84. Ⓐ Ⓑ Ⓒ Ⓓ   114. Ⓐ Ⓑ Ⓒ Ⓓ
25. Ⓐ Ⓑ Ⓒ Ⓓ   55. Ⓐ Ⓑ Ⓒ Ⓓ   85. Ⓐ Ⓑ Ⓒ Ⓓ   115. Ⓐ Ⓑ Ⓒ Ⓓ
26. Ⓐ Ⓑ Ⓒ Ⓓ   56. Ⓐ Ⓑ Ⓒ Ⓓ   86. Ⓐ Ⓑ Ⓒ Ⓓ   116. Ⓐ Ⓑ Ⓒ Ⓓ
27. Ⓐ Ⓑ Ⓒ Ⓓ   57. Ⓐ Ⓑ Ⓒ Ⓓ   87. Ⓐ Ⓑ Ⓒ Ⓓ   117. Ⓐ Ⓑ Ⓒ Ⓓ
28. Ⓐ Ⓑ Ⓒ Ⓓ   58. Ⓐ Ⓑ Ⓒ Ⓓ   88. Ⓐ Ⓑ Ⓒ Ⓓ   118. Ⓐ Ⓑ Ⓒ Ⓓ
29. Ⓐ Ⓑ Ⓒ Ⓓ   59. Ⓐ Ⓑ Ⓒ Ⓓ   89. Ⓐ Ⓑ Ⓒ Ⓓ   119. Ⓐ Ⓑ Ⓒ Ⓓ
30. Ⓐ Ⓑ Ⓒ Ⓓ   60. Ⓐ Ⓑ Ⓒ Ⓓ   90. Ⓐ Ⓑ Ⓒ Ⓓ   120. Ⓐ Ⓑ Ⓒ Ⓓ

ANSWER SHEET
Practice Test 2

121. Ⓐ Ⓑ Ⓒ Ⓓ
122. Ⓐ Ⓑ Ⓒ Ⓓ
123. Ⓐ Ⓑ Ⓒ Ⓓ
124. Ⓐ Ⓑ Ⓒ Ⓓ
125. Ⓐ Ⓑ Ⓒ Ⓓ
126. Ⓐ Ⓑ Ⓒ Ⓓ
127. Ⓐ Ⓑ Ⓒ Ⓓ
128. Ⓐ Ⓑ Ⓒ Ⓓ

129. Ⓐ Ⓑ Ⓒ Ⓓ
130. Ⓐ Ⓑ Ⓒ Ⓓ
131. Ⓐ Ⓑ Ⓒ Ⓓ
132. Ⓐ Ⓑ Ⓒ Ⓓ
133. Ⓐ Ⓑ Ⓒ Ⓓ
134. Ⓐ Ⓑ Ⓒ Ⓓ
135. Ⓐ Ⓑ Ⓒ Ⓓ
136. Ⓐ Ⓑ Ⓒ Ⓓ

137. Ⓐ Ⓑ Ⓒ Ⓓ
138. Ⓐ Ⓑ Ⓒ Ⓓ
139. Ⓐ Ⓑ Ⓒ Ⓓ
140. Ⓐ Ⓑ Ⓒ Ⓓ
141. Ⓐ Ⓑ Ⓒ Ⓓ
142. Ⓐ Ⓑ Ⓒ Ⓓ
143. Ⓐ Ⓑ Ⓒ Ⓓ
144. Ⓐ Ⓑ Ⓒ Ⓓ

145. Ⓐ Ⓑ Ⓒ Ⓓ
146. Ⓐ Ⓑ Ⓒ Ⓓ
147. Ⓐ Ⓑ Ⓒ Ⓓ
148. Ⓐ Ⓑ Ⓒ Ⓓ
149. Ⓐ Ⓑ Ⓒ Ⓓ
150. Ⓐ Ⓑ Ⓒ Ⓓ

Practice Test 2

AANPCB-Style

DIRECTIONS: You have 3 hours to answer the following 150 questions.

1. All the following are causative bacteria associated with acute otitis media, EXCEPT:

    (A) *Pseudomonas aeruginosa.*
    (B) *Streptococcus pneumoniae.*
    (C) *Haemophilus influenzae.*
    (D) *Moraxella catarrhalis.*

2. All the following are risk factors associated with lung cancer, EXCEPT:

    (A) working in a furniture factory.
    (B) a history of working in a paint shop for 30 years.
    (C) a patient receiving five chest ultrasounds within the past 3 years.
    (D) a patient receiving three rounds of radiation to the chest for the past 4 years.

3. Per Joint National Committee (JNC 8) recommendations, which of the following scenarios should prompt the nurse practitioner to initiate blood pressure therapy?

    (A) a 59-year-old patient with history of type 2 diabetes and an average blood pressure of 140/90 for the past three clinical visits
    (B) a 93-year-old patient with a history of gastroesophageal reflux (GERD) and an average blood pressure of 140/90 for the past three clinical visits
    (C) a 33-year-old patient with a BMI of 25 with an average blood pressure of 140/90 for the past two clinical visits
    (D) a 45-year-old patient with no health problems who had an average blood pressure of 140/90 for the past three clinical visits

4. Which of the following is the most common cause of gynecomastia among the male teenage population?

    (A) puberty
    (B) drugs
    (C) cirrhosis or malnutrition
    (D) testicular failure

5. The majority of uncomplicated urinary tract infections are caused by:

   (A) *Staphylococcus saprophyticus.*
   (B) *Escherichia coli.*
   (C) *Proteus mirabilis.*
   (D) *Klebsiella.*

6. Which of the following is the recommended diagnostic test for an adult presenting with heartburn, dysphagia, and weight loss?

   (A) esophagogastroduodenoscopy (EGD)
   (B) ambulatory esophageal pH monitoring
   (C) chest X-ray
   (D) CT scan

7. Which of the following types of seizure is seen most commonly in children?

   (A) status epilepticus
   (B) febrile seizures
   (C) partial-onset seizures
   (D) absence seizures

8. A five-year-old child is brought into the clinic by a parent who reports that the child refuses to use his right arm after a fall from playing on a merry-go-round. The parent thinks his child may have hyperextended his arm during the fall. The child is sitting calmly with his right arm held close to the body. Vital signs are stable. The nurse practitioner notes some superficial scratches on the arm, but no deformity is observed. The child can move his arm freely in all range of motion positions except supination. What should the nurse practitioner do first?

   (A) order an X-ray of the arm
   (B) contact the local department of human resources for suspected child abuse
   (C) advise the parent to take the child to the emergency department
   (D) gently attempt to hyper-pronate the arm with a combination of supination and flexion movements

9. In an ambulatory care setting, fever of unknown origin (FUO) is defined as:

   (A) fever of greater than 101.3°F.
   (B) fever of greater than 101.3°F that occurs on at least three occasions over a three week period.
   (C) fever of greater than 101.3°F persisting for a one-week period.
   (D) fever of greater than 101.3°F that occurs on at least three occasions over a one-week period.

10. Which of the following statements is true about squamous cell carcinoma in situ?

   (A) The condition is also known as Bowen's disease.
   (B) It is the most common skin cancer.
   (C) This is a benign lesion.
   (D) It is more invasive than other skin cancer types.

11. A nurse practitioner is evaluating a six-year-old child who presents with complaints of severe pain in his scrotal area. Examination reveals a unilateral painful swelling in the left testicle with a lack of cremasteric reflex. Elevation of the scrotum does not relieve the pain. What should the nurse practitioner do next?

    (A) apply a cold compress
    (B) order a testicular ultrasound
    (C) order an X-ray of the scrotal area
    (D) order complete blood count (CBC)

12. A 32-year-old female presents to the clinic with concerns of urinary frequency. She is currently 27 weeks pregnant. She read an article online that said that pregnant women should get a gestational diabetes screening. What is the current recommendation regarding gestational diabetes screening?

    (A) perform an oral glucose tolerance test (OGTT) between 24 and 28 weeks gestation
    (B) order a fasting plasma glucose (FPG) test
    (C) order a hemoglobin A1c test
    (D) perform an in-office finger stick blood glucose test

13. Which of the following individuals is most likely to abuse prescription medications?

    (A) a 13-year-old boy
    (B) a 20-year-old female
    (C) a 35-year-old male
    (D) a 60-year-old female

14. The current average age of menarche in the United States is:

    (A) 11 years.
    (B) 12 years.
    (C) 13 years.
    (D) 14 years.

15. A nurse practitioner may function in all the following roles in hospice care, EXCEPT:

    (A) prescribe supportive medications.
    (B) supervise team care members.
    (C) bill for hospice services.
    (D) recertify for hospice care for a patient with a terminal illness.

16. A nurse practitioner should utilize all the following resources in making clinical decisions, EXCEPT:

    (A) National Guideline Clearinghouse.
    (B) American Academy of Pediatrics.
    (C) Google Health.
    (D) Advisory Committee on Immunization Practices (ACIP).

17. Which of the following encounters can be considered as a new patient visit?

    (A) An out-of-town patient presents to the clinic for the first time and has a primary care provider at home.
    (B) A patient presents for a follow-up appointment concerning blood pressure.
    (C) A patient returns to the clinic for his monthly B12 injection.
    (D) A patient, who has not been to the clinic in two years, presents for care.

18. While reviewing the recommendation guidelines, the nurse practitioner will offer clinical services aligned with the following grades recommended by the USPSTF:

    (A) grade A only.
    (B) grades A and B.
    (C) grades A, B, and C.
    (D) grades A, B, C, and D.

19. The most common bacterial pathogen isolated in acute sinusitis during the summer months is:

    (A) *Streptococcus pneumoniae.*
    (B) *Haemophilus influenzae.*
    (C) *Moraxella catarrhalis.*
    (D) *Staphylococcus aureus.*

20. Which of the following drugs may be a better choice for smoking cessation therapy for a patient presenting with signs and symptoms of depression?

    (A) Nicorette polacrilex (gum)
    (B) bupropion hydrochloride (Zyban)
    (C) varenicline (Chantix)
    (D) Nicoderm CQ

21. The first-line pharmacological treatment for hypertension among the African American population is a thiazide diuretic and:

    (A) a central agonist.
    (B) an angiotensin-converting enzyme (ACE) inhibitor.
    (C) a calcium channel blocker.
    (D) an angiotensin receptor blocker (ARB).

22. Which of the following insulins has a gradual onset with no peak time and a duration of up to 24 hours?

    (A) insulin isophane suspension (NPH)
    (B) insulin glargine
    (C) insulin isophane suspension (NPH)/regular insulin
    (D) regular insulin

23. Which of the following drugs may cause hematuria?

   (A) rifampin
   (B) erythromycin
   (C) glimepiride
   (D) lansoprazole

24. A 16-year-old male presents to the clinic with a complaint of pain and discomfort in his stomach. The symptoms usually subside after meals. According to medical history, the patient had a cholecystectomy when he was 7 years old. Vital signs are within normal limits. Patient denies episodes of nausea or vomiting. During the assessment, the patient reports tenderness on palpation of the epigastric region. What should the nurse practitioner suspect?

   (A) gastroesophageal reflux disease (GERD)
   (B) peptic ulcer disease (PUD)
   (C) gallbladder disease
   (D) angina

25. What are the common manifestations of Parkinson's disease (PD)?

   (A) tremor at rest
   (B) hypotonia
   (C) ptosis
   (D) hyperhidrosis

26. A young couple presents to the clinic with their newly adopted eight-month-old infant for a wellness visit. During the assessment, the nurse practitioner is able to elicit positive Ortolani's and Barlow's signs. The nurse practitioner tells the parents that a referral is warranted for possibility of hip displacement. What type of treatment should the nurse practitioner anticipate for the infant?

   (A) The infant may need surgical intervention.
   (B) The infant may need a Pavlik harness.
   (C) The infant may need a spica cast.
   (D) No treatment is needed at this time.

27. What is the current recommended international normalized ratio (INR) for patients taking warfarin (Coumadin)?

   (A) between 1.0 and 2.0
   (B) between 2.0 and 3.0
   (C) between 3.0 and 4.0
   (D) between 4.0 and 5.0

28. A 15-year-old male athlete presents to the office with acne concerns. The nurse practitioner notes papulopustular, cystic acne on his forehead and chin. The nurse practitioner decides to initiate therapy. Which of the following is the most appropriate choice?

   (A) oral retinoid
   (B) topical clindamycin
   (C) topical benzoyl peroxide
   (D) oral tetracycline

29. All the following medications can be used to treat chronic pelvic pain syndrome (CPPS) in a male patient, EXCEPT:

    (A) terazosin (Hytrin).
    (B) doxazosin (Cardura).
    (C) nitrofurantoin (Macrobid).
    (D) tamsulosin (Flomax).

30. What is the current recommended calcium supplement dosage during pregnancy for a healthy 28-year-old patient?

    (A) 1,300 mg
    (B) 1,000 mg
    (C) 2,000 mg
    (D) 3,000 mg

31. The "party drug" flunitrazepam may produce:

    (A) amnesia.
    (B) seizures.
    (C) delusions.
    (D) agitation.

32. On a physical exam, a child is found to have 10–15 medium-brown-colored café au lait spots that are greater than 1 cm in diameter. Based on this finding, the differential diagnoses should include:

    (A) vitiligo.
    (B) tinea corporis.
    (C) eczema.
    (D) neurofibromatosis (NF).

33. A 67-year-old patient presents for her wellness exam. The nurse practitioner is reviewing her pneumococcal immunization history. The patient received a Prevnar 13 immunization two years ago. Which immunization is due during this visit?

    (A) PCV13
    (B) PPSV23
    (C) PCV13 and PPSV23
    (D) patient's pneumococcal vaccination is up to date

34. Which organization publishes the "Standard of Practice for Nurse Practitioners?"

    (A) Board of Nursing (BON)
    (B) American Nurses Association (ANA)
    (C) Nurse Practice Act (NPA)
    (D) American Association of Nurse Practitioners (AANP)

35. A seven-year-old patient presents to the clinic with pain in her left ear. The nurse practitioner evaluates the patient and determines that she needs a left ear irrigation. Upon completion of the procedure, the nurse practitioner further diagnoses the patient with a left ear infection. The patient is given an antibiotic prescription with instructions to return to the clinic for ear recheck in two weeks. What is the E/M code for this visit?

    (A) 99212
    (B) 99213
    (C) 99211
    (D) 99214

36. A two-year-old is diagnosed with acute bronchiolitis. Which of the measures below would not be part of the management plan?

    (A) humidification/nebulizer treatments
    (B) antipyretics
    (C) antibiotics
    (D) oral steroids

37. All the following common symptoms are present in a patient with cataracts, EXCEPT:

    (A) loss of peripheral vision.
    (B) night vision problem.
    (C) sensitivity to sunlight.
    (D) cloudy lens.

38. Your patient is an 80-year-old male presenting with respiratory symptoms. Pulmonary function studies give the following results:
    Total lung capacity: normal
    PaO_2: decreased
    $PaCO_2$: increased
    On physical examination, you note coarse crackles and forced expiratory wheezes bilaterally. Based on these findings, which diagnosis is most likely?

    (A) chronic asthma
    (B) influenza
    (C) community acquired pneumonia (CAP)
    (D) emphysema

39. Your patient is a young woman with a diagnosis of community-acquired pneumonia (CAP). She was in the office seven days ago and received a prescription for azithromycin. She calls the office to report that she is still having fever and is not feeling much better. What should the nurse practitioner do next?

    (A) increase the dose of azithromycin and continue for another week
    (B) stop the azithromycin and prescribe amoxicillin/clavulanate
    (C) continue the same dose of azithromycin for another seven days
    (D) stop the antibiotic, as the illness must be viral

40. A 34-year-old patient has an average blood glucose of 180 mg/dL and A1c 8%. The nurse practitioner and the patient agree to initiate monotherapy, with a plan to reduce the A1c from 8% to 7% within the next three months. The patient has a glucose meter at home. The nurse practitioner encourages the patient to maintain an average daily glucose of:

(A) 171–186 mg/dL.

(B) 156–170 mg/dL.

(C) 140–155 mg/dL.

(D) 125–139 mg/dL.

41. Which of the following is the most common type of mineral causing renal calculi?

(A) calcium

(B) struvite

(C) uric acid

(D) cysteine

42. A nurse practitioner suspects that a patient may have acute pancreatitis. Which of the following lab tests should be ordered?

(A) serum lipase and amylase

(B) alanine aminotransferase (ALT) and aspartate aminotransferase (AST)

(C) basic metabolic panel (BMP)

(D) serum uric acid measurement

43. A 19-year-old college student presents to the clinic with his roommate. The patient complains of lethargy, mild neck pain, and nausea and vomiting. Symptoms started upon returning from a field trip. During the examination, the nurse practitioner flexes the patient's hips and knees. At the same time, the patient's neck is also passively flexed.
What is the name of this test?

(A) Brudzinski

(B) Kernig

(C) Tinel

(D) Phalen

44. A 55-year-old female patient with stage 3 renal disease is seen for an injury on her right hand and arm. Upon reviewing the X-ray, the nurse practitioner diagnoses her with comminuted fracture of the right radius. What should the nurse practitioner do next?

(A) immobilize the hand, refer the patient to an orthopedic surgeon

(B) order a bone mineral density test

(C) immobilize the hand, prescribe non-steroidal anti-inflammatory drug (NSAID)

(D) prescribe NSAID, follow up in three days

45. A nurse practitioner is readjusting a dosage of warfarin (Coumadin) for a 54-year-old patient. How soon should the nurse practitioner reevaluate the prothrombin time (PT) and international normalized ratio (INR)?

(A) within 48 hours

(B) within three to five days

(C) in two weeks

(D) in one month

46. A 31-year-old patient presents with a pruritic rash that has been present around his waist area for the past two weeks. The nurse practitioner obtained skin scrapings from the affected area and performed a KOH test. Multiple pseudohyphae were noted under the microscope. Based on the findings, which is the appropriate diagnosis?

    (A) candidiasis
    (B) cellulitis
    (C) psoriasis
    (D) folliculitis

47. A 21-year-old male presents with a chief complaint of a "sore" under his scrotum. The patient first noticed a small red bump on his scrotum about a week ago. The lesion then became an open sore. What test should the nurse practitioner order?

    (A) labs to check for other STIs
    (B) CBC
    (C) CMP
    (D) scrotal ultrasound

48. What is the current recommended calcium supplement dosage during pregnancy for a healthy 18-year-old patient?

    (A) 1,300 mg
    (B) 1,000 mg
    (C) 2,000 mg
    (D) 3,000 mg

49. Acute alcohol withdrawal is associated with a multitude of symptoms including delirium tremens, which presents as uncontrollable shaking and tachycardia with mental status changes including agitation and delirium. Which of the following is used in the management of tremors associated with alcohol withdrawal?

    (A) carbamazepine
    (B) Dilantin
    (C) codeine
    (D) clonidine

50. Which of the following will likely decrease the risk for acute otitis media (AOM) in an infant?

    (A) iron supplementation
    (B) daily orange juice
    (C) breastfeeding
    (D) vitamin D supplementation

51. Falls related to hypotension are fairly common in older adults. Medications that may be implicated in orthostatic hypotension include all the following, EXCEPT:

    (A) loop diuretics.
    (B) tricyclic antidepressants.
    (C) calcium channel blockers.
    (D) aminoglycoside antibiotics.

52. The most common bacterial pathogen isolated in acute bacterial rhinosinusitis during the winter months is:

    (A) *Streptococcus pneumoniae.*
    (B) *Haemophilus influenzae.*
    (C) *Moraxella catarrhalis.*
    (D) *Staphylococcus aureus.*

53. The International Classification of Diseases (ICD) was developed to promote international comparability in the collection, classification, processing, and presentation of mortality statistics. Which organization is responsible for updating the classifications?

    (A) Healthy People 2020
    (B) World Health Organization (WHO)
    (C) Centers for Disease Control and Prevention (CDC)
    (D) The North Atlantic Treaty Organization (NATO)

54. Recommended monotherapy for management of community-acquired pneumonia caused by *Streptococcus pneumonia* is:

    (A) IV ceftriaxone.
    (B) IV vancomycin.
    (C) amoxicillin/clavulanate.
    (D) doxycycline.

55. Your patient is a six-month-old male who is brought to the clinic by his mother. Mother reports the baby has had a fever for a day or two and does not want to eat. She tells you he only sleeps a couple of hours at a time and wakes up crying. Upon physical examination, you note mild rhinitis, clear oropharynx, and eyes without redness or drainage. Otoscopic exam of the ears demonstrates a bright red, bulging, tympanic membrane (TM) in the right ear. The left TM is pearly gray with fluid noted behind the TM. Based on this presentation, the diagnosis is most likely:

    (A) acute otitis externa (AOE).
    (B) acute otitis media (AOM).
    (C) acute upper respiratory infection (URI).
    (D) none of the above.

56. The most common presenting symptom of bronchitis is:

    (A) fever.
    (B) cough.
    (C) purulent sputum.
    (D) wheezing.

57. Your patient has a diagnosis of aortic stenosis. Which of the following statements is true regarding this diagnosis?

    (A) Aortic stenosis usually presents acutely with disabling symptoms of dyspnea and angina.
    (B) Life expectancy following diagnosis is usually 10 years.
    (C) Aortic stenosis is diagnosed most often in the fourth decade of life.
    (D) Cardinal symptoms of aortic stenosis include syncope, heart failure, and dyspnea on exertion (which progresses to dyspnea at rest).

58. What is a common side effect of metformin (Glucophage)?

   (A) weight gain
   (B) swelling of legs
   (C) headache
   (D) gastrointestinal disturbance

59. Your patient is a 24-year-old female with a chief complaint of dysuria. Urine dip in the office is positive for bacteria, with a small amount of blood. The patient has no other medical problems and has no allergies. She has not been prescribed antibiotics in at least one year. First-line recommendation for treatment of uncomplicated cystitis includes all the following, EXCEPT:

   (A) nitrofurantoin.
   (B) trimethoprim-sulfamethoxazole.
   (C) cephalexin.
   (D) azithromycin.

60. Which of the following lab results may help the nurse practitioner confirm a diagnosis of appendicitis in patients with an atypical presentation?

   (A) total WBCs, 11,000/mm^3; neutrophils, 30%; lymphocytes, 40%; bands, 2%
   (B) total WBCs, 17,000/mm^3; neutrophils, 80%; lymphocytes, 20%; bands, 9%
   (C) total WBCs, 12,000/mm^3; neutrophils, 60%; lymphocytes, 45%; bands, 3%
   (D) total WBCs, 16,000/mm^3; neutrophils, 55%; lymphocytes, 30%; bands, 4%

61. Which of the following is the most sensitive method in the evaluation of a patient with encephalitis caused by herpes simplex virus?

   (A) computed tomography (CT) scan
   (B) magnetic resonance imaging (MRI)
   (C) electroencephalography (EEG)
   (D) cerebrospinal fluid (CSF)

62. Your patient is a 62-year-old female with a chief complaint of foot pain. On examination, you note focal tenderness on palpation over the area of the plantar fascia. This is suggestive of:

   (A) a ligamentous injury.
   (B) plantar fasciitis.
   (C) a bone spur.
   (D) gout.

63. A six-year-old child comes to the clinic for follow-up with a nurse practitioner for an evaluation of iron deficiency. Previous clinical labs show hemoglobin is 8.3 g/dL and a hematocrit of 30%. The patient was prescribed 3 mg/kg/day of elemental iron for four weeks. The current lab work shows hemoglobin of 9.8 g/dL and hematocrit of 34%. What should the nurse practitioner do next?

   (A) increase the ferrous sulfate to 6 mg/kg/day and recheck labs in two months
   (B) continue the ferrous sulfate 3 mg/kg/day and recheck labs in two months
   (C) reduce the ferrous sulfate to 1 mg/kg/day and recheck labs in two months
   (D) discontinue the ferrous sulfate and recheck labs in two months

64. A six-year-old child presents to the clinic accompanied by a parent, who reports the child has been complaining of itchiness on both hands. The child has recently returned from a sleepover party. The nurse practitioner notices several erythematous papules and linear burrows in the interdigital web spaces on both hands. What is the appropriate diagnosis?

   (A) lice
   (B) tinea manuum
   (C) scabies
   (D) atopic dermatitis

65. All the following options are risk factors for prostate cancer, EXCEPT:

   (A) long-distance cycling.
   (B) positive family history.
   (C) African American ethnicity.
   (D) commercial truck driving.

66. All the following medications are only taken *once a month* for treatment of osteoporosis, EXCEPT:

   (A) zoledronic acid (Reclast)
   (B) ibandronate sodium (Boniva).
   (C) alendronate sodium (Fosamax).
   (D) risedronate sodium (Actonel).

67. Your patient is a 35-year-old male who presents with persistent thoughts about being dirty and becoming contaminated. He is constantly washing his hands, and he takes showers and changes his clothes several times a day. This behavior is consistent with:

   (A) generalized anxiety disorder (GAD).
   (B) post-traumatic stress disorder (PTSD).
   (C) bipolar disorder (BD).
   (D) obsessive-compulsive disorder (OCD).

68. Your patient is a seven-month-old male who is in for his episodic well-child visit. He is sitting in his mother's lap. You begin the exam with:

   (A) palpating the abdomen.
   (B) auscultating the heart and lungs.
   (C) examining the head and eyes.
   (D) checking reflexes.

69. An elderly patient presents to your office with a new diagnosis of iron-deficiency anemia. What is your next step?

   (A) prescribe iron and follow up in three months
   (B) refer to GI for a colonoscopy
   (C) order a repeat CBC to confirm results
   (D) take a detailed diet history

70. A certification candidate failed his family nurse practitioner certification exam recently. There is a 60-day waiting period before the candidate can retake the exam. During this waiting period, the candidate started to use his APRN title. This is inappropriate because family nurse practitioner title protection is held through the:

    (A) Board of Nursing (BON).
    (B) American Nurses Association (ANA).
    (C) Nurse Practice Act (NPA).
    (D) American Association of Nurse Practitioners (AANP).

71. The International Classification of Diseases (ICD)-9 is based on data collected between 1979 and 1998. What is the current accepted version of ICD to use in coding?

    (A) ICD-12
    (B) ICD-11
    (C) ICD-10
    (D) ICD-13

72. A family nurse practitioner is reviewing the efficacy of a new drug in managing the reduction of blood pressure for one of her patients. The report states the following:
    "Following oral administration of Drug X, the onset of diuresis occurs in 15–30 minutes. Peak activity is reached between 1 and 2 hours. The diuretic action lasts for 8–10 hours."
    Based on the statement, and assuming that this is a once-a-day fixed dose oral drug, what would be a good time for a patient to take this medication?

    (A) 8:00 A.M.
    (B) 12:00 P.M.
    (C) 4:00 P.M.
    (D) 8:00 P.M.

73. A patient reporting a gradual, painless, progressive loss of vision with complaints of glare at night and photophobia should be evaluated for:

    (A) glaucoma.
    (B) cataracts.
    (C) macular degeneration.
    (D) retinopathy.

74. Which of the following antithrombotic medications requires lab monitoring?

    (A) apixaban (Eliquis)
    (B) rivaroxaban (Xarelto)
    (C) warfarin (Coumadin)
    (D) dabigatran (Pradaxa)

75. The definitive test to confirm the diagnosis of acute gout attack is:

    (A) synovial fluid analysis.
    (B) serum uric acid level.
    (C) complete blood count (CBC).
    (D) C-reactive protein.

76. Your patient is a 23-year-old female with complaints of burning with urination, frequency, and urgency. On urine dip, leukocytes are positive, and nitrites are negative. Which of the following should you consider?

(A) The patient is taking antibiotics.
(B) The patient has a sexually transmitted infection (STI).
(C) The patient has a kidney stone.
(D) The patient is pregnant.

77. All the following are common causes of sensorineural hearing loss, EXCEPT:

(A) presbycusis.
(B) acoustic neuroma.
(C) otitis externa.
(D) Meniere's disease.

78. Gastroesophageal reflux disease (GERD) may present with atypical symptoms. Which of the following would NOT likely be associated with GERD?

(A) cough
(B) rhinitis
(C) pneumonia
(D) wheezing

79. A tumor of the eighth cranial nerve may cause which of the following?

(A) loss of sense of smell
(B) inability to open and close the eyes
(C) taste abnormalities
(D) dizziness

80. Your patient is a 26-year-old male who presents with complaints of aching pain in the neck and the cervical paraspinal muscles of the back. He tells you he has been having muscle spasms and stiffness of the upper back and shoulder for about four to five weeks. This presentation may indicate:

(A) cervical myelopathy.
(B) cervical radiculopathy.
(C) mechanical neck pain.
(D) mechanical neck pain with whiplash.

81. Iron deficiency anemia is the most prevalent cause of:

(A) microcytic anemia.
(B) macrocytic anemia.
(C) pernicious anemia.
(D) normocytic anemia.

82. A 47-year-old patient presents with fever, chills, severe malaise, headache, and butterfly rash over the cheeks. The FNP suspects that the patient may have erysipelas. What should the nurse practitioner do next?

(A) order permethrin cream 1% (Nix)
(B) refer the patient to the emergency department
(C) order topical metronidazole
(D) order oral tetracycline

83. A 35-year-old male comes to the clinic with a chief complaint of scrotal pain that radiates to the left flank. On examination, you note swelling of the left testicle with thick, indurated scrotal skin. Based on this presentation, what is the diagnosis?

(A) Peyronie's disease
(B) orchitis
(C) testicular torsion
(D) epididymitis

84. A nurse practitioner is evaluating an inconclusive mammogram report on her 31-year-old obese patient. The patient presented with a nodule on her right breast and has a two-generation family history of breast cancer. What should the nurse practitioner do next?

(A) order a follow-up mammogram
(B) order a breast biopsy
(C) order breast ultrasound
(D) order a complete blood count (CBC)

85. All the following diagnoses are considered mood disorders, EXCEPT:

(A) bipolar disorder.
(B) schizoaffective disorder.
(C) seasonal affective disorder (SAD).
(D) agoraphobia.

86. A two-week-old infant is brought in for his well-child exam. Upon physical examination, you notice a dimple right above the sacral area. There is a small tuft of hair in the dimple. This finding is suggestive of:

(A) hirsutism.
(B) Arnold-Chiari malformation.
(C) spina bifida occulta.
(D) neurofibromatosis.

87. The United States Preventive Services Task Force (USPSTF) recommends screening for hepatitis C in which age group?

(A) those born before 1935
(B) those born between 1935 and 1955
(C) those born between 1945 and 1965
(D) those born between 1965 and 1985

88. Which of the following acts was enacted to ensure that only individuals with a legitimate reason to do so will have access to patient information?

    (A) Health Insurance for Patient Access and Availability
    (B) Health Insurance Portability and Accountability Act
    (C) Health Insurance Protection of Access and Availability
    (D) Health Insurance Protection, Access, and Accountability

89. A nurse practitioner is performing a wellness exam on a 65-year-old Medicare patient. The nurse practitioner is expected to be reimbursed at which percentage of the physician rate for the same medical services provided.

    (A) 85%
    (B) 100%
    (C) 80%
    (D) 90%

90. For a clinical question about a medical intervention, what is considered the highest level of evidence?

    (A) meta-analysis
    (B) synthesis of evidence
    (C) randomized controlled trial
    (D) systematic review

91. Mark is an 86-year-old male who is on chronic digoxin therapy. His family reports that Mark is having increasing problems with memory. His chief complaint today is, "I'm just not feeling well." Mark has not had labs in 12 months and the nurse practitioner is concerned about his digoxin level. Common symptoms of digoxin toxicity include:

    (A) tingling in the extremities.
    (B) nausea and vomiting.
    (C) generalized rash.
    (D) headache.

92. A patient with a diagnosis of Graves' disease will likely have:

    (A) an elevated alkaline phosphatase level.
    (B) an elevated T3 level.
    (C) an elevated thyroid stimulating hormone (TSH) level.
    (D) elevated liver function studies.

93. Renal artery stenosis may lead to renal failure if untreated or undiagnosed. One early indicator of possible renal artery stenosis is the presence of:

    (A) coarctation of the aorta (COA).
    (B) decreased glomerular filtration rate (GFR).
    (C) increased blood pressure.
    (D) decreased urine production.

94. Which of the following components is most important in the diagnosis of acute appendicitis?

    (A) serum sedimentation rate
    (B) CBC with differential
    (C) kidney, ureter, and bladder (KUB) X-ray
    (D) history and physical

95. On examination of a two-week-old infant, you note irritability, poor appetite, and rapid head growth. Distended veins are seen on the scalp. This presentation suggests:

    (A) hydrocephalus.
    (B) meningitis.
    (C) cerebral palsy.
    (D) Reye's syndrome

96. A 56-year-old male reports a burning, stinging pain around the buttocks area, with extension down the back of the right leg and some numbness and tingling. This presentation suggests:

    (A) sciatica.
    (B) herniated disc.
    (C) osteoarthritis.
    (D) cervical radiculopathy.

97. A family nurse practitioner is reviewing a hematology report on a 39-year-old patient with beta-thalassemia minor and notes a hemoglobin level of 10 g/dL. What should the nurse practitioner do next?

    (A) refer the patient back to the oncologist
    (B) check the serum ferritin level
    (C) give a fluid bolus with IV normal saline
    (D) prescribe ferrous sulfate 300 mg/day PO

98. What is the first line treatment for rosacea manifesting as inflammatory papules, pustules, and telangiectasias located on the central third of the face?

    (A) oral tetracycline
    (B) oral doxycycline
    (C) oral minocycline
    (D) topical metronidazole

99. A 40-year-old male is seen with symptoms of fever, chills, low back pain, myalgia, and tenesmus (painful anal contractions). Your evaluation should include all the following, EXCEPT:

    (A) urinalysis.
    (B) CBC.
    (C) prostatic massage.
    (D) rectal exam.

100. A 15-year-old patient asks the nurse practitioner to initiate a pain management plan for her fibrocystic breast disease with danazol (Danocrine). How should the nurse practitioner respond to the patient?

   (A) Many patients do not like the side effects of danazol.
   (B) Danazol is the drug of choice for fibrocystic breast disease.
   (C) A short-term course of seven-day treatment is preferred.
   (D) Danazol is not the right medication for you.

101. The usual first-line recommendation for management of major depressive disorder (MDD) is:

   (A) tricyclic antidepressants (TCA).
   (B) monoamine oxidase inhibitors (MAOIs).
   (C) selective serotonin reuptake inhibitors (SSRIs).
   (D) all of the above.

102. During growth and development, an infant learns to move the shoulder before learning to control finger movement. This is an example of which type of development?

   (A) proximodistal
   (B) cephalocaudal
   (C) general to specific
   (D) central to peripheral

103. Current requirements for patient hospice care reimbursement by Medicare include eligibility for Medicare Part A, physician and hospice medical director certification of terminal illness with a prognosis of six months or less, care provided by a Medicare-approved program, and:

   (A) patient-given informed consent for palliative care instead of cure.
   (B) availability of a family or support-caregiver.
   (C) requirement of intensive pain management.
   (D) all of the above.

104. What is the pedigree sign for a healthy male?

   (A) empty square
   (B) empty circle
   (C) filled in square
   (D) filled in circle

105. Which of the following is true concerning evidence-based practice (EBP)?

   (A) Decision-making is shared.
   (B) The process begins with a clinical question.
   (C) The process is used to improve patient care.
   (D) All of the above

106. The discovery of an S3 heart sound in an elderly patient may indicate:

   (A) aortic stenosis.
   (B) mitral stenosis.
   (C) heart failure.
   (D) hypertensive heart disease.

107. The most appropriate screening test for diabetic nephropathy is:

    (A) creatinine clearance.

    (B) serum creatinine level.

    (C) BUN/creatinine ratio.

    (D) microalbuminuria level.

108. Acute kidney injury (AKI) is the rapid deterioration of renal function with an inability to maintain fluid and electrolyte balance and prevent the accumulation of toxic waste products. The definition of AKI requires a rise in the serum creatinine level or a significant decrease in urine output for more than six hours. Injury may occur prerenal, renal, and postrenal. All of the following are prerenal causes of AKI, EXCEPT:

    (A) hemorrhage.

    (B) radiocontrast agents.

    (C) cardiac failure.

    (D) sepsis.

109. Your patient is a 24-year-old male with a diagnosis of giardia after an extended backpacking trip. Which of the following is recommended for management of giardia?

    (A) vancomycin

    (B) metronidazole

    (C) penicillin

    (D) trimethoprim-sulfamethoxazole

110. Prophylactic treatment for migraine headaches may include all of the following classes of medications, EXCEPT:

    (A) beta blockers (BBs).

    (B) tricyclic antidepressants (TCAs).

    (C) anticonvulsants.

    (D) 5-HT-1 agonists.

111. The clinical presentation of fatigue and symmetrical stiffness and pain of multiple joints that is severe in the morning and persists for several hours is consistent with:

    (A) osteoarthritis.

    (B) rheumatoid arthritis.

    (C) systemic lupus erythematosus.

    (D) gouty arthritis.

112. Which of the following is the most sensitive method for diagnosing sickle cell disease?

    (A) bone marrow biopsy

    (B) hemoglobin and hematocrit

    (C) CBC with peripheral smear

    (D) hemoglobin electrophoresis

113. A 27-year-old woman who is three months pregnant recently spent time in a hot tub while on vacation. The patient has discrete, erythematous 1–2 mm papules that are centered around hair follicles around the abdomen and trunk area. How will the nurse practitioner manage this condition?

   (A) prescribe topical keratolytics and topical antibiotics
   (B) order a culture
   (C) prescribe sulfamethoxazole/trimethoprim (Bactrim)
   (D) prescribe tetracycline (Sumycin)

114. Your patient is a 68-year-old who has been taking finasteride for the past six months for a diagnosis of benign prostatic hyperplasia (BPH). When you check his PSA level today, you notice that there is no change. Your initial expectation would be that:

   (A) his PSA level should have gone down if the elevation was due to BPH.
   (B) it is normal for there to be no change in his PSA level at this time.
   (C) you need to increase his dose of finasteride.
   (D) his PSA should have gone up because of the effect of the alpha-adrenergic antagonist.

115. The highest incidence and mortality rates for lung cancer are found in:

   (A) African American men.
   (B) Caucasian women.
   (C) Asian men.
   (D) Caucasian men.

116. In screening for alcohol abuse in elderly adults, which screen is appropriate?

   (A) PHQ 2
   (B) CAGE
   (C) PHQ 9
   (D) MMSE

117. A two-year-old child with sickle cell anemia (SCA) should receive which immunizations?

   (A) all routine immunizations, but at an accelerated schedule
   (B) all routine immunizations, but at a decelerated schedule
   (C) all routine immunizations according to CDC schedule
   (D) individualized and limited immunizations

118. Patient confidentiality may be breached when:

   (A) medical information is provided to an adult child.
   (B) medical records are sent to the public health department.
   (C) medical records are given to insurance companies.
   (D) medical records are subpoenaed for a legal proceeding.

119. A patient report of severe cramping and pain in his legs while walking or running that is relieved by rest suggests a diagnosis of:

   (A) intermittent claudication.
   (B) Raynaud's disease.
   (C) atherosclerotic disease.
   (D) neurogenic claudication.

120. A patient has a differential diagnosis of primary adrenal insufficiency. His 8:00 A.M. cortisol level is low. What is expected with regard to his other lab results?

    (A) elevated aldosterone level
    (B) elevated plasma ACTH level
    (C) decreased plasma ACTH level
    (D) decreased aldosterone level

121. You receive an endoscopic pathology report on a patient with gastroesophageal reflux disease (GERD). The report notes the presence of Barrett's epithelium. In discussing the results with the patient, which of the following is correct?

    (A) Barrett's epithelium is premalignant tissue.
    (B) Barrett's epithelium supports esophageal healing.
    (C) Barrett's epithelium is resistant to erosive effects of gastric acid.
    (D) All of the above

122. An elderly male patient presents with an abrupt onset of a unilateral headache located around the right temple area. He describes the pain as excruciating and marked tenderness is noted on gentle palpation of the area. This presentation is suggestive of:

    (A) Bell's palsy.
    (B) temporal arteritis.
    (C) cerebrovascular accident (CVA).
    (D) transient ischemic attack (TIA).

123. A nurse practitioner is evaluating a patient with complaints of flu-like symptoms. The patient has a mild elevation of fever (100.3°F). Physical assessment is inconclusive. The patient underwent a splenectomy two months ago. Which of the following supports initiation of empiric antibiotic therapy?

    (A) The patient is at high risk of bleeding disorders.
    (B) The patient is more likely to demonstrate worsening anemia.
    (C) The patient is at increased risk of hepatomegaly.
    (D) The patient is susceptible to infection.

124. A furuncle is usually caused by which of the following pathogens?

    (A) *Staphylococcus aureus*
    (B) *Streptococcus pneumoniae*
    (C) *Haemophilus influenzae*
    (D) *Moraxella catarrhalis*

125. A 17-year-old female presents to your office with a chief concern about never having a period. She reports that she has never had any menstrual bleeding and she is worried something is wrong. You discuss with her some of the causes of primary amenorrhea. Which of the following is NOT a cause of primary amenorrhea?

    (A) ovarian dysfunction
    (B) pregnancy
    (C) imperforate hymen
    (D) type 1 diabetes mellitus

126. Nurse practitioners obtain their legal right to practice from:

    (A) Centers for Medicare and Medicaid Services (CMS).
    (B) the board of nursing where they practice.
    (C) laws of the state where they practice.
    (D) the Nurse Practice Act.

127. Your patient is a six-year-old who has type 1 DM. Her mother brought her in today because of an area of cellulitis on her lower leg. While examining her, you notice the patient has deep, rapid respirations and a fruity odor to her breath. You suspect:

    (A) hypoglycemia.
    (B) Stevens-Johnson syndrome (SJS).
    (C) ketoacidosis.
    (D) sepsis.

128. A nurse practitioner diagnoses a nine-year-old patient with mononucleosis. There is no medication prescribed during the visit. The nurse practitioner warns the patient and parent of the danger of participating in contact sports during this time. How long should the patient wait before being able to participate in sports?

    (A) one week
    (B) two weeks
    (C) three weeks
    (D) four weeks

129. A nurse practitioner diagnoses a college student with varicella. How soon can the student return to class?

    (A) one week
    (B) two weeks
    (C) three days without a fever
    (D) once all vesicles have crusted over

130. A 15-year-old female who has been prescribed combined oral contraceptives for birth control is seen in the clinic for a prescription refill. While discussing how she is doing, the patient tells you her acne has become a lot worse since she started the pill. To address this problem, you prescribe a combined oral contraceptive with:

    (A) increased estrogen content.
    (B) increased estrogen and progestin content.
    (C) the same levels of estrogen and progestin, but a different brand name.
    (D) decreased progestin content.

131. The ethical concept of autonomy refers to:

    (A) the nurse practitioner's right to autonomous practice.
    (B) the patient's right to make decisions about his or her own health care.
    (C) the provider's right to accept or deny patient admittance to their practice.
    (D) none of the above.

132. The drug of choice for management of acute anaphylaxis is:

    (A) diphenhydramine IV or 25–100 mg PO QID for adults.
    (B) epinephrine 1:1,000 0.3–0.5 mL SubQ for adults.
    (C) prednisone 2 mg/kg/day PO in a single dose and then a prednisone taper for one to two weeks.
    (D) amlodipine besylate 5 mg QID for four weeks.

133. Your patient is a 42-year-old man who presents with concerns about a lesion on his face. He reports that it has been there awhile but does seem to be getting bigger. On exam, you find a lesion with a depressed center, firm elevated border, and telangiectatic vessels throughout. This finding is most consistent with:

    (A) squamous cell carcinoma.
    (B) basal cell carcinoma.
    (C) malignant melanoma.
    (D) Kaposi's sarcoma.

134. Your patient is a 26-year-old female who is 12 hours postpartum. Amniotic fluid embolism is a devastating complication associated with childbirth. All of the following symptoms are consistent with a diagnosis of amniotic fluid embolism, EXCEPT:

    (A) respiratory distress.
    (B) fever.
    (C) hypotension.
    (D) seizures.

135. What is the primary purpose of professional licensure?

    (A) to protect the public by ensuring a minimum level of competence
    (B) to regulate professional practice
    (C) to monitor numbers of professionals in an area
    (D) to ensure academic equality

136. Polycythemia vera is an acquired myeloproliferative disease that causes excessive production of all blood cell lines. Patients present with headache, dizziness, blurred vision, and fatigue. Treatment of choice for this condition is:

    (A) oral ferrous sulfate TID.
    (B) systemic corticosteroids.
    (C) chemotherapy.
    (D) repeated phlebotomy.

137. Permethrin lotion is applied over the entire body from the neck down and left on for 8–14 hours before showering off. This is recommended in the treatment of:

    (A) scabies.
    (B) eczema.
    (C) herpes simplex.
    (D) psoriasis.

138. Condyloma acuminata is a genital condition that presents with wart-like growths in the ano-genital region. The cause of the disease is human papillomavirus, which has several types. Genital warts are usually caused by which types?

    (A) 6 and 11
    (B) 11 and 16
    (C) 19 and 24
    (D) 31 and 33

139. A nurse practitioner was able to manage a patient's weight loss without the intervention of conventional medication treatment. She plans to disseminate her patient's treatment outcome with the community members. The nurse practitioner should write a:

    (A) case study.
    (B) prospective population study.
    (C) meta-analysis.
    (D) retrospective population study.

140. Folate acid deficiency produces which of the following RBC indices?

    (A) microcytic, hypochromic
    (B) macrocytic, hypochromic
    (C) microcytic, normochromic
    (D) macrocytic, normochromic

141. A patient presents with silvery, scaly plaques on the extensor surfaces of both arms. This finding is consistent with:

    (A) hyperthyroidism.
    (B) scleroderma.
    (C) psoriasis.
    (D) eczema.

142. Which of the following genital conditions is associated with increased vaginal discharge that contains numerous white blood cells?

    (A) herpes simplex virus type 2
    (B) chlamydia
    (C) vaginitis
    (D) vaginosis

143. Problem-focused outpatient visits require documentation of:

    (A) chief complaint and brief HPI.
    (B) chief complaint, brief HPI, focused ROS, and PMH.
    (C) chief complaint, HPI, ROS, PMH, and FMH.
    (D) chief complaint, HPI, expanded ROS, PMH, and FMH.

144. Your patient is a 24-year-old male with HIV. He comes to the clinic for routine labs. The results indicate that his viral load is decreasing. What does this indicate?

(A) disease progression

(B) the need for increased doses of antiretroviral medications

(C) that the medications are working

(D) that the patient can no longer transmit the virus

145. Your patient is a six-year-old girl with a cluster of vesicles with weeping, honey-colored crusts just beneath her nostrils. The diagnosis is most likely:

(A) varicella.

(B) impetigo.

(C) herpes simplex.

(D) shingles.

146. Your patient is a 21-year-old female with a recent diagnosis of endometriosis. During the visit today, you discuss the condition along with causes. The primary symptom of endometriosis is:

(A) amenorrhea.

(B) hypermenorrhea.

(C) recurrent pelvic pain.

(D) fever.

147. Which type of malpractice insurance will cover a nurse practitioner for a lawsuit brought sometime in the future, even if the NP no longer carries that insurance?

(A) claims-based malpractice

(B) occurrence-type malpractice

(C) comprehensive malpractice

(D) tail coverage

148. Your female patient presents with a chief complaint of vaginal discharge. On pelvic examination, you note profuse, odorous, frothy, green discharge. Based on these findings, which diagnosis is most likely?

(A) trichomoniasis

(B) chlamydia

(C) syphilis

(D) primary HSV2

149. The method of billing Medicare in which outpatient services are rendered by non-physician providers and billed under the physician's billing number is called:

(A) secondary billing.

(B) Medicare fraud.

(C) "incident-to" billing.

(D) third-party billing.

150. An 11-year-old out of town patient presents to the clinic with concerns of pain in his left ear. He has never been to this clinic. According to his father, the patient was diagnosed with a left ear infection two weeks ago in their hometown. He completed all of his medication without any adverse effects. The nurse practitioner evaluates the patient's left ear and concludes that there is no sign of new infection. The NP further suggests that the patient take ibuprofen to relieve the pain symptoms. The NP spends approximately 20 minutes in the room with the patient. What is the E/M code for this visit?

(A) 99202

(B) 99204

(C) 99205

(D) 99203

ANSWER KEY
Practice Test 2

AANPCB-Style

1. **(A)**	36. **(C)**	71. **(C)**	106. **(C)**	141. **(C)**
2. **(C)**	37. **(A)**	72. **(A)**	107. **(D)**	142. **(C)**
3. **(A)**	38. **(D)**	73. **(B)**	108. **(B)**	143. **(A)**
4. **(A)**	39. **(B)**	74. **(C)**	109. **(B)**	144. **(C)**
5. **(B)**	40. **(B)**	75. **(A)**	110. **(D)**	145. **(B)**
6. **(A)**	41. **(A)**	76. **(B)**	111. **(B)**	146. **(C)**
7. **(B)**	42. **(A)**	77. **(C)**	112. **(D)**	147. **(B)**
8. **(D)**	43. **(A)**	78. **(B)**	113. **(A)**	148. **(A)**
9. **(B)**	44. **(A)**	79. **(D)**	114. **(A)**	149. **(C)**
10. **(A)**	45. **(B)**	80. **(C)**	115. **(A)**	150. **(D)**
11. **(B)**	46. **(A)**	81. **(A)**	116. **(B)**	
12. **(A)**	47. **(A)**	82. **(B)**	117. **(C)**	
13. **(B)**	48. **(A)**	83. **(D)**	118. **(A)**	
14. **(C)**	49. **(D)**	84. **(B)**	119. **(A)**	
15. **(D)**	50. **(C)**	85. **(D)**	120. **(B)**	
16. **(C)**	51. **(D)**	86. **(C)**	121. **(A)**	
17. **(A)**	52. **(B)**	87. **(C)**	122. **(B)**	
18. **(B)**	53. **(B)**	88. **(B)**	123. **(D)**	
19. **(A)**	54. **(D)**	89. **(A)**	124. **(A)**	
20. **(B)**	55. **(B)**	90. **(A)**	125. **(D)**	
21. **(C)**	56. **(B)**	91. **(B)**	126. **(D)**	
22. **(B)**	57. **(D)**	92. **(B)**	127. **(C)**	
23. **(A)**	58. **(D)**	93. **(C)**	128. **(D)**	
24. **(B)**	59. **(D)**	94. **(D)**	129. **(D)**	
25. **(A)**	60. **(B)**	95. **(A)**	130. **(D)**	
26. **(A)**	61. **(B)**	96. **(A)**	131. **(B)**	
27. **(B)**	62. **(B)**	97. **(B)**	132. **(B)**	
28. **(C)**	63. **(B)**	98. **(D)**	133. **(B)**	
29. **(C)**	64. **(C)**	99. **(C)**	134. **(B)**	
30. **(B)**	65. **(D)**	100. **(A)**	135. **(A)**	
31. **(A)**	66. **(A)**	101. **(C)**	136. **(D)**	
32. **(D)**	67. **(D)**	102. **(A)**	137. **(A)**	
33. **(B)**	68. **(B)**	103. **(A)**	138. **(A)**	
34. **(D)**	69. **(B)**	104. **(A)**	139. **(A)**	
35. **(D)**	70. **(C)**	105. **(D)**	140. **(D)**	

Answer Explanations

1. **(A)** *Pseudomonas aeruginosa* is commonly found in acute otitis externa. The causative bacteria associated with acute otitis media are *Streptococcus pneumoniae* (40–50% in adult), *Haemophilus influenzae* (10–30%), and *Moraxella* (*Branhamella*) *catarrhalis* (a majority of which express the beta-lactamase gene and are resistant to first-line penicillin and cephalosporin antibiotics).

2. **(C)** Ultrasound uses high-frequency sound waves to evaluate internal organs and structures. Unlike X-ray, ultrasound does not expose the patient to radiation. Risk factors associated with lung cancer include exposure to benzopyrene and radon, mustard gas, uranium mining (nickel and chromium particles), asbestos, arsenic fumes, nuclear bombs, and radiation, either intentional exposure via medical procedure/treatment or unintentional exposure from the environment.

3. **(A)** In the general population, pharmacological treatment for hypertension should be initiated at: 60 years and older: > 150/90. Younger than 60: > 140/90. In patients 18 or older with diabetes or CKD, pharmacological treatment should be initiated at > 140/90. A majority of the aging population will have GERD symptoms. Taking age into consideration, the 93-year-old does not need antihypertensive therapy. The 33-year-old has a blood pressure of 140/90 and a BMI of 25. Antihypertensive pharmacotherapy is not indicated at this point for this patient.

4. **(A)** The most common causes of gynecomastia in male teenagers are puberty (25%), idiopathic (25%), drug related (15%), cirrhosis or malnutrition (10%), and testicular failure (10%). Gynecomastia is enlargement of breast tissue in males. The condition may present unilaterally or bilaterally and is often a source of shame or embarrassment for teenage boys. The condition, occurring during puberty, usually resolves without intervention within a year or two. The condition affects 12–40% of males in the United States general population and the majority (40–60%) of men after the age of 50.

5. **(B)** The majority of urinary tract infections are caused by *Escherichia coli* (60–80%), with *Staphylococcus saprophyticus* (5–20%) as the second most common pathogen. Complicated urinary tract infections are caused by *Proteus mirabilis*, *Klebsiella*, *Enterobacter*, *Serratia*, and *Pseudomonas*.

6. **(A)** Esophagogastroduodenoscopy (EGD) is recommended by the College of Physicians as part of the best practice in primary care to screen adult patients presenting with heartburn, dysphagia, and weight loss. Ambulatory esophageal pH monitoring is suggested when a patient is unresponsive to four weeks of empiric therapy for GERD. This is the most accurate method to diagnose GERD, as it involves placing a pH probe 5 cm above the lower esophageal sphincter. Chest X-ray and CT scan are not the recommended diagnostic tests with the presented symptoms.

7. **(B)** Febrile seizures are the most common type of seizures in children. They are usually brief, presenting concurrently with other illnesses associated with rapid changes of body temperature. Status epilepticus is a condition during which seizures occur continuously without recovery between episodes. Partial-onset seizures involve a loss of awareness and/or consciousness along with changes in sensory and muscular systems. Absence seizures may last between 15 and 30 seconds. The patient abruptly stops whatever activity they are doing (and may appear to stare into space). The person will recover without any lingering confusion or other ill effects.

8. **(D)** Based on the description, this may be a case of nursemaid elbow, where an annular liga-ment was displaced due to trauma. A reduction technique can be used, as described. If this fails to move the ligament back into place, the arm should be immobilized and the patient referred to orthopedics. An X-ray may not provide any information about this type of injury. There is no information provided that indicates contacting DHR is appropriate.

9. **(B)** In an ambulatory care setting, fever of unknown origin (FUO) is defined as fever of greater than 101.3°F that occurs on at least three occasions over a three-week period. In a hospital setting, FUO is defined as fever of greater than 101.3°F that persists for a one-week period.

10. **(A)** Squamous cell carcinoma in situ is also known as Bowen's disease and is an early stage of skin cancer that develops from squamous cells. It is slow-growing and less invasive than other types of skin cancer. Basal cell carcinoma is the most common skin cancer.

11. **(B)** A patient suspected of having testicular torsion requires an immediate testicular ultra-sound. If an ultrasound cannot be obtained, refer the patient to the emergency department. Urologist detorsion of the organ and restoration of testicular blood flow are crucial within the first six hours or testicle loss will occur.

12. **(A)** The oral glucose tolerance test is used to screen pregnant women for gestational diabetes between 24 and 28 weeks of pregnancy. Other options may provide the status of the glucose level, but they are not the recommended screening method for gestational diabetes.

13. **(B)** Research indicates that young adults between the ages of 18 and 25 are more likely to abuse prescription medications than other age groups.

14. **(C)** Menarche usually occurs between ages 11 and 15. The current (2020) average menarche age in the United States is 13 years.

15. **(D)** The nurse practitioner may prescribe medications or treatments, supervise or manage medical care, and bill for services associated with hospice care just as a physician would. However, a nurse practitioner may not recertify hospice care for a patient who is terminally ill. Only medical physicians (MD, DO) can certify or recertify hospice service for a patient who is terminally ill.

16. **(C)** Google Health is utilizing artificial intelligence algorithms that are presumably accurate to promote data sharing. However, nurse practitioners should refer to the conventional, cred-ible websites for making informed medical decisions.

17. **(A)** According to the 2018 CPT manual, a new patient is one who has not received any face-to-face professional services from the physician/qualified health care professional or another physician/qualified health care professional, who belongs to the same group practice, within the past three years.

18. **(B)** In a primary care setting, nurse practitioners should offer clinical services aligned with recommendation of grades A and B by the USPSTF. Grade C services should only be offered to patients with individual circumstances, as the net benefit is small. Grade D interventions should not be offered.

19. **(A)** The most common bacterial pathogens isolated in acute sinusitis are *Streptococcus pneu-moniae* (40%, particularly during summer and fall), *Haemophilus influenzae* (30%, especially during winter and spring), and, to a lesser extent, *Moraxella catarrhalis* (more common in children). *Staphylococcus aureus* (less than 5%) is seen less often.

20. **(B)** Bupropion (Zyban) is an antidepressant and also a smoking deterrent. This would be a great adjunct therapy for a patient with symptoms of depression without requiring additional medications. There are other options for smoking cessation that do not have the antidepressant effects of bupropion hydrochloride.

21. **(C)** In the African American population, a thiazide diuretic and/or a calcium channel blocker is the preferred choice for initial treatment. An angiotensin-converting enzyme inhibitor is less effective in treating hypertension in this population. A centrally acting agonist, such as clonidine, is not recommended first-line therapy for hypertension.

22. **(B)** Insulin glargine has a gradual onset with no peak time and a duration of up to 24 hours.

Types of Insulin	(Onset, Peak, Duration)
Lispro insulin	> 15 min, 30–60 min, 3–4 hr
Regular insulin	30–60 min, 2–6 hr, 6–8 hr
Insulin isophane suspension (NPH)	1–1.5 hr, 4–12 hr, 18–24 hr
Insulin isophane suspension (NPH)/regular insulin	30–60 min, 2–12 hr, 24 hr
Insulin glargine	gradual onset, no peak, 24 hr
Insulin detemir	gradual onset, 6–10 hr, 24 hr

23. **(A)** Rifampin is an antitubercular drug used in the treatment of tuberculosis. Adverse effects include hematuria, acute renal failure, and hemoglobinuria. The other three medications are not associated with hematuria.

24. **(B)** Peptic ulcer disease usually produces pain when the epigastric area is palpitated; pain symptoms are usually relieved after food. Gastroesophageal reflux disease does not produce pain when palpating the epigastric area, and usually symptoms worsen with/after food. Gallbladder disease is not the correct option, as the patient had a cholecystectomy (gallbladder removal) when he was seven years old. Nausea and possible vomiting are more common with cholelithiasis (gallstones) and cholecystitis (inflammation of the gallbladder). There are no signs or symptoms to indicate a cardiac etiology.

25. **(A)** Common manifestations of Parkinson's disease include tremor at rest, muscular rigidity, difficulty maintaining body posture, slow movements (bradykinesia), and repetitive slow movement of the thumb and forefinger (pill rolling).

26. **(A)** Pavlik harness and spica cast are two of the treatments for hip dysplasia for infants younger than 6 months old. The 6-to-8-month-old infant may need closed/open reduction intervention. Untreated hip dysplasia will reduce the mobility of the hip, resulting in difficulties learning to walk.

27. **(B)** The current recommended international normalized ratio for patients taking warfarin (Coumadin) is between 2.0 and 3.0.

28. **(C)** The two most common anti-acne agents are topical benzoyl peroxide and retinoic acid. These are usually the first-line treatment for mild acne. The oral retinoid is effective on nodulocystic acne, and it requires monitoring by a dermatologist. Topical antibiotics may be effective to control the acne. Oral tetracycline is also an alternate route, but caution the patient of the side effects on teeth and hyperpigmentation of the skin.

29. **(C)** A male patient diagnosed with chronic pelvic pain syndrome is usually treated with alpha blockers to reduce bladder, neck, and urethral spasms. The most common drugs are terazosin, doxazosin, and tamsulosin. Antibiotics have no role in the management of CPPS.

30. **(B)** The American College of Obstetricians and Gynecologists (ACOG) recommends 1,000 mg of calcium per day for pregnant or breastfeeding women. Women 19 years old or younger require additional calcium and should take 1,300 mg as their daily supplement.

31. **(A)** Flunitrazepam (also known as Rohypnol) is a benzodiazepine used as a "party drug" in the United States. The agent has a rapid onset, and effects are severe. Sexual disinhibition is one of the side effects of the drug, thus it has become known as the "date rape drug." Because of its propensity to cause amnesia, individuals are at risk for sexual assault and may be given the drug without being aware.

32. **(D)** NF is a neurocutaneous disorder that is often diagnosed during childhood. The most common form is called von Recklinghausen's NF. Children with NF have cognitive deficits, learning disabilities, and other neuro-related problems. These children should be referred for diagnosis and management.

33. **(B)** CDC recommends pneumococcal vaccination (PCV13 or Prevnar 13 *and* PPSV23 or Pneumovax 23) for all adults 65 years and older. Administer a dose of PCV13, then a dose of PPSV23 at least one year later. If the patient has already received one or more doses of PPSV23, administer the dose of PCV13 at least one year after the administration of PPSV23.

34. **(D)** The "Standard of Practice for Nurse Practitioners" is published by the American Association of Nurse Practitioners.

35. **(D)** For established patients, the common service codes are 99212 (10 minutes), 99213 (15 minutes), 99214 (25 minutes), and 99215 (40 minutes). In this scenario, the nurse practitioner irrigated the ear, diagnosed, and treated the patient. Thus, 99214 is the appropriate choice.

36. **(C)** Bronchiolitis is a viral upper respiratory infection affecting infants and young children. Because the etiology is viral, antibiotics should not be prescribed. Humidified air, nebulizer treatments, antipyretics, and oral steroids are helpful in relieving symptoms in this self-limiting illness.

37. **(A)** Loss of peripheral vision and eye pain are more commonly present in patients with glaucoma. Patients with cataracts may report night vision problems (inability to drive at night), sensitivity to sunlight, seeing halos around lights, having double vision, and cloudy lenses.

38. **(D)** Emphysema is an irreversible obstructive lung disease. Airflow is restricted due to the disease process itself. Emphysema causes destruction of the walls of the alveoli. Predisposing factors include cigarette smoking, which causes chronic inflammation with repeated, prolonged WBC recruitment to the alveoli. The alveoli become hyper-distended and are unable to recoil appropriately, resulting in increased residual lung volume, increased carbon dioxide retention, and reduced expiratory volume. Influenza presents as an acute systemic illness with body aches, fever, and chills predominating. Respiratory symptoms are usually not pronounced unless secondarily infected with bacteria. Chronic asthma is considered a partially reversible respiratory disorder. CAP is an acute infection of the lungs, usually caused by *S. pneumoniae* in adults.

39. **(B)** Appropriate management of CAP should produce an improvement in symptoms within 24–48 hours. This patient is not improving and continues to have a fever. This indicates a resistant organism. The nurse practitioner should prescribe amoxicillin/clavulanate because the most likely pathogen is *S. pneumoniae*, which is susceptible to penicillin therapy.

40. **(B)** Each 1% change in A1c represents a change of approximately 35 mg/dL in average blood glucose. In the management of diabetes, a small step in the reduction of A1c is key to success and further reduction. 171–186 mg/dL A1c% (7.6–8.1); 156 mg/dL A1c% (7.1–7.6); 140 mg/dL A1c% (6.5–7.0); 125 mg/dL A1c% (6.0–6.5)

41. **(A)** The most common stones found in nephrolithiasis are calcium (75–80%). This is followed by struvite (15%), uric acid (7%), and cystine (< 1%).

42. **(A)** Patients with acute pancreatitis often have elevated serum lipase and amylase levels. Alanine aminotransferase is most concentrated in the liver. The liver will release the enzyme into the bloodstream when there is damage or injury to the organ. Therefore, it is a more specific indicator to determine the well-being of the liver. Aspartate aminotransferase is normally found in a variety of tissues, including liver, heart, muscle, kidney, and the brain. It is released into the serum when any one of these tissues is damaged. Thus, it is not a specific indicator for the liver or pancreas. Basic metabolic panel evaluates the status of the kidneys, level of blood glucose, and serum electrolyte levels. A uric acid blood test determines how much uric acid is present in the bloodstream. This test is usually ordered to support a diagnosis of gout.

43. **(A)** Brudzinski's sign. The Brudzinski's and Kernig's maneuvers are used to evaluate for possible meningitis, and the Tinel's and Phalen's maneuvers are used to assess carpal tunnel impingement associated with carpal tunnel syndrome.

44. **(A)** Colles fracture usually results from impact or fall on an outstretched hand. It is often seen in post-menopausal women or individuals with osteoporosis. Comminuted fracture means the break is in more than two pieces. The patients should be referred to an orthopedic surgeon or emergency department as soon as possible. While drawing labs for bone mineral density test is appropriate due to the possibility of osteoporosis, the comminuted fracture is the main issue to focus on during the visit. The nurse practitioner should avoid NSAIDs in patients with preexisting renal disease.

45. **(B)** The prothrombin time and international normalized ratio need to be reevaluated within three to five days for dosage adjustment of warfarin, if indicated.

46. **(A)** A candida yeast infection can also be identified in other areas of the body by performing a KOH test by obtaining samples from the mouth (oral thrush), vagina (vaginitis), and skin (candidiasis). Pseudohyphae are a type of filament that form pseudomycelia, most commonly in polymorphic fungi like *Candida spp.* Cellulitis is usually caused by Gram-positive bacteria, with the infection involving the dermis and subcutaneous tissue of the limb. Psoriasis is a chronic skin condition that is immune-mediated and characterized by erythematous areas with silvery scales, patches, and plaques. Folliculitis is a benign skin disorder that appears as pinpoint red bumps from the hair follicle commonly seen on the face, scalp, chest, back, buttock, and legs.

47. **(A)** This patient is presenting with symptoms suggestive of chancroid. Chancroid is caused by *Haemophilus ducreyi*, and the lesion may be accompanied by painful lymphadenopathy. Patients who present with chancroid should also be tested for other STIs such as HIV, syphilis, gonorrhea, chlamydia, and hepatitis B and C. A CBC, CMP, and ultrasound will not be helpful in managing this illness.

48. **(A)** The American College of Obstetricians and Gynecologists (ACOG) recommends 1,000 mg of calcium per day for pregnant or breastfeeding women. Women 19 years old or younger require additional calcium and should take 1,300 mg as their daily supplement.

49. **(D)** Clonidine is an alpha-adrenergic agonist and is very effective in treating tachycardia and tremors associated with alcohol withdrawal. Carbamazepine and Dilantin are anti-epileptic medications, while codeine is used as an analgesic and cough suppressant.

50. **(C)** Of the choices given, breastfeeding is most likely to decrease an infant's risk for developing AOM. Risk factors for the development of AOM include exposure to cigarette smoke, supine feeding, daycare attendance, and use of a pacifier.

51. **(D)** Aminoglycosides are a class of antibiotics used for infections caused by *Escherichia coli*, *Klebsiella* species, *Proteus mirabilis*, *Enterobacter* species, *Acinetobacter* species, and *Pseudomonas aeruginosa*. These medications are poorly absorbed from the gastrointestinal tract and must be given parenterally. Aminoglycosides may cause nephrotoxicity and ototoxicity but have not been associated with hypotension. Loop diuretics, TCAs, and CCBs all have the potential to cause or exacerbate postural hypotension; therefore, these agents should be used with caution in older adults.

52. **(B)** The most common bacterial pathogen isolated in acute bacterial rhinosinusitis during winter months is *Haemophilus influenzae* (30%, especially during winter and spring), *Streptococcus pneumoniae* (40%, particularly during summer and fall), and, to a lesser extent, *Moraxella catarrhalis* (more common in children). *Staphylococcus* is seen less often (less than 5%).

53. **(B)** The International Classification of Diseases was developed by the World Health Organization. The ICD is used to identify a patient's diagnosis and reasons for seeking care. The ICD codes also provide a systemic mechanism for classifying morbidity and mortality cases through clustering specific recorded ICDs. Healthy People is not a worldwide program. It is only available in the United States, and it identifies the nation's health improvement priorities through utilizing evidence-based national health objectives. The Centers for Disease Control and Prevention is the leading public health institute in the United States. It plays a significant role in monitoring public health, fostering and promoting health safety, health research, and providing leadership, education, and training to enhance public health. The North Atlantic Treaty Organization is an international alliance that consists of 29 member states from North American and Europe.

54. **(D)** Recommended treatment of community acquired pneumonia (CAP) caused by *S. pneumoniae* is doxycycline or azithromycin. This recommendation is appropriate for individuals who are otherwise healthy and have no recent history of antibiotic use.

55. **(B)** This presentation is suggestive of acute otitis media, which is an infection of the middle ear space and a common complication of upper respiratory infection. Environmental risk factors for AOM include daycare attendance, exposure to tobacco smoke, exposure to older siblings, bottle feeding in a supine position, and pacifier use. The most common pathogens associated with AOM include *Streptococcus pneumoniae*, *Haemophilus influenzae*, and *Moraxella catarrhalis*.

56. **(B)** A cough is the presenting symptom in most cases of bronchitis. Fever is unusual, and, while occasional wheezes may be present, they are not the most common finding. Purulent sputum may or may not be associated with this illness and is not diagnostic of etiology.

57. **(D)** Aortic stenosis presents with a classic triad of progressive dyspnea on exertion, heart failure, and syncope. In adults with AS, cardiac output is maintained until late in the disease course. Patients are then usually between 60 and 70 years of age. Development of symptoms associated with AS is gradual following an asymptomatic latent period of 20 years.

58. **(D)** The common side effects of metformin are weight loss, GI disturbance, and metallic taste. Fluid retention and headaches are not common side effects of metformin.

59. **(D)** Patients with uncomplicated cystitis present with irritative voiding symptoms without fever. The cause is usually *E. coli.* No systemic toxicity is present. Recommended first-line management includes the use of cephalexin 250–500 mg PO q6hr for 1–3 days, nitrofurantoin 100 mg PO q12hr for 5–7 days, and trimethoprim-sulfamethoxazole 160/800 PO BID for 3 days. Azithromycin is a macrolide antibiotic used to treat bacterial infections such as sinusitis, bronchitis, pneumonia, and STIs.

60. **(B)** White blood cells (WBCs) with a differential will provide better data to support a diagnosis of acute appendicitis. During an episode of acute appendicitis, elevation of leucocytes, neutrophilia, and bands will be observed. Research shows that 80–85% of adults with appendicitis have a WBC count greater than 10,500 cells/μL. Approximately 80% of patients will also have neutrophilia greater than 75%. Less than 4% of patients with appendicitis have a WBC count less than 10,500 cells/μL and neutrophils less than 75%. The presence of bands indicates severe infection and requires emergency department referral. Since appendicitis is also an inflammatory disease, C-reactive protein (CRP) is another test to determine the presence of inflammation to support the diagnosis if needed.

61. **(B)** Magnetic resonance imaging is the most sensitive method in the evaluation of a patient with encephalitis caused by herpes simplex virus. Computed tomograph scan (with or without contrast) should be used if MRI is not available.

62. **(B)** Plantar fasciitis is a condition of the hind foot (back portion of the foot), and patients often report subcalcaneal pain that may radiate to the arch of the foot. Pain usually occurs when the patient is walking or running and is worse in the morning. A ligamentous injury is commonly seen in the knee joint. These injuries decrease the stability of the knee and can severely impact ambulation. A bone spur may be felt as a focal area of pain that is consistent over time and is worse when standing or walking. Gout is an acute condition affecting the synovium of the joints. Patients report acute, severe pain in the associated area, often with redness and warmth over the affected joint.

63. **(B)** The nurse practitioner should continue the ferrous sulfate 3 mg/kg/day and recheck labs in two months. The iron deficiency treatment is improving per the lab result. Increasing the dosage will not speed up the progression but, rather, may increase risk of constipation. It is premature to stop the treatment or decrease the dosage.

64. **(C)** Scabies is a highly contagious skin infection caused by *Sarcoptes scabiei* itch mite and is usually seen in individuals within crowded living conditions, in long-term care facilities, or in hospitals. Scabies is transmitted through close physical contact and through shared bedding and linens. Tineas affect most parts of the body and are classified according to location. Tinea manuum is a hand fungus. It is a skin condition that is caused by a certain type of fungi called dermatophytes. Atopic dermatitis (eczema) presents as an itchy, dry eruption that occurs on the face, neck, trunk, hands, and wrists and in the antecubital and popliteal folds. Patients present with severe itching and multiple excoriated areas from scratching. Nits may be seen on the hair shaft and actual lice seen on the scalp, skin, or clothes. Based on the assessment data, there is no data to support lice infection.

65. **(D)** Risk factors for prostate cancer include age > 50 years old, avid long-hour cyclists, positive family history, obesity, and African American ethnicity. Commercial long-distance truck drivers may be prone to prostatitis due to limited bathroom breaks during the long-distance drives, but not prostate cancer.

66. **(A)** Bisphosphonate medications are used to treat osteoporosis to increase bone strength and reduce fractures. Risedronate sodium has *multiple dosing* forms. It may be used daily, weekly, twice monthly, and once monthly. Ibandronate sodium is a *once-monthly* treatment. Alendronate sodium are *once-weekly* treatments. Zoledronic acid (Reclast, Zometa) is a *once-yearly* IV infusion treatment.

67. **(D)** OCD presents as persistent, recurrent, irrational, obsessive thoughts and the performance of uncontrollable compulsive behavior. The disorder often begins during childhood, adolescence, or young adulthood. It may also present acutely following a stressful life event. These obsessions and compulsions cause the person severe anxiety and distress. Often these patients present to primary care with complaints of anxiety or depression. They express distress over their inability to stop the obsessions and compulsions. Management begins with a strong, trusting relationship between patient and provider. Behavioral therapy is often the mainstay of treatment. Generalized anxiety disorder is characterized by persistent, pervasive anxiety that has been present for at least six months. Post-traumatic stress disorder is associated with exposure to a traumatic event or situation. Symptoms include recurrent flashbacks and hypervigilance. Bipolar disorder presents with periods of mania or hypomania alternating with depressive symptoms.

68. **(B)** When assessing an infant who is quiet, start with auscultating the heart and lungs. This is a noninvasive procedure that can be performed best when the infant is not crying. Other parts of the exam will likely cause crying, so save them for later.

69. **(B)** An elderly patient with iron-deficiency anemia likely has an occult GI bleed. This should be ruled out quickly and the cause of the anemia determined.

70. **(C)** The title protection is maintained through the Nurse Practice Act. The purpose of title protection is to protect the public from unlicensed nurses or fraudulent use of unapproved credentials: RN, NP, APRN.

71. **(C)** The current version accepted in coding is ICD-10; however, ICD-11 is currently available online (2018). There is no version 12 or 13 at this point. The International Classification of Diseases was developed to promote international comparability in the collection, classification, processing, and presentation of mortality statistics.

72. **(A)** The best option is 8:00 A.M. The diuretic action lasts for 8–10 hours, which may result in frequent bathroom visits. Thus, the earlier the better. The nurse practitioner wants to promote uninterrupted sleep for the patient.

73. **(B)** A cataract is an opacity of the lens of the eye that commonly develops with aging. Other causes or risk factors for cataract development include congenital lens dysphoria, excessive exposure to UVB light, and trauma. Cataracts may be unilateral; however, most progress to bilateral involvement. Cataract surgery is the most common surgery covered by Medicare in the United States. Open-angle glaucoma presents with slow, painless vision loss, usually beginning with peripheral vision and often with increased intraocular pressure. Macular degeneration is an age-related progressive loss of central vision. The disorder may present with gradual vision loss or acutely as a result of leaking of retinal vessels. Retinopathy associated with diabetes also contributes to vision loss over time. On fundoscopic exam, diabetic retinopathy appears as microaneurysms, exudates, dilated and tortuous vessels, and neovascularization of the retina and optic disc.

74. **(C)** All the listed medications are treatment options for stroke prevention in a nonvalvular atrial fibrillation. Only warfarin requires INR testing. The goal INR is between 2.0 and 3.0.

75. **(A)** The definitive test to confirm the diagnosis of acute gout attack is urate crystals in joint fluid aspirate. Normal synovial fluid appears clear to light yellow. The synovial fluid will be turbid during an acute attack. C-reactive protein is to identify the presence of an inflammatory process. Initial testing for gout includes evaluating the serum uric acid level. However, research suggests that uric acid may be normal (15%) during an acute gout attack. Clinicians should look for other laboratory findings. The erythrocyte sedimentation rate and white blood cells will be elevated during an acute attack.

76. **(B)** Although the patient presents with symptoms characteristic of a UTI, that response is not an option in this question. Based on the patient's age and symptoms, consider an STI as the cause. A patient on antibiotics would likely not be experiencing dysuria unless the organism was resistant to the antibiotic. In any case, antibiotics would not cause the symptoms. A kidney stone usually presents with an acute onset of excruciating flank pain and possibly blood in the urine. This presentation does not fit that scenario. Although the patient could be pregnant (and this should be ruled out), her symptoms do not correspond to early pregnancy symptoms, which include frequency without dysuria.

77. **(C)** Common causes of sensorineural hearing loss are presbycusis, Meniere's disease, and acoustic neuroma. Common causes of conductive hearing loss are cerumen impaction, otitis externa, and tympanic membrane rupture.

78. **(B)** The pathophysiology of GERD involves the reflux of acidic stomach contents from the stomach to the esophagus. Reflux often increases during the night when the patient is lying down. Because of this, some degree of aspiration is common, and patients may present with symptoms pointing to a respiratory diagnosis; however, the underlying cause is GERD. Rhinitis is seen in allergic rhinitis and upper respiratory infections but is not associated with GERD.

79. **(D)** CN VIII is the vestibulocochlear nerve, which is responsible for hearing and balance; therefore, a tumor on this nerve may cause dizziness. An acoustic neuroma produces hearing loss and tinnitus. An inability to open and close the eyes indicates a problem with CN VII, which is the facial nerve. The cranial nerves responsible for taste include CN VII and X. CN I is the olfactory nerve, controlling the sense of smell.

80. **(C)** Mechanical neck pain presents as aching pain in the paraspinal muscles in the cervical area and stiffness of the ligaments and muscles throughout the shoulder area. This may last up to six weeks. Cervical myelopathy, cervical cord compression, presents with neck pain and bilateral weakness and paresthesia in the upper and lower extremities. Cervical radiculopathy, nerve root compression, causes sharp burning or tingling pain in the neck and one arm. Mechanical pain with whiplash usually begins the day after the injury and is usually accompanied by headaches, dizziness, and malaise.

81. **(A)** Iron deficiency anemia is the most common anemia worldwide and continues to affect millions across the globe each year. This type of anemia is occasionally seen in infants as they expend maternal stores of iron they had at birth and is often related to diet. Iron deficiency anemia is a hypochromic (pale RBCs), microcytic (small RBCs) anemia. Macrocytic anemia is seen in folate deficiency, vitamin B12 deficiency. Pernicious anemia is one of the vitamin B12 deficiency anemias. Normocytic anemia is seen in hypothyroidism (most commonly), acute blood loss, early iron deficiency anemia, acquired pure red blood cell aplasia, or chronic renal insufficiency.

82. **(B)** Patients with erysipelas should be referred to the ED immediately for management. Rapid progression may lead to death.

83. **(D)** Epididymitis may be sexually transmitted—usually in men younger than 40—and caused by *Chlamydia trachomatis* or *Neisseria gonorrhoeae*. A non-sexually transmitted form occurs in men older than 40 and is associated with urinary tract infections and prostatitis. Patients present with irritative voiding symptoms, fever, and painful epididymis swelling. Peyronie's disease is a fibrotic disorder of the penis, which results in varying degrees of pain, curvature, or deformity. This may disrupt normal sexual functioning. Orchitis is inflammation of one or both testes, causing swelling and pain. Testicular torsion is an acute condition in which the testes become twisted within the scrotum causing severe pain. Torsion requires surgical correction within six hours to save the testis.

84. **(B)** A mammogram is usually the first step in screening for breast cancer. One of the limitations of a mammogram is that it may not be able to provide a clear image on a patient with dense tissue, such as fibrocystic breast disease. Breast ultrasound will differentiate a cystic mass or solid mass. The definitive diagnostic procedure is a breast biopsy. This patient has a strong family history of breast cancer and will be a good candidate for breast biopsy.

85. **(D)** Mood disorders are chronic or prolonged in nature and affect all aspects of a patient's life. Many times, during an exacerbation of a mood disorder, there is a distinct change in the individual's engagement with the world. They often become isolated or manic. Agoraphobia is a fear of heights and is present only when the patient is exposed to heights.

86. **(C)** Spina bifida presents in four ways: occulta, meningocele, closed neural tube defects, and myelomeningocele. The most common form is occulta, which develops when one or more vertebrae are not formed properly. A layer of skin covers the defect, thus the name "occulta." This type of spina bifida rarely causes problems. Hirsutism is an excess growth of body hair, usually due to elevated androgen levels. Arnold-Chiari malformation presents as a cyst-like growth in the fourth ventricle, the cerebellum, or the brain stem. Neurofibromatosis is a neurocutaneous disease developing from the epithelial layer of the embryo. There are two types. Type 1 is characterized by multiple hyperpigmented neurofibromas. Type 2 presents with bilateral CN VIII tumors, often with other intraspinal tumors.

87. **(C)** The Task Force is recommending a one-time hepatitis C screen to individuals born between 1945 and 1965 because of the increased risk of the disease in this age group. People receiving blood or blood products before universal screening was in place are at risk for potential prior exposure.

88. **(B)** The Health Insurance Portability and Accountability Act (HIPAA) was enacted in 1996 and provides guidelines for the management of confidential medical information. This act ensures that only individuals with a legitimate reason to do so will have access to patient information. Some legitimate reasons for accessing patient information include treatment, health care entities/operations, and payment organizations.

89. **(A)** The 1997 Balanced Budget Act (BBA), signed by President Bill Clinton, allows nurse practitioners to be reimbursed at 85% of the physician rate for medical services provided to patients.

90. **(A)** A meta-analysis reviews all quantitative findings from multiple studies relating to the topic of interest. Synthesis of evidence is an evidence review with critical appraisal of findings. A randomized controlled trial is a quantitative study design. Systematic review is a literature review based on a specific topic.

91. **(B)** The most common symptoms associated with digoxin toxicity are nausea and vomiting. Other side effects and adverse effects that occur less commonly include diarrhea, headache, abdominal pain, anorexia, fatigue, drowsiness, confusion, slow heart rate, and vision changes such as seeing halos around lights.

92. **(B)** Graves' disease is an autoimmune form of hyperthyroidism. It is the most common etiology related to thyrotoxicosis. This disorder is much more common in women than men and usually occurs between 20 and 40 years of age. T3 is a very metabolically active form of thyroid hormone and will be elevated in Graves' disease. Thyroid stimulating hormone is produced in response to low thyroid activity. A patient with Graves' disease has a hyperactive thyroid gland; therefore, the TSH will be low. Alkaline phosphatase is an enzyme that is seen in all tissues of the body and may be elevated with bone and liver disease. It is not usually elevated in Graves' disease unless another disorder is present. Liver function studies measure the liver's ability to perform necessary processes and are a good indication of overall liver condition.

93. **(C)** Approximately 5% of adults in the United States who have hypertension also have renal artery stenosis. This is usually seen in individuals over the age of 45 who have a history of atherosclerotic disease. Other risk factors include diabetes, smoking, and chronic kidney disease. These individuals may have refractory hypertension that is difficult to control, pulmonary edema with high blood pressure, and acute kidney injury (AKI) upon starting an ACE inhibitor.

94. **(D)** A thorough history and focused physical exam are the most important components of assessment for acute appendicitis. The presentation is classic, with onset of periumbilical abdominal pain localized to the right lower quadrant, possible low-grade fever, nausea, and constipation or mild diarrhea reported. The physical exam usually reveals rebound tenderness and guarding with palpation of the right lower abdominal quadrant. Signs of visceral irritation may be present. As the condition progresses, the patient experiences pain when extending the right leg. The sedimentation rate may be elevated with acute appendicitis, but this is not specific as the level rises with many infectious processes. A CBC with differential will likely demonstrate an elevated white count with a "left shift" indicating bacterial infection. However, this finding is not specific for acute appendicitis. A KUB X-ray is not diagnostic for this disorder and would not normally be part of the workup.

95. **(A)** This grouping of signs and symptoms suggests hydrocephalus. Other signs include a high-pitched cry and tense, bulging fontanels due to increased amount of CSF producing cranial pressure. Meningitis in an infant usually presents with signs of sepsis such as increased temperature and poor feeding. Cerebral palsy is seen with a persistence of primitive reflexes, delayed growth and development, and lack of movement through developmental milestones. Reye's syndrome is seen following a viral infection with symptoms such as malaise, vomiting, and progressive neurologic deterioration.

96. **(A)** The presentation of sciatica frequently includes pain in the buttocks area, which radiates down the leg along with paresthesia. The pain may occur suddenly and resolve or may persist for a few days. Inflammation of the sciatic nerve causes pain. This condition may be associated with a herniated disc, spinal stenosis, osteoarthritis, and direct injury to the nerve. Cervical radiculopathy occurs in the neck and shoulder area innervated by the cervical spinal nerves.

97. **(B)** A patient with beta-thalassemia minor may have low hemoglobin without iron deficiency. The nurse practitioner should check the serum ferritin level before concluding that the patient may have an iron deficiency. Fluid IV bolus with normal saline can be helpful for sickle cell crises. If the patient needs further lab tests, refer the patient back to the oncologist.

98. **(D)** Rosacea manifesting as inflammatory with this description should be treated with topical therapies such as metronidazole, azelaic acid, topical ivermectin, or sulfacetamide-sulfur. Oral/systemic agents are typically used in patients who present with multiple lesions or fail to respond satisfactorily to topical agents.

99. **(C)** Acute bacterial prostatitis is usually caused by *E. coli* or pseudomonas. Patients present with fever, irritative voiding symptoms, perineal, sacral, or suprapubic pain. Obstructive symptoms may occur as the prostate enlarges. Hospitalization may be required for this condition. During workup, a CBC, urinalysis, and rectal exam may all be appropriate. However, prostatic massage should not be done in a patient with symptoms of prostatitis, as this could cause the infection to spread.

100. **(A)** Danazol is a synthetic steroid (androgen derivative that suppresses pituitary gonadotropins) that may be used to treat breast pain, endometriosis, pelvic pain, and infertility. However, many patients report that side effects are worse than the symptoms. Examples of common side effects include weight gain, acne, hair loss, vaginal dryness, and hirsutism. The nurse practitioner needs to respond to a 15-year-old with direct, yet open ended, statements allowing an opportunity for the teenager to ask questions about the side effects. The statement "danazol is not the right medication for you" sounds authoritative and will prevent the patient from asking any questions that she may have.

101. **(C)** All of these classes of medication may be used to treat MDD, however the SSRIs are the usual recommendation for initial management. This class is associated with fewer side effects and less potential for toxicity with overdose. MOAIs have many drug and food interactions. TCAs often cause drowsiness and may be fatal in overdose.

102. **(A)** Development of motor skills begins in the central part of the body and moves outward toward the periphery. This is proximodistal development. Growth and development also occur in a cephalocaudal direction, meaning head control occurs before walking.

103. **(A)** Hospice care provides end-of-life care to patients with a terminal illness. Medicare will reimburse for these services if requirements have been met. One component for eligibility is that the patient must sign an informed consent specifying that they are agreeing to palliative care instead of curative care. New legislation is being drafted to include a broader range in patients for eligibility for palliative care which provides services to individuals with chronic, life-altering disease, even if they have a longer (or unknown) prognosis for survival.

104. **(A)** An empty square represents a healthy male, and an empty circle represents a healthy female. A filled in square or circle indicates an affected male or female.

105. **(D)** Evidence-based practice consists of six steps: creating a clinical question, searching for relevant evidence in the literature, appraising the evidence critically, integrating the patient goals and values into the decision, evaluating the outcome, and disseminating the evidence.

106. **(C)** A finding of an S3 heart sound in an older patient suggests enlargement of the left ventricle because of heart failure or a cardiomyopathy. The extra heart sound is produced by blood hitting a compliant left ventricle and is commonly associated with fluid overload. An S3 may be a normal finding in children and women who are pregnant.

107. **(D)** Microalbuminuria is a sensitive and early measure of diabetic nephropathy. It is an appropriate screening test for undiagnosed renal disease. A screen for microalbuminuria should be performed annually in patients with T2DM who are at least 21 years old. Creatinine clearance measures the rate at which the kidney clears creatinine from the blood and is also used to evaluate renal function. Creatinine is formed as a result of muscle, bone, and urine metabolism. Serum levels vary between males and females and are usually decreased in elderly individuals. BUN/creatinine ratio measures levels of blood urea nitrogen, which is a byproduct of protein metabolism and creatinine. Evaluating the ratio between these levels in the serum is another measure of renal function. However, the most sensitive test is for microalbuminuria.

108. **(B)** Prerenal causes of AKI include fluid and electrolyte depletion, sepsis, hemorrhage, cardiac or liver failure, heat stroke, and burns. Renal causes of AKI include toxins, ischemia, acute glomerulonephritis, pyelonephritis, myoglobinuria, and radiocontrast agents. Postrenal causes of AKI include prostate disease, bladder tumor, renal calculi, or pelvic tumor.

109. **(B)** Giardiasis is a protozoal infection caused by *Giardia lamblia*. This parasite is found all over the world but is most prevalent in countries with poor, unsanitary water supply. Risk factors for giardia include travel to endemic areas, drinking contaminated water, men who have sex with men, and individuals with impaired immunity. About 50% of individuals who are infected have no symptoms, but in those who do, acute diarrheal syndrome is reported most often. This acute period may be followed by a period of chronic diarrhea. Most people seek treatment after they have been sick for at least a week and have lost about 5 kg or more. Management is with metronidazole 250 mg PO TID for 5–7 days. The other medications listed are not indicated for giardia.

110. **(D)** 5-HT-1 agonists include sumatriptan, which is used in abortive management of an established migraine headache. This medication should not be used in individuals who have a history of cardiovascular or ischemic disease, CVA, uncontrolled hypertension, or transient ischemic attacks (TIAs). Patients should be advised that they may experience flushing, tingling, or discomfort of the chest, neck, or jaw area. First dose of this medication should be supervised because of the cardiovascular risks. Other medications used for abortive treatment include NSAIDs or narcotics. Prophylactic management includes the use of BBs, TCAs, and anticonvulsants.

111. **(B)** Rheumatoid arthritis is a systemic autoimmune disorder that is seen more often in women than men. The disease manifests as multiple, symmetric joint involvement with inflammation, synovitis, and joint deformities. Important to remember is that RA produces systemic symptoms along with joint pain. Systemic symptoms may include low-grade fever, fatigue, and normocytic anemia. Management is with disease-modifying antirheumatic drugs (DMARDs), of which methotrexate is the mainstay. Methotrexate is contraindicated during pregnancy; therefore, women who require this medication must receive a contraceptive prescription as well, with verbalization of patient adherence to contraception while taking methotrexate.

112. **(D)** Hemoglobin electrophoresis is the most sensitive method for diagnosing sickle cell disease/anemia. Complete blood count (CBC) with peripheral smear will identify anemia based on hemoglobin and hematocrit levels but is unable to differentiate the type of hemoglobin present. Bone marrow biopsy is indicated if presentation is suggestive of myelodysplastic disorder such as anemia. Hemoglobin and hematocrit will indicate serum percentage/levels of these two components of the blood.

113. **(A)** The patient has pseudomonas folliculitis, also known as hot-tub folliculitis, that is superficial at this point and may be treated with topical keratolytics and topical antibiotics. Culture is indicated if the lesions are resistant to treatment. Since the patient is three months pregnant, both oral antibiotics (category D) would not be a safe choice.

114. **(A)** BPH is the most common benign tumor in men. Symptoms usually occur as obstructive or irritative symptoms. When pharmacological therapy is indicated, finasteride is a 5-alpha-reductase inhibitor that produces a decrease in gland hypertrophy but must be taken for six months before clinical improvement is seen. Symptomatic improvement with this medication is usually seen only in men with marked prostate enlargement. Side effects include decreased libido, erectile dysfunction, and reduced ejaculate. Serum PSA levels are usually reduced by around 50% with this medication.

115. **(A)** According to recent statistics published by the American Lung Association, African American men and women have the highest rates of lung cancer; however, African American men have the highest mortality rates. Lung cancer is a disease of aging and is associated with several environmental factors, the primary one being cigarette smoking. Although more men are diagnosed with lung cancer, more women are living with lung cancer.

116. **(B)** CAGE questionnaire is a validated screening tool for alcohol abuse in adults of all ages. The questions included are: "Have you ever felt like you should **C**ut down on your drinking?" "Do you get **A**nnoyed when other people criticize your drinking?" "Have you ever felt **G**uilty about drinking?" "Have you ever had a drink in the morning as an **E**ye opener?" The PHQ 2 and PHQ 9 are screening tools for depression. The MMSE is a screen for cognitive decline.

117. **(C)** Children with SCA should receive all immunizations according to schedule. Sickle cell crises occur when children become ill and thus prevention of illness is important.

118. **(A)** Patient confidentiality is breached when medical information is given to another person without the express permission of the patient.

119. **(A)** Intermittent claudication is characteristically described as cramping and pain in the legs that is relieved by rest. Raynaud's disease affects the fingers and hands and is triggered by cold or heat as well as emotional distress. Atherosclerotic disease is associated with atherosclerotic heart disease and is part of the continuum of that disorder. Symptoms are limb ischemia with exertion. Neurogenic claudication presents as pain with walking or standing that radiates from the spine to the buttocks, thighs, lower legs, and feet.

120. **(B)** Pathophysiology of primary adrenal insufficiency involves a deficiency of adrenal hormone produced by the adrenal glands. ACTH secreted by the pituitary gland will be elevated in an effort to increase cortisol levels via negative feedback. Aldosterone is a mineralocorticoid steroid hormone produced by the adrenal gland to increase renal retention of sodium.

121. **(A)** Barrett's epithelium, also known as Barrett's esophagus, is a condition in which squamous epithelial tissue of the esophagus is replaced by metaplastic epithelium, often a result of chronic reflux. Barrett's esophagus is considered to be premalignant for esophageal adenocarcinoma. Regular endoscopic surveillance is recommended. The other choices are incorrect.

122. **(B)** Temporal arteritis (giant cell arteritis) affects individuals over the age of 50 and presents with severe headache, jaw claudication, and polymyalgia rheumatica. The cause is unknown; however, herpes zoster is suspected. There is scalp tenderness with visual problems such as amaurosis fugax or diplopia. Jaw claudication as a presenting symptom has a high predictive

value in diagnosis of temporal arteritis. The temporal artery is indurated and often hardened upon physical exam. Bell's palsy presents as painless loss of sensation and control of one side of the face. A CVA and TIA are both related to areas of infarction in the brain that present symptoms related to the area impacted and are usually unilateral. Treatment of temporal arteritis includes high-dose steroid therapy and requires referral to a rheumatology specialist for management.

123. **(D)** The spleen plays an active part in removing bacteria and aging RBCs from the bloodstream. A patient who has had a splenectomy will, therefore, have a higher risk for serious infection without this line of defense in place. *Streptococcus pneumoniae* is a serious pathogen that is seen in patients who are asplenic. These patients should receive the pneumococcal vaccine. Removal of the spleen is not associated with enlargement of the liver (hepatomegaly), does not increase bleeding risk, and does not contribute to more pronounced expression of anemia.

124. **(A)** An abscess (furuncle or boil) is a localized inflammatory area that is the result of a more deep-seated infection, usually by *Staphylococcus aureus* (rarely by other pathogens). These lesions drain pus and are autoinoculable, meaning the patient can spread the infection to other areas. A carbuncle is an area consisting of several abscesses that have merged.

125. **(D)** Several physiologic factors may cause primary amenorrhea. These include ovarian failure or dysfunction, disorders of the anterior pituitary gland, anatomic defects, chronic anovulation, and disorders of the nervous system. Pregnancy is the number one cause of amenorrhea in women and should be ruled out in every case. Girls who have never had a regular menstrual cycle may still ovulate and have the potential to become pregnant (although rare).

126. **(D)** The Nurse Practice Act is a statute implemented by the state legislature. This act spells out legal scope of practice, and the purpose of the act is to protect the public. The nurse practice act is enforced by the state board of nursing.

127. **(C)** The patient is presenting with signs of DKA, which include Kussmaul respirations (deep, rapid), fruity odor to the breath, and ketonuria. The blood glucose is usually very high, and the patient may have symptoms of dehydration. Hypoglycemia produces sweating, tachycardia, nervousness, and hunger. SJS often results from a drug reaction and presents with skin lesions that are erythematous macules on the head and neck that spread to the trunk and extremities with formation of blisters. The rash becomes confluent and often involves the mucosa. Sepsis presents with hypotension, fever, decreased level of consciousness, and multi-organ involvement.

128. **(D)** The patient should wait a minimum of four weeks after symptoms resolve before participating in sports. The spleen, as a lymphoid organ, becomes enlarged during infectious mononucleosis. This hypertrophy places the patient at risk for splenic rupture. The spleen will return to its normal size after the illness, but this may take several weeks.

129. **(D)** The average incubation period of varicella infection is 14–16 days. The period of infectivity is 48 hours prior to the onset of rashes until all skin lesions have fully crusted.

130. **(D)** Acne may be improved when a patient is taking combined oral contraceptives. However, a patient with worsening acne may need a lower dose of progestin. Progestins are androgenic hormones which increase sebaceous gland activity, leading to clogged follicles.

131. **(B)** The ethical term autonomy refers to a patient's inherent right to make decisions about health care without undue influence by anyone else, including the provider.

132. **(B)** The drug of choice for acute anaphylaxis is epinephrine given immediately subcutaneously and repeated in five minutes if needed. Diphenhydramine IV is a second-line drug; PO diphenhydramine is an antihistamine. Prednisone is beneficial for severe or refractory urticaria. Amlodipine may be helpful in treating chronic urticaria in those unresponsive to other treatments.

133. **(B)** Appearance of a basal cell carcinoma (BCC) is a lesion with a depressed center and raised border with telangiectasia. These lesions are seen most often in adults over age 40 and rarely metastasize. Squamous cell carcinoma (SCC) appears on sun-exposed areas of the body and appear as scaly, red patches; open sores; warts; or elevated lesions that may crust or bleed. Malignant melanoma appears as a dark, variegated lesion with irregular borders and elevation. Kaposi's sarcoma forms abnormal blotches or tumors on the skin that are purple, red, or brown.

134. **(B)** Amniotic fluid embolism occurs when amniotic fluid (including fetal tissue, cells, etc.) enter the maternal bloodstream and travel to the heart or lungs. This complication usually occurs during delivery or immediately after delivery. Signs and symptoms associated with amniotic fluid embolism include acute onset of shortness of breath, pulmonary edema, hypotension, cardiovascular collapse, disseminated intravascular coagulation (DIC), altered level of consciousness, bleeding, seizures, and coma. Fever is not a presenting factor in the acute development of this condition, which has a high mortality rate.

135. **(A)** The primary purpose for professional licensing is to protect the public by ensuring at least a minimum level of professional competence.

136. **(D)** Polycythemia vera is a disorder of the bone marrow causing overproduction of blood cells, mostly red blood cells. This causes increased blood viscosity and associated symptoms such as headache, dizziness, and blurred vision. Patients often have generalized pruritus and recurrent epistaxis. There are engorged retinal veins on the fundoscopic exam. Splenomegaly is extremely common and is palpable in most individuals. This disorder carries a very high risk of thrombosis following surgery and a high rate of peptic ulcer disease. Management is repeated phlebotomy with 500 mL removed every week until the hematocrit drops to less than 45%. Because this repeated phlebotomy depletes the body's iron stores, which then decreases RBC production, it is important that these patients do not take iron supplementation as this will reverse any progress made.

137. **(A)** Permethrin is the recommended first-line treatment for scabies. Although resistance is increasing, this agent continues to eradicate most cases; however, a repeat application is advised after one week. Eczema outbreaks may be treated with topical hydrocortisone cream. Herpes simplex may respond to topical antivirals, but most often oral antiviral medication is needed. Psoriasis is treated with disease-modifying agents such as the new biologic medications.

138. **(A)** Human papillomavirus (HPV) is the most common sexually transmitted infection (STI) in the United States; however, statistics are estimates, as this infection is not a reportable one. Most HPV infections produce no symptoms and clear spontaneously. However, HPV can cause genital warts. HPV types 6 and 11 are responsible for most cases of genital warts and have less propensity to become cancer than other types. HPV types 16 and 18 cause most cases of cervical cancer.

139. **(A)** Case studies usually consist of interesting or unusual presentations. This is the best choice in this scenario as there is only one patient. The other options require multiple research participants. A meta-analysis is an intense, comprehensive review of published research studies about a specific topic or disease in health care. Prospective studies look at populations and develop hypotheses regarding a certain topic in relation to a certain population. Retrospective studies look back in time and gain information from things that have already occurred.

140. **(D)** Folic acid works with vitamin B12 in the production of mature red blood cells. Without folic acid, the bone marrow destroys the abnormal cells, leading to a characteristic macrocytic anemia. This type of anemia is clinically indistinguishable from vitamin B12 anemia. Folic acid deficiency is almost always due to diet. Folic acid is found in dark green leafy vegetables, citrus fruits, and animal proteins. An adequate dietary intake is 50–100 mcg/day, except for women who are pregnant, who require 800 mcg/day. Current recommendations are for all women of childbearing age to take a folic acid supplement every day to prevent neural tube defects in a developing fetus.

141. **(C)** Psoriasis presents with classic silvery scales on extensor surfaces. Hyperthyroidism often gives the skin a velvety appearance, and it is often warm to the touch. Scleroderma gives the skin a taut, shiny, thickened appearance. Eczema presents variably as erythematous patches that may appear on extensor surfaces, the face, the trunk, and extremities.

142. **(C)** Vaginitis is inflammation of vaginal tissue presenting with increased discharge with large numbers of white blood cells present. Vaginosis is inflammation without leukocytosis. Herpes simplex type 2 (genital herpes) presents with an initial infection consisting of systemic and local symptoms, lasting about three weeks. Patients report fatigue, flu-like symptoms, and fever. Multiple lesions erupt at the site of exposure and begin as small blisters, which are very painful. Lymphadenopathy is also present with primary infection. As the lesions begin to resolve, they crust over and disappear. Subsequent outbreaks are usually milder without systemic symptoms. Lesions usually resolve faster as well. Chlamydia is an STI that presents with vaginal spotting, post-coital bleeding, purulent vaginal discharge, urinary symptoms, and lower abdominal pain. Physical examination may reveal abdominal tenderness, cervical friability, and mucopurulent vaginal discharge.

143. **(A)** A problem-focused visit involves a chief complaint and requires straightforward decision making. Required documentation for a problem-focused visit includes chief complaint and brief HPI. No ROS or family history.

144. **(C)** A decreasing viral load suggests that his antiretroviral therapy is working as intended. A decreased viral load indicates efficacy of the treatment plan. Although HIV cannot be cured, viral loads can be managed, and the disease may be followed as a chronic condition. Although low viral loads decrease the risk of transmitting the virus, it does not eliminate this risk. Patients should be advised that they are still able to pass the disease to someone else and safe sexual practices should be used consistently. When the viral load has fallen to undetectable levels, the risk for transmitting the virus is less than 1%; however, the risk is not zero.

145. **(B)** Impetigo is a bacterial skin infection caused by *Staphylococcus aureus*, *Streptococcus pyogenes*, or a mix of the two. Impetigo is seen most commonly in children between the ages of two and five. Predisposing factors are a break in the skin, warm climate, and poor hygiene.

Varicella is chickenpox, which presents with crops of vesicular lesions quickly becoming pustular and then scabbing over. Herpes simplex is a related disorder that causes groups of vesicular lesions that burst and then scab over. Shingles is reactivation of latent varicella zoster that causes a painful, erythematous, vesicular rash along a dermatome. The rash usually does not cross the midline of the body.

146. **(C)** Endometriosis is the implantation of endometrial tissue in areas outside the uterus. Affected sites include the fallopian tubes, the ovaries, myometrium, colon, appendix, and pelvic ligaments. Risk factors include genetic factors, early menarche, being Caucasian, and short menstrual cycles. The presentation of endometriosis is widely variable and may include severe dysmenorrhea, dysuria, dyspareunia, and recurrent (cyclic) pelvic pain, which is the most common symptom. Endometriosis may also be asymptomatic. Fever is not usually associated with endometriosis.

147. **(B)** Occurrence-type malpractice insurance policies protect an NP in the event of a lawsuit brought in the future if the event occurred during a covered period. Claims-based malpractice covers claims only if the NP is currently enrolled in the plan when the suit is filed.

148. **(A)** Trichomoniasis is a sexually transmitted infection that, in women, present with copious vaginal discharge. In men, the presentation is nongonococcal urethritis. Trichomoniasis is caused by a protozoan organism. Examination of discharge under microscope will demonstrate motile organisms. Tests for bacterial vaginosis (seen with a pH > 4.5 and a fishy odor occurring when potassium hydroxide is added to the slide) are often positive for trichomonas. Management is with tinidazole or metronidazole 2 g PO x 1. All infected persons, including sexual partners, should be treated. Chlamydia is a sexually transmitted infection caused by a bacterium *Chlamydia trachomatis*. Women with chlamydia often report vaginal spotting, postcoital bleeding, purulent vaginal discharge, dysuria, and lower abdominal pain. Syphilis is a systemic, sexually transmitted disease caused by *Treponema pallidum*, and presents initially as a primary lesion (or chancre) at the site of infection. Untreated syphilis may progress to systemic disease. Herpes simplex 2 is genital herpes. Primary infection usually involves a prodrome of malaise, low-grade fever, and fatigue a few days before a vesicular rash develops. This rash is extremely painful; however, lesions clear on their own. The virus remains latent until reactivation occurs. Secondary or subsequent outbreaks are less severe than the initial one.

149. **(C)** "Incident-to" billing is a method for reimbursement of outpatient services provided by a non-physician provider and billed under the physician's number. With this type of billing, the agency will receive 100% of the physician fee. Location of the services may be in the physician's primary office, an off-site location, an institution, or the patient's home. With this arrangement, the physician is required to make the first patient visit and develop a plan of care. Follow-up services are billed as "incident-to" the physician services.

150. **(D)** For new patients, the common level service code with the approximate amount of time spent with a patient includes 99202 (10 minutes), 99203 (15 minutes), 99204 (25 minutes), and 99205 (40 minutes). With new patient care, the nurse practitioner will need additional time to evaluate the coding components. The presented scenario does not require additional workup, decision-making is not complex, and time spent in the room was 20 minutes. Thus, 99203 is the appropriate choice.

References

Chapter 1

Burns, C. E., Barber Starr, N., Dunn, A. M., Blosser, C. G., Brady, M. A., & Garzon, D. L. (2017). *Pediatric Primary Care* (6 ed.). St. Louis, Missouri Elsevier.

Buttaro, T. M., Trybulski, J., Polgar-Bailey, P., & Sandberg-Cook, J. (2017). *Primary Care: A Collaborative Practice* (6 ed.). St. Louis, Missouri: Elsevier.

Domino, F. J., Baldor, R. A., Golding, J., & Stephens, M. B. (2023). *The 5-Minute Clinical Consult Premium 2023* (31 ed.). Philadelphia, PA: Wolters Kluwer.

Dunphy, L. M. H., Winland-Brown, J. E., Porter, B. O., & Thomas, D. J. (2019). *Primary Care: The Art and Science of Advanced Practice Nursing* (5 ed.). Philadelphia, PA: F.A. Davis Company.

Pathanapitoon, K., Dodds, E. M., Cunningham, E. T., & Rothova, A. (2017). Clinical Spectrum of HLA-B27-Associated Ocular Inflammation. *Ocular Immunology and Inflammation*, 25(4), 569-576. doi:10.1080/09273948.2016.1185527.

Chapter 2

Burns, C. E., Barber Starr, N., Dunn, A. M., Blosser, C. G., Brady, M. A., & Garzon, D. L. (2017). *Pediatric Primary Care* (6 ed.). St. Louis, Missouri Elsevier.

Buttaro, T. M., Trybulski, J., Polgar-Bailey, P., & Sandberg-Cook, J. (2017). *Primary Care: A Collaborative Practice* (6 ed.). St. Louis, Missouri: Elsevier.

Domino, F. J., Baldor, R. A., Golding, J., & Stephens, M. B. (2023). *The 5-Minute Clinical Consult Premium 2023* (31 ed.). Philadelphia, PA: Wolters Kluwer.

Dunphy, L. M. H., Winland-Brown, J. E., Porter, B. O., & Thomas, D. J. (2019). *Primary Care: The Art and Science of Advanced Practice Nursing* (5 ed.). Philadelphia, PA: F.A. Davis Company.

Maxine, A. P., Stephen, J. M., Michael, W. R., McPhee, S. J., Papadakis, M. A., & Rabow, M. W. (2018). *Current Medical Diagnosis & Treatment 2022* (61 ed.). New York, NY: McGraw Hill Medical.

McCance, K. L., & Huether, S. E. (2019). *Pathophysiology: The Biologic Basis for Disease in Adults and Children* (8 ed.). St. Louis, Missouri: Elsevier.

Chapter 3

Bugge, C., Sether, E. M., Pahle, A., Halvorsen, S., & Sonbo Kristiansen, I. (2018). Diagnosing heart failure with NT-proBNP point-of-care testing: lower costs and better outcomes. A decision analytic study. *BJGP Open*. doi:10.3399/bjgpopen18X101596.

Burns, C. E., Barber Starr, N., Dunn, A. M., Blosser, C. G., Brady, M. A., & Garzon, D. L. (2017). *Pediatric Primary Care* (6 ed.). St. Louis, Missouri Elsevier.

Buttaro, T. M., Trybulski, J., Polgar-Bailey, P., & Sandberg-Cook, J. (2021). *Primary Care: A Collaborative Practice* (6 ed.). St. Louis, Missouri: Elsevier.

Dionne, J. M. (2017). Updated Guideline May Improve the Recognition and Diagnosis of Hypertension in Children and Adolescents; Review of the 2017 AAP Blood Pressure Clinical Practice Guideline. *Current Hypertension Reports*, 19(10), 84. doi:10.1007/s11906-017-0780-8.

Domino, F. J., Baldor, R. A., Golding, J., & Stephens, M. B. (2023). *The 5-Minute Clinical Consult Premium 2023* (31 ed.). Philadelphia, PA: Wolters Kluwer.

Dunphy, L. M. H., Winland-Brown, J. E., Porter, B. O., & Thomas, D. J. (2019). *Primary Care: The Art and Science of Advanced Practice Nursing* (5 ed.). Philadelphia, PA: F.A. Davis Company.

Iyengar, A., Sanaiha, Y., Aguayo, E., Seo, Y.-J., Dobaria, V., Toppen, W., . . . Benharash, P. Comparison of Frequency of Late Gastrointestinal Bleeding with Transcatheter Versus Surgical Aortic Valve Replacement. *American Journal of Cardiology*. doi:10.1016/j.amjcard.2018.07.047.

Maxine, A. P., Stephen, J. M., Michael, W. R., McPhee, S. J., Papadakis, M. A., & Rabow, M. W. (2022). *Current Medical Diagnosis & Treatment 2022* (61 ed.). New York, NY: McGraw Hill Medical.

McCance, K. L., & Huether, S. E. (2019). *Pathophysiology: The Biologic Basis for Disease in Adults and Children* (8 ed.). St. Louis, Missouri: Elsevier.

McKee, G., Mooney, M., O'Donnell, S., O'Brien, F., Biddle, M. J., & Moser, D. K. A cluster and inferential analysis of myocardial infarction symptom presentation by age. *European Journal of Cardiovascular Nursing*, 0(0), 1474515118772824. doi:10.1177/1474515118772824.

Whelton, P. K., Carey, R. M., Aronow, W. S., Casey, D. E., Collins, K. J., Dennison Himmelfarb, C., . . . Wright, J. T. (2017). Guideline for the Prevention, Detection, Evaluation, and Management of High Blood Pressure in Adults. *Journal of the American College of Cardiology*. doi:10.1016/j.jacc.2017.11.006.

Yancy, C. W., Jessup, M., Bozkurt, B., Butler, J., Casey, D. E., Colvin, M. M., . . . Westlake, C. (2017). 2017 ACC/AHA/HFSA Focused Update of the 2013 ACCF/AHA Guideline for the Management of Heart Failure. *Journal of the American College of Cardiology*, 70(6), 776-803. doi:10.1016/j.jacc.2017.04.025.

Chapter 4

Burns, C. E., Barber Starr, N., Dunn, A. M., Blosser, C. G., Brady, M. A., & Garzon, D. L. (2017). *Pediatric Primary Care* (6 ed.). St. Louis, Missouri Elsevier.

Buttaro, T. M., Trybulski, J., Polgar-Bailey, P., & Sandberg-Cook, J. (2021). *Primary Care: A Collaborative Practice* (6 ed.). St. Louis, Missouri: Elsevier.

Domino, F. J., Baldor, R. A., Golding, J., & Stephens, M. B. (2023). *The 5-Minute Clinical Consult Premium 2023* (31 ed.). Philadelphia, PA: Wolters Kluwer.

Dunphy, L. M. H., Winland-Brown, J. E., Porter, B. O., & Thomas, D. J. (2019). *Primary Care: The Art and Science of Advanced Practice Nursing* (5 ed.). Philadelphia, PA: F.A. Davis Company.

Habif, T. P. (2016). *Clinical Dermatology: A Color Guide to Diagnosis and Therapy* (6 ed.). St. Louis, Missouri: Elsevier.

Pharmacologic approaches to glycemic treatment: *Standards of Medical Care in Diabetes*—(2021). *Diabetes Care*. 2021;44(Suppl 1):S111-S124. doi:10.2337/dc21-S009.

Chapter 5

Burns, C. E., Barber Starr, N., Dunn, A. M., Blosser, C. G., Brady, M. A., & Garzon, D. L. (2017). *Pediatric Primary Care* (6 ed.). St. Louis, Missouri Elsevier.

Dunphy, L. M. H., Winland-Brown, J. E., Porter, B. O., & Thomas, D. J. (2019). *Primary Care: The Art and Science of Advanced Practice Nursing* (5 ed.). Philadelphia, PA: F.A. Davis Company.

KDIGO Workgroup. (2013). KDIGO 2012 Clinical Practice Guideline for the Evaluation and Management of Chronic Kidney Disease. *International Society of Nephrology*, 3(1), 19-62. doi:*https://doi.org/10.1038/kisup.2012.64*.

Nicolle, L. E., Bradley, S., Colgan, R., Rice, J. C., Schaeffer, A., & Hooton, T. M. (2005). Infectious Diseases Society of America guidelines for the diagnosis and treatment of asymptomatic bacteriuria in adults. *Clin Infect Dis, 40*(5), 643-654. doi:10.1086/427507.

Schuiling, K. D., & Likis, F. E. (2017). *Women's Gynecologic Health* (3 ed.). Burlington, Massachusetts: Jones & Bartlett Learning.

Chapter 6

Burns, C. E., Barber Starr, N., Dunn, A. M., Blosser, C. G., Brady, M. A., & Garzon, D. L. (2017). *Pediatric Primary Care* (6 ed.). St. Louis, Missouri Elsevier.

Buttaro, T. M., Trybulski, J., Polgar-Bailey, P., & Sandberg-Cook, J. (2021). *Primary Care: A Collaborative Practice* (6 ed.). St. Louis, Missouri: Elsevier.

Chey, W. D., Kurlander, J., & Eswaran, S. (2015). Irritable bowel syndrome: A clinical review. *JAMA,* 313(9), 949-958. doi:10.1001/jama.2015.0954.

Domino, F. J., Baldor, R. A., Golding, J., & Stephens, M. B. (2023). *The 5-Minute Clinical Consult Premium 2023* (31 ed.). Philadelphia, PA: Wolters Kluwer.

Dunphy, L. M. H., Winland-Brown, J. E., Porter, B. O., & Thomas, D. J. (2019). *Primary Care: The Art and Science of Advanced Practice Nursing* (5 ed.). Philadelphia, PA: F.A. Davis Company.

Lacy, B. E., Mearin, F., Chang, L., Chey, W. D., Lembo, A. J., Simren, M., & Spiller, R. (2016). Bowel Disorders. *Gastroenterology,* 150(6), 1393-1407.e1395. doi:10.1053/j.gastro.2016.02.031.

Wolf, A. M. D., Fontham, E. T. H., Church, T. R., Flowers, C. R., Guerra, C. E., LaMonte, S. J., ... Smith, R. A. (2018). Colorectal cancer screening for average-risk adults: 2018 guideline update from the American Cancer Society. *CA: A Cancer Journal for Clinicians*, 68(4), 250-281. doi:10.3322/caac.21457.

Chapter 7

Centers for Disease Control and Prevention. (2015). Lyme Disease: Two-step Laboratory Testing Process. Retrieved from *https://www.cdc.gov/lyme/diagnosistesting/labtest/twostep/*.

Greeniee, J. E. (2018). Overview of Meningitis. Retrieved from *https://www.merckmanuals.com/professional/neurologic-disorders/meningitis/overview-of-meningitis*.

Jackson, J. L., Mancuso, J. M., Nickoloff, S., Bernstein, R., & Kay, C. (2017). Tricyclic and Tetracyclic Antidepressants for the Prevention of Frequent Episodic or Chronic Tension-Type Headache in Adults: A Systematic Review and Meta-Analysis. *Journal of General Internal Medicine*, 32(12), 1351-1358. doi:10.1007/s11606-017-4121-z.

Kirthi, V., Derry, S., & Moore, R. A. (2013). Aspirin with or without an antiemetic for acute migraine headaches in adults. *Cochrane Database Syst Rev,* 4, Cd008041. doi:10.1002/14651858.CD008041.pub3.

Law, S., Derry, S., & Moore, R. A. (2016). Sumatriptan plus naproxen for the treatment of acute migraine attacks in adults. *Cochrane Database Syst Rev,* 4, Cd008541. doi:10.1002/14651858.CD008541.pub3

Marmura, M. J., Silberstein, S. D., & Schwedt, T. J. (2015). The acute treatment of migraine in adults: the American Headache Society evidence assessment of migraine pharmacotherapies. *Headache, 55*(1), 3-20. doi:10.1111/head.12499.

Probyn, K., Bowers, H., Mistry, D., Caldwell, F., Underwood, M., Patel, S., ... Pincus, T. (2017). Non-pharmacological self-management for people living with migraine or tension-type headache: a systematic review including analysis of intervention components. *BMJ Open*, 7(8). doi:10.1136/bmjopen-2017-016670.

U.S. Preventive Services Task Force. (2016). Aspirin Use to Prevent Cardiovascular Disease and Colorectal Cancer: Preventive Medication. Retrieved from *https://www.uspreventiveservicestaskforce.org/Page/Document/UpdateSummaryFinal/aspirin-to-prevent-cardiovascular-disease-and-cancer*.

Chapter 8

Buttaro, T. M., Trybulski, J., Polgar-Bailey, P., & Sandberg-Cook, J. (2021). *Primary Care: A Collaborative Practice* (6 ed.). St. Louis, Missouri: Elsevier.

Carpintero, P., Caeiro, J. R., Carpintero, R., Morales, A., Silva, S., & Mesa, M. (2014). Complications of hip fractures: A review. *World Journal of Orthopedics*, 5(4), 402-411. doi:10.5312/wjo.v5.i4.402.

Domino, F. J., Baldor, R. A., Golding, J., & Stephens, M. B. (2023). *The 5-Minute Clinical Consult Premium 2023* (31 ed.). Philadelphia, PA: Wolters Kluwer.

Dunphy, L. M. H., Winland-Brown, J. E., Porter, B. O., & Thomas, D. J. (2019). *Primary Care: The Art and Science of Advanced Practice Nursing* (5 ed.). Philadelphia, PA: F.A. Davis Company.

Lamba, N., Lee, S., Chaudhry, H., & Foster, C. S. (2016). A review of the ocular manifestations of rheumatoid arthritis. *Cogent Medicine*, 3(1), 1243771. doi:10.1080/2331205X.2016.1243771.

Maxine, A. P., Stephen, J. M., Michael, W. R., McPhee, S. J., Papadakis, M. A., & Rabow, M. W. (2022). *Current Medical Diagnosis & Treatment 2022* (61 ed.). New York, NY: McGraw Hill Medical.

Ramiro, S., Gaujoux-Viala, C., Nam, J. L., Smolen, J. S., Buch, M., Gossec, L., ... Landewé, R. (2014). Safety of synthetic and biological DMARDs: a systematic literature review informing the 2013 update of the EULAR recommendations for management of rheumatoid arthritis. *Annals of the Rheumatic Diseases*, 73(3), 529-535. doi:10.1136/annrheumdis-2013-204575.

Smolen, J. S., Landewe, R., Bijlsma, J., Burmester, G., Chatzidionysiou, K., Dougados, M., ... van der Heijde, D. (2017). EULAR recommendations for the management of rheumatoid arthritis with synthetic and biological disease-modifying antirheumatic drugs: 2016 update. *Ann Rheum Dis*, 76(6), 960-977. doi:10.1136/annrheumdis-2016-210715.

Chapter 9

Buttaro, T. M., Trybulski, J., Polgar-Bailey, P., & Sandberg-Cook, J. (2021). *Primary Care: A Collaborative Practice* (6 ed.). St. Louis, Missouri: Elsevier.

Domino, F. J., Baldor, R. A., Golding, J., & Stephens, M. B. (2023). *The 5-Minute Clinical Consult Premium 2023* (31 ed.). Philadelphia, PA: Wolters Kluwer.

Dunphy, L. M. H., Winland-Brown, J. E., Porter, B. O., & Thomas, D. J. (2019). *Primary Care: The Art and Science of*

Advanced Practice Nursing (5 ed.). Philadelphia, PA: F.A. Davis Company.

Ho, L., & John, R. M. (2015). Understanding and Managing Glucose-6-Phosphate Dehydrogenase Deficiency. *The Journal for Nurse Practitioners*, 11(4), 443-450. doi:*https://doi.org/10.1016/j.nurpra.2015.01.007.*

Matsumoto, T., Nogami, K., & Shima, M. (2017). A combined approach using global coagulation assays quickly differentiates coagulation disorders with prolonged aPTT and low levels of FVIII activity. *International Journal of Hematology*, 105(2), 174-183. doi:10.1007/s12185-016-2108-x.

Maxine, A. P., Stephen, J. M., Michael, W. R., McPhee, S. J., Papadakis, M. A., & Rabow, M. W. (2022). *Current Medical Diagnosis & Treatment 2022* (61ed.). New York, NY: McGraw Hill Medical.

Chapter 10

Ball, J. W., Dains, J. E., Flynn, J. A., Solomon, B., & Stewart, R. W. (2019). *Physical Examination and Health Assessment Online for Seidel's Guide to Physical Examination* (9 ed.). Philadelphia, PA: Mosby Inc.

Burns, C. E., Barber Starr, N., Dunn, A. M., Blosser, C. G., Brady, M. A., & Garzon, D. L. (2017). *Pediatric Primary Care* (6 ed.). St. Louis, Missouri: Elsevier.

Buttaro, T. M., Trybulski, J., Polgar-Bailey, P., & Sandberg-Cook, J. (2022). *Primary Care: A Collaborative Practice* (6 ed.). St. Louis, Missouri: Elsevier.

Camarero-Mulas, C., Delgado Jiménez, Y., Sanmartín-Jiménez, O., Garcés, J. R., Rodríguez-Prieto, M. A., Alonso-Alonso, T., . . . Descalzo, M. A. (2018). Mohs micrographic surgery in the elderly: comparison of tumours, surgery and first-year follow-up in patients younger and older than 80 years old in REGESMOHS. *Journal of the European Academy of Dermatology and Venereology*, 32(1), 108-112. doi:10.1111/jdv.14586.

Domino, F. J., Baldor, R. A., Golding, J., & Stephens, M. B. (2023). *The 5-Minute Clinical Consult Premium 2023* (31 ed.). Philadelphia, PA: Wolters Kluwer.

Dunphy, L. M. H., Winland-Brown, J. E., Porter, B. O., & Thomas, D. J. (2019). *Primary Care: The Art and Science of Advanced Practice Nursing* (5 ed.). Philadelphia, PA: F.A. Davis Company.

Habif, T. P. (2016). *Clinical Dermatology: A Color Guide to Diagnosis and Therapy* (6 ed.). St. Louis, Missouri: Elsevier.

Maxine, A. P., Stephen, J. M., Michael, W. R., McPhee, S. J., Papadakis, M. A., & Rabow, M. W. (2022). *Current Medical Diagnosis & Treatment 2022* (61 ed.). New York, NY: McGraw Hill Medical.

McCance, K. L., & Huether, S. E. (2019). *Pathophysiology: The Biologic Basis for Disease in Adults and Children* (8 ed.). St. Louis, Missouri: Elsevier.

Chapter 11

Almont, T., Farsi, F., Krakowski, I., El Osta, R., Bondil, P., & Huyghe, E. (2018). Sexual health in cancer: the results of a survey exploring practices, attitudes, knowledge, communication, and professional interactions in oncology healthcare providers. *Support Care Cancer*. doi:10.1007/s00520-018-4376-x.

Borelli, S., & Lautenschlager, S. (2015). Differential diagnosis and management of balanitis. *Hautarzt*, 66(1), 6-11. doi:10.1007/s00105-014-3554-0.

Dimitrov, D. T., Masse, B. R., & Donnell, D. (2016). PrEP Adherence Patterns Strongly Affect Individual HIV Risk and Observed Efficacy in Randomized Clinical Trials. *J*

Acquir Immune Defic Syndr, 72(4), 444-451. doi:10.1097/qai.0000000000000993.

DiNenno, E. A., Prejean, J., Irwin, K., Delaney, K. P., Bowles, K., Martin, T., . . . Lansky, A. (2017). Recommendations for HIV Screening of Gay, Bisexual, and Other Men Who Have Sex with Men—United States, 2017. *MMWR Morb Mortal Wkly Rep*, 66(31), 830-832. doi:10.15585/mmwr.mm6631a3.

Menon-Johansson, A. S. (2018). Proven prevention tools for addressing STI epidemics. *Isr J Health Policy Res*, 7(1), 47. doi:10.1186/s13584-018-0242-z.

Merriel, S. W. D., Funston, G., & Hamilton, W. (2018). Prostate Cancer in Primary Care. *Adv Ther*. doi:10.1007/s12325-018-0766-1.

Ng, Y. C., Caires, A., & Mayeux, J. (2018). Message from an Urgent Care PrEP Provider for Health Care Professionals. *J Assoc Nurses AIDS Care*, 29(1), 130-132. doi:10.1016/j.jana.2017.09.010.

Rosser, B. R. S., Capistrant, B., Torres, M. B., Konety, B., Merengwa, E., Mitteldorf, D., & West, W. (2016). The effects of radical prostatectomy on gay and bisexual men's sexual functioning and behavior: qualitative results from the restore study. *Sex Relation Ther*, 31(4), 432-445. doi:10.1080/14681994.2016.1217985.

Rosu, M. B., Oliffe, J. L., & Kelly, M. T. (2017). Nurse Practitioners and Men's Primary Health Care. *American Journal of Men's Health, 11*(5), 1501-1511. doi:10.1177/1557988315617721.

Workowski, K. A., & Bolan, G. A. (2015). Sexually transmitted diseases treatment guidelines, 2015. *MMWR Recomm Rep*, 64(Rr-03), 1-137.

Chapter 12

Buttaro, T. M., Trybulski, J., Polgar-Bailey, P., & Sandberg-Cook, J. (2021). *Primary Care: A Collaborative Practice* (6 ed.). St. Louis, Missouri: Elsevier.

Centers for Disease Control and Prevention. (2017a). Genital HPV Infection—Fact Sheet. Retrieved from *https://www.cdc.gov/std/HPV/STDfact-HPV.htm.*

Daniele, N. D., Carbonelli, M. G., Candeloro, N., Iacopino, L., De Lorenzo, A., & Andreoli, A. (2004). Effect of supplementation of calcium and vitamin D on bone mineral density and bone mineral content in peri- and post-menopause women: A double-blind, randomized, controlled trial. *Pharmacological Research, 50*(6), 637-641. doi:*https://doi.org/10.1016/j.phrs.2004.05.010.*

Dimmock, P. W., Wyatt, K. M., Jones, P. W., & O'Brien, P. M. S. (2000). Efficacy of selective serotonin-reuptake inhibitors in premenstrual syndrome: a systematic review. *The Lancet*, 356(9236), 1131-1136. doi:*https://doi.org/10.1016/S0140-6736(00)02754-9.*

Domino, F. J., Baldor, R. A., Golding, J., & Stephens, M. B. (2023). *The 5-Minute Clinical Consult Premium 2023* (31 ed.). Philadelphia, PA: Wolters Kluwer.

Dunphy, L. M. H., Winland-Brown, J. E., Porter, B. O., & Thomas, D. J. (2019). *Primary Care: The Art and Science of Advanced Practice Nursing* (5 ed.). Philadelphia, PA: F.A. Davis Company.

Fassbender, A., Vodolazkaia, A., Saunders, P., Lebovic, D., Waelkens, E., De Moor, B., & D'Hooghe, T. (2013). Biomarkers of endometriosis. *Fertil Steril*, 99(4), 1135-1145. doi:10.1016/j.fertnstert.2013.01.097.

Gordon, C. M., Ackerman, K. E., Berga, S. L., Kaplan, J. R., Mastorakos, G., Misra, M., . . . Warren, M. P. (2017). Functional Hypothalamic Amenorrhea: An Endocrine Society Clinical Practice Guideline. *J Clin Endocrinol Metab, 102*(5), 1413-1439. doi:10.1210/jc.2017-00131.

Habibi, N., Huang, M. S. L., Gan, W. Y., Zulida, R., & Safavi, S. M. (2015). Prevalence of Primary Dysmenorrhea and Factors Associated with Its Intensity Among Undergraduate Students: A Cross-Sectional Study. *Pain Management Nursing,* 16(6), 855-861. doi:*https://doi.org/10.1016/j.pmn.2015.07.001.*

Kanwal, R., Haider, S. I., Soomro, K., & Butt, H. (2017). Association between primary dysmenorrhea and depression level among students. *The Rehabilitation Journal,* 1(02), 13-16.

Maxine, A. P., Stephen, J. M., Michael, W. R., McPhee, S. J., Papadakis, M. A., & Rabow, M. W. (2022). *Current Medical Diagnosis & Treatment 2022* (61 ed.). New York, NY: McGraw Hill Medical.

Maza, M., & Gage, J. C. (2017). Considerations for HPV primary screening in lower-middle income countries. *Preventive Medicine,* 98, 39-41. doi:*https://doi.org/10.1016/j.ypmed.2016.12.029.*

Murray, S. S., McKinney, E. S., Holub, K. S., & Jones, R. (2019). *Foundations of Maternal-Newborn and Women's Health Nursing* (7 ed.). St. Louis, Missouri: Elsevier.

Naheed, B., Kuiper, J. H., Uthman, O. A., O'Mahony, F., & O'Brien, P. M. S. (2017). Non-contraceptive oestrogen-containing preparations for controlling symptoms of premenstrual syndrome. *Cochrane Database of Systematic Reviews* (3). doi:10.1002/14651858.CD010503.pub2.

Nose-Ogura, S., Yoshino, O., Dohi, M., Kigawa, M., Harada, M., Kawahara, T., . . . Saito, S. (2018). Low Bone Mineral Density in Elite Female Athletes With a History of Secondary Amenorrhea in Their Teens. *Clinical Journal of Sport Medicine,* published ahead of print. doi:10.1097/jsm.0000000000000571.

Posner, G. D., Foote, W. R., & Oxorn, H. (2013). *Oxorn-Foote Human Labor & Birth* (6 ed.). New York, NY: McGraw Hill Medical.

Schuiling, K. D., & Likis, F. E. (2017). *Women's Gynecologic Health* (3rd ed.). Burlington, Massachusetts: Jones & Bartlett Learning.

Chapter 13

American Psychiatric, A., American Psychiatric, A., & Force, D. S. M. T. (2013). *Diagnostic and Statistical Manual of Mental Disorders: DSM-5.* Arlington, VA: American Psychiatric Association.

Bandoli, G., Campbell-Sills, L., Kessler, R. C., Heeringa, S. G., Nock, M. K., Rosellini, A. J., . . . Stein, M. B. (2017). Childhood adversity, adult stress, and the risk of major depression or generalized anxiety disorder in US soldiers: a test of the stress sensitization hypothesis. *Psychol Med,* 47(13), 2379-2392. doi:10.1017/s0033291717001064.

Blair, K. S., Otero, M., Teng, C., Geraci, M., Ernst, M., Blair, R. J. R., . . . Grillon, C. (2017). Reduced optimism and a heightened neural response to everyday worries are specific to generalized anxiety disorder, and not seen in social anxiety. *Psychol Med,* 47(10), 1806-1815. doi:10.1017/S0033291717000265.

Burns, C. E., Barber Starr, N., Dunn, A. M., Blosser, C. G., Brady, M. A., & Garzon, D. L. (2017). *Pediatric Primary Care* (6 ed.). St. Louis, Missouri: Elsevier.

Buttaro, T. M., Trybulski, J., Polgar-Bailey, P., & Sandberg-Cook, J. (2021). *Primary Care: A Collaborative Practice* (6 ed.). St. Louis, Missouri: Elsevier.

Cipriani, A., Furukawa, T. A., Salanti, G., Chaimani, A., Atkinson, L. Z., Ogawa, Y., . . . Geddes, J. R. (2018). Comparative efficacy and acceptability of 21 antidepressant drugs for the acute treatment of adults with major depressive disorder: a systematic review and network meta-analysis. *The Lancet,* 391(10128), 1357-1366. doi:*https://doi.org/10.1016/S0140-6736(17)32802-7.*

Dunphy, L. M. H., Winland-Brown, J. E., Porter, B. O., & Thomas, D. J. (2019). *Primary Care: The Art and Science of Advanced Practice Nursing* (5 ed.). Philadelphia, PA: F.A. Davis Company.

Gureje, O., & Thornicroft, G. (2015). Health equity and mental health in post-2015 sustainable development goals. *The Lancet Psychiatry,* 2(1), 12-14. doi:10.1016/S2215-0366(14)00094-7.

Hasan, A., Falkai, P., Wobrock, T., Lieberman, J., Glenthøj, B., Gattaz, W. F., . . . Möller, H. J. (2017). World Federation of Societies of Biological Psychiatry (WFSBP) guidelines for biological treatment of schizophrenia—a short version for primary care. *International Journal of Psychiatry in Clinical Practice,* 21(2), 82-90. doi:10.1080/13651501.2017.1291839.

Chapter 14

Benito-Fernández, J., Vázquez-Ronco, M. A., Morteruel-Aizkuren, E., Mintegui-Raso, S., Sánchez-Etxaniz, J., & Fernández-Landaluce, A. (2006). Impact of Rapid Viral Testing for Influenza A and B Viruses on Management of Febrile Infants Without Signs of Focal Infection. *The Pediatric Infectious Disease Journal,* 25(12), 1153-1157. doi:10.1097/01.inf.0000246826.93142.b0.

Burns, C. E., Barber Starr, N., Dunn, A. M., Blosser, C. G., Brady, M. A., & Garzon, D. L. (2017). *Pediatric Primary Care* (6 ed.). St. Louis, Missouri: Elsevier.

Dow, D., Guthrie, W., Stronach, S. T., & Wetherby, A. M. (2017). Psychometric analysis of the Systematic Observation of Red Flags for autism spectrum disorder in toddlers. *Autism,* 21(3), 301-309. doi:10.1177/1362361316636760.

Filatova, S., Koivumaa-Honkanen, H., Hirvonen, N., Freeman, A., Ivandic, I., Hurtig, T., . . . Miettunen, J. (2017). Early motor developmental milestones and schizophrenia: A systematic review and meta-analysis. *Schizophrenia Research,* 188, 13-20. doi:*https://doi.org/10.1016/j.schres.2017.01.029.*

Nunes, M., & Madhi, S. (2018). Prevention of influenza-related illness in young infants by maternal vaccination during pregnancy [version 1; referees: 2 approved]. *F1000Research,* 7(122). doi:10.12688/f1000research.12473.1.

Peyre, H., Charkaluk, M.-L., Forhan, A., Heude, B., & Ramus, F. (2017). Do developmental milestones at 4, 8, 12 and 24 months predict IQ at 5–6 years old? Results of the EDEN mother–child cohort. *European Journal of Pediatric Neurology,* 21(2), 272-279. doi:*https://doi.org/10.1016/j.ejpn.2016.11.001.*

Piaget, J. (1979). *Science of Education and the Psychology of the Child.* New York: Penguin Books.

Piaget, J., Grize, J.-B., & Szeminska, A. (1977). *Epistemology and Psychology of Functions.* Dordrecht; Boston: D. Reidel.

Poehling, K. A., Szilagyi, P. G., Staat, M. A., Snively, B. M., Payne, D. C., Bridges, C. B., . . . Edwards, K. M. (2011). Impact of maternal immunization on influenza hospitalizations in infants. *American Journal of Obstetrics and Gynecology,* 204(6, Supplement), S141-S148. doi:*https://doi.org/10.1016/j.ajog.2011.02.042.*

Scharf, R. J., Scharf, G. J., & Stroustrup, A. (2016). Developmental Milestones. *Pediatrics in Review,* 37(1), 25-38. doi:10.1542/pir.2014-0103.

Sheldrick, R. C., & Perrin, E. C. (2013). Evidence-Based Milestones for Surveillance of Cognitive, Language, and Motor Development. *Academic Pediatrics,* 13(6), 577-586. doi:*https://doi.org/10.1016/j.acap.2013.07.001.*

Chapter 15

Centers for Disease Control and Prevention. (2018b). Recommended Immunization Schedule for Adults Aged 19 Years or Older, United States, 2018. Retrieved from *https://www.cdc.gov/vaccines/schedules/downloads/adult/adult-combined-schedule.pdf.*

Centers for Medicare & Medicaid Services. (2018). Prescription Drug Coverage—General Information. Retrieved from *https://www.cms.gov/Medicare/Prescription-Drug-Coverage/PrescriptionDrugCovGenIn/index.html.*

Cubanski, J., Casillas, G., & Damico, A. (2015). *Poverty Among Seniors: An Updated Analysis of National and State Level Poverty Rates Under the Official and Supplemental Poverty Measures.* Retrieved from *http://files.kff.org/attachment/issue-brief-poverty-among-seniors-an-updated-analysis-of-national-and-state-level-poverty-rates-under-the-official-and-supplemental-poverty-measures.*

National Hospice and Palliative Care Organization. (2009). Tip Sheet for ADRs and Medicare Appeals. Retrieved from *https://www.nhpco.org/2009-alertsround-archive/new-tip-sheet-adrs-and-medicare-appeals.*

National Hospice and Palliative Care Organization. (2018). Hospice Eligibility Requirements. Retrieved from *https://www.nhpco.org/hospice-eligibility-requirements.*

Chapter 16

Al-Aama, T. (2011). Falls in the elderly: Spectrum and prevention. *Canadian Family Physician, 57*(7), 771-776.

American Nurses Association. (2010). *Nursing's Social Policy Statement: The Essence of the Profession* (3 ed.). Silver Spring, Maryland: American Nurses Association.

American Nurses Association, & National Association of School Nurses. (2017). *School Nursing: Scope and Standards of Practice.* Retrieved from *https://www.r2library.com/Resource/Title/1558107193.*

Boltz, M. (2016). *Evidence-Based Geriatric Nursing Protocols for Best Practice* (5 ed.). New York, NY: Springer.

Buppert, C. (2018). *Nurse Practitioner's Business Practice and Legal Guide* (6 ed.). Burlington, Massachusetts: Jones & Bartlett Learning.

Fowler, M. D. M., & American Nurses Association. (2015). *Guide to the Code of Ethics for Nurses with Interpretive Statements: Development, Interpretation, and Application* (2 ed.). Silver Spring, Maryland: American Nurses Association.

Goguen, D. (2018). Medical Malpractice State Laws: Statutes of Limitations. Retrieved from *http://www.alllaw.com/articles/nolo/medical-malpractice-state-laws-statutes-limitations.html.*

Iowa Institute of Human Genetics. (2018). How to Draw a Pedigree. Retrieved from *https://medicine.uiowa.edu/humangenetics/resources/how-draw-pedigree/basic-pedigree-symbols.*

Joel, L. A. (2018). *Advanced Practice Nursing: Essentials for Role Development* (4 ed.). Philadelphia, PA: F.A. Davis Company.

Power, T. A. (1989). *Family Matters: A Layperson's Guide to Family Functioning* (2 ed.). Meredith, New Hampshire: Hathaway Press.

Scherzer, R., Dennis, M. P., Swan, B. A., Kavuru, M. S., & Oxman, D. A. (2017). A Comparison of Usage and Outcomes Between Nurse Practitioner and Resident-Staffed Medical ICUs. *Critical Care Medicine, 45*(2).

Sonenberg, A., & Knepper, H. J. (2017). Considering disparities: How do nurse practitioner regulatory policies, access to care, and health outcomes vary across four states? *Nursing Outlook, 65*(2), 143-153. doi:*https://doi.org/10.1016/j.outlook.2016.10.005.*

Stewart, J. G., & DeNisco, S. M. (2019). *Role Development for the Nurse Practitioner* (2 ed.). Burlington, MA: Jones & Bartlett.

Timmons, E. J. (2017). The effects of expanded nurse practitioner and physician assistant scope of practice on the cost of Medicaid patient care. *Health Policy, 121*(2), 189-196. doi:*https://doi.org/10.1016/j.healthpol.2016.12.002.*

Traczynski, J., & Udalova, V. (2018). Nurse practitioner independence, health care utilization, and health outcomes. *Journal of Health Economics, 58,* 90-109.

U.S. Department of Health & Human Services. (2013). Summary of the HIPAA Privacy Rule. Retrieved from *https://www.hhs.gov/hipaa/for-professionals/privacy/laws-regulations/index.html.*

Xue, Y., Kannan, V., Greener, E., Smith, J. A., Brasch, J., Johnson, B. A., & Spetz, J. (2018). Full Scope-of-Practice Regulation Is Associated With Higher Supply of Nurse Practitioners in Rural and Primary Care Health Professional Shortage Counties. *Journal of Nursing Regulation, 8*(4), 5-13. doi:10.1016/S2155-8256(17)30176-X.

Chapter 17

American Academy of Professional Coders. (2018). What is HCPCS? Retrieved from *https://www.aapc.com/resources/medical-coding/hcpcs.aspx.*

American Medical Association. (2018). *CPT 2017 Professional Edition* (4 ed.). Illinois, Chicago: American Medical Association.

Dunphy, L. M. H., Winland-Brown, J. E., Porter, B. O., & Thomas, D. J. (2019). *Primary Care: The Art and Science of Advanced Practice Nursing* (5 ed.). Philadelphia, PA: F.A. Davis Company.

Goroll, A. H., & Mulley, A. G. (2014). *Primary Care Medicine: Office Evaluation and Management of the Adult Patient* (7 ed.). Philadelphia, PA: Wolters Kluwer/Lippincott Williams & Wilkins Health.

Chapter 18

Alligood, M. R. (2018). *Nursing Theorists and Their Work* (9 ed.). St. Louis, Missouri: Elsevier.

Butts, J. B. (2019). *Nursing Ethics: Across the Curriculum and into Practice* (5 ed.). Burlington, MA: Jones & Bartlett Learning.

Centers for Disease Control and Prevention. (2016a). Guidelines and Recommendations. Retrieved from *https://stacks.cdc.gov/cbrowse/?parentId=cdc:100&pid=cdc:100&type=1&facetRange=960.*

Centers for Disease Control and Prevention. (2016b). Prevention of HIV/AIDS, Viral Hepatitis, STDs, and TB Through Health Care. Retrieved from *https://www.cdc.gov/nchhstp/preventionthroughhealthcare/index.htm.*

Centers for Disease Control and Prevention. (2017). Prevention Status Report. Retrieved from *https://www.cdc.gov/psr/index.html.*

Centers for Disease Control and Prevention. (2018). Advisory Committee on Immunization Practices (ACIP). Retrieved from *https://www.cdc.gov/vaccines/acip/index.html.*

Hughes, R., & Agency for Healthcare Research Quality. (2008). Patient safety and quality: an evidence-based handbook for nurses. Rockville, MD: Agency for Healthcare Research and Quality.

JAMA Network. (2015). The 2014 JNC 8 and 2017 AHA/ACA Guidelines for Management of High Blood Pressure in Adults. Retrieved from *https://sites.jamanetwork.com/jnc8/*.

LoBiondo-Wood, G., & Haber, J. (2018). *Nursing Research: Methods and Critical Appraisal for Evidence-Based Practice* (9 ed.). St. Louis, Missouri: Elsevier.

McGonigle, D., & Mastrian, K. G. (2018). *Nursing Informatics and the Foundation of Knowledge* (4 ed.). Burlington, MA: Jones & Bartlett Learning.

Polit, D. F., & Beck, C. T. (2017). *Nursing Research: Generating and Assessing Evidence for Nursing Practice* (10 ed.). Philadelphia, Pennsylvania: Wolters Kluwer.

Trust for America's Health. (2013). A Compendium of Proven Community-Based Prevention Programs. Retrieved from *http://healthyamericans.org/report/110*.

U.S. Preventive Services Task Force. (2012). Grade Definitions. Retrieved from *https://www.uspreventiveservicestaskforce.org/Page/Name/grade-definitions*.

Index